# Ethical Decisions in Medicine

*Margaret Holmes*

# Ethical Decisions in Medicine
## Second Edition

**Howard Brody, M.D., Ph.D.**

Assistant Professor of Family Practice and Philosophy, and Assistant Coordinator, Medical Humanities Program, Michigan State University College of Human Medicine, East Lansing

Little, Brown and Company     Boston

Library of Congress Catalog Card No. 80-84250

ISBN 0-316-10899-5

Printed in the United States of America

ALP

# Preface

Like the first edition, this book is designed as an introductory text in medical ethics. It features a programmed-text format that enhances its use as a self-instructional unit. It can also be used as a primary textbook in medical ethics for classes taught to students in the health professions. As a case study book, it can supplement more philosophically oriented texts, many of which have appeared since the first edition was published. There are, however, numerous revisions in this second edition which deserve special mention.

Since 1976, many events have had an impact on the field of medical ethics: the Quinlan trial, the passage of the California Natural Death Act, and the birth of the first "test tube baby" are several examples. A text that made no mention of these events would appear out of date even if its basic principles were sound, and so portions of this book have been revised to reflect these recent occurrences. Of more importance, the literature on medical ethics has grown and improved tremendously. Many of the works listed in the References to this edition had not yet appeared when the first edition was published. Within philosophy, medical dilemmas are no longer viewed merely as problems in applied ethics but are seen as suitable challenges for the theoretical philosopher, and the published literature is much richer as a result. Special effort was devoted to including in this edition the best from this recent literature.

I also have tried to take advantage of lessons gleaned from the reception given to the first edition. The programmed-text format has been retained and, I hope, strengthened. Many readers of the first edition found it helpful; those who did not generally found that it was not a hindrance. Case studies continue to be used as the major teaching device in this edition. Several cases from the previous edition have been revised or replaced, and the total number of cases has been increased slightly. While the original text was intended for use by medical students, some of the most enthusiastic response came from classes in nursing, pharmacy, and other allied health sciences. I have reworded some of the cases and much of the text in recognition of this broader audience.

In the first edition, I attempted to outline an ethical method that could be accepted without reliance on a single religious tradition and that could accommodate a variety of religious values. I was surprised to find that some readers perceived this as a rejection of religion and religious values. I am pleased, therefore, to include here an appendix by Martin Benjamin, Professor of Philosophy at Michigan State University, that speaks directly to the role of religion in ethics.

Finally, over the past four years I have modified my own thoughts on several of the topics presented in this book. I hope that the sections on informed consent, terminal care and quality of life, abortion, resource allocation, euthanasia, and the social responsibility of health professionals each reflect a more carefully reasoned approach compared to the earlier edition. The main arguments on the concepts of health and disease in Chapter 17 are the same substantively but have been rearranged in a more logical sequence. Chapter 18, formerly titled Bioethics, is now called The Foundations of Values and incorporates mostly new material.

H. B.

# Acknowledgments

While this book still bears the imprint of all of those whose ideas and assistance contributed to the first published edition, a number of significant departures from that earlier work mark this second edition. Many of these changes arose from my productive contacts with members of the Medical Humanities Program and the Department of Philosophy at Michigan State University, most notably Martin Benjamin, who has been kind enough to contribute an appendix to this edition. On many topics included in this book, my own thinking has been so much influenced by Dr. Benjamin's that it is difficult to single out his contributions for proper recognition. I hope he will accept this general acknowledgment in lieu of specific citations in the following chapters.

Among the gratifying responses to the publication of the first edition were detailed communications from many teachers who used the book in the classroom setting and who made many pertinent criticisms. Jack Hanford of Ferris State College, Michigan; Dr. Edmund Pellegrino, then Vice-President for Health Affairs of the University of Tennessee, now President of the Catholic University of America, Washington, D.C.; Carol Gilbert of the School of Nursing, University of Michigan; and Dr. Glenn Graber of the Philosophy Department, University of Tennessee; all devoted special efforts to compiling their reactions. Many others also passed on helpful suggestions.

The actual task of revising the manuscript took place during my residency at the University of Virginia Medical Center. I am grateful to Dr. B. Lewis Barnett and the faculty of the Department of Family Practice, and to Dr. Thomas Hunter and Joseph Fletcher of the Program in Human Biology and Society, for their support and encouragement.

I wish finally to amend an unfortunate omission from the Acknowledgments in the first edition and express my thanks to the past and present editorial staff of Little, Brown and Company for their valuable assistance, especially Jon Paul Davidson, Nancy Shapiro, William Patrick, Curtis Vouwie, and Lois Hall.

# Contents

x

# List of Cases for Discussion

# Key to Symbols

**26** ↓                      The text is continued in Frame 26. (If no num-
                              ber, the text is continued in the next frame be-
                              low.)

UNCLEAR *43                   If this statement is unclear, go to Frame 43 for
                              more discussion.

LEGAL                         If you are curious about the legal implications
IMPLICATIONS? *19             of this point, go to Frame 19. If not, continue
                              the main body of text as directed.

**32** ↑                      Resume your reading of the main body of the
                              text at Frame 32.

SKIP TO CASES ↓ 83            If you are not interested in what is to follow
                              immediately, you may skip ahead and start
                              reading about the sample cases in Frame 83.

REVIEW RIGHTS ↑ 12–15         If you would like to review the concept of
                              "rights," which is mentioned in this frame, re-
                              turn to the original discussion in Frames 12–15.
                              Then resume reading the main body of text
                              with the next frame below this one.

Whenever possible, a frame referred to by an asterisk (footnote frame) will
be located at the bottom of that page, preceded itself by an asterisk, and
separated from the main text by a solid line. When the arrows direct you to
other frames to check your answers to a list of questions, those frames will
be on the next several pages, also separated by solid lines from the main
text. (These frames will be in numerical order so that you can locate them
easily.) Portions of the text that you may skip without loss of continuity will
be set off by broken lines.

Remember that all direction numbers refer to frame numbers, not page
numbers. The only exceptions are references to the material in an appendix
or in the suggested readings at the back of the book and numbers in the
table of contents and list of cases.

Some text material is italicized for review purposes, and some is under-
scored for emphasis.

When an author's name is mentioned in the text, the full reference can be found in the References and Suggested Readings for that chapter in the back of the book.

In many places in the book, the pronouns "he," "him," and "his," to refer to persons of both sexes, are used for purposes of brevity only.

# Objectives

After completing this self-instructional book, the student should be able to:

1. Given an appropriate clinical case or cases as examples, outline a problem-solving method for dealing with the ethical questions involved. Such a method should include:
   a) identification of the key ethical questions
   b) formulation of an ethical statement of what ought to be done, in a form specific enough to allow for constructive debate and discussion
   c) determination of both short-range and long-range consequences of the proposed ethical statement, including consequences on the physiologic, psychological, and social levels
   d) assignment of weights to these consequences according to their relative probabilities of occurrence
   e) comparison of these consequences with one's own set of values, to determine the acceptability of the ethical statement
   f) provision for dealing with a contradiction between one's values and the predicted consequences, either through a revision of the ethical statement or through a reordering of the priorities of one's values
   g) provision for testing one's personal values for their acceptability by reference to commonly accepted morality or by comparison with a set of basic ethical principles

2. Given a clinical case as an example, identify which aspects of the medical decision to be made are technical in nature and which are ethical, and explain how the technical aspects and the ethical aspects are related to each other.

3. Given either a case example or an issue area in medical ethics, discuss the ethical questions raised in terms of:
   a) the nature of the doctor–patient relationship
   b) informed consent
   c) quality of life or "personhood"
   d) determination of the right of participation in the decision-making process; or whatever combination of these is applicable

4. Given a hypothetical argument on a medical-ethical topic, detect any common errors in ethical argument and explain how the thoughts of the speaker could be better restated. The common errors include:
   a) appealing to empirical data to settle an ethical question (e.g., "Everybody does it, so I ought to also.")

b) arguing backward from results to the original ethical questions, called retrospective ethics (e.g., "The operation was a success, so it doesn't matter now that the surgeon didn't get the patient's informed consent.")

c) assuming that a person will have good motives because of his social or professional role, and assuming that good motives will lead to good actions (e.g., "As a doctor, I always have the best interest of my patient at heart, so I don't have to ask the patient what he wants done in a particular case.")

d) arguing the ethics of a position by definition, without reference to actual consequences (e.g., "Euthanasia is nothing but a form of suicide; therefore it is wrong.")

e) basing one's ethical claims on a "right" without stating where the right originates, on what authority it is based, or who has the responsibility to fulfill it (e.g., "As a woman I have a right to bear normal children of my own.")

f) arguing that an ethical statement or action is wrong because it may lead to bad consequences, without showing that those consequences are in fact probable (the "domino theory") (e.g., "Abortion on demand is wrong because if you allow it, the next thing you know there'll be total promiscuity and a breakdown of the family.")

g) arguing on the basis of a "catch phrase" that is either inherently devoid of meaning or so general and vague as to be inapplicable to specific instances (e.g., "playing God," *"primum non nocere"*)

h) placing great weight on a possible consequence of very low probability, to the exclusion of more probable consequences (e.g., "You should never allow a patient to die without doing everything possible to prolong life, because tomorrow a new miracle cure might be discovered.")

# Not Objectives

Because the nature of medical ethics is often misunderstood and is often confused with what is now referred to as "medical etiquette" or rules of intraprofessional conduct, these "not objectives" are mentioned here for clarification.

After completing this book, the student will *not* be able to:

1. Recite a set of rules of proper medical conduct, the application of which will assure that one does the ethical thing in any instance.
2. State an ethical decision-making method that, for any specific case, will yield one and only one "right" answer as to the ethical thing to do.
3. Cite a code of ethics that will guide one's behavior in all problematic cases.
4. Discuss some aspect of medical law, and state how the law would view any action taken in a specific case.

# Ethical Decisions in Medicine

# Why Study Medical Ethics? 1

L.W., a 54-year-old computer designer, is now in the eighth day of his recu- **1**
peration from abdominal surgery to repair an ulcer, and he is being cared
for by his surgeon. While a likable person, L.W. has a history of neuroses
and gives the impression of being a chronic complainer, possibly with a
touch of the hypochondriac about him as well. The nurses note that he
always requests his pain shot of Demerol, which the surgeon has ordered
"every 4 hours prn," and that he regularly complains of recurring pain
about $\frac{1}{2}$ hour before his next shot is due. ↓

This morning, the surgeon examines L.W. and finds that all outward signs **2**
point to a routine postoperative recovery. The surgeon reminds L.W. that
Demerol, while a very potent pain drug, nevertheless has a high addiction
potential if used regularly over too long a period. Noting that "most of my
patients" are relatively pain-free by the eighth day after surgery, the surgeon suggests that if the order for Demerol were discontinued, L.W. would
find that he could really do without it just as well.

L.W. objects. He insists that regardless of how the other patients respond,
he is having real pain and thinks he could not stand it without medication.
He doesn't like the idea of addiction any more than the surgeon does, but
he asks that he be kept on Demerol "at least for a few more days."

After a bit more discussion along this line, the surgeon tells L.W. that he
is changing the order to Talwin, a less potent pain drug but one with much
less potential for addiction. ↓

Cases like this one occur every day in all hospitals. Decisions such as the **3**
one made by the surgeon to change medications are made many times each
day with no more than a moment's thought. If asked to elaborate upon the
nature of the above decision, the surgeon would most likely compare the
pharmacologic properties of the two drugs and conclude that "I made the
decision according to my clinical judgment." The topic of "ethics" would
never arise. ↓

4    Is the decision really "clinical judgment"? Surely that is a large part of it; the surgeon could not have acted as he did without a purely technical knowledge of the actions of the drugs, augmented by his own experience with large numbers of patients who have used them. But notice that this way of looking at the decision leaves a lot which is assumed but never stated. The surgeon seems to be assuming that L.W. is not feeling as much pain as he thinks, although he has no way to prove this one way or the other. He has judged L.W. to be a less reliable reporter in this regard than some of his other patients. Also, implicit in his decision is the judgment that it is better to suffer a certain amount of pain than to become addicted to a narcotic
↓    drug.

5    Let's examine that last judgment more closely. If the person in fact knows both what it is like to suffer pain and what it is like to be addicted to a drug, as best as he could based on the reported experiences of others, is there any technical knowledge or data that will help him to choose one alternative over the other? In fact, this is a kind of decision to which factual knowledge can contribute, but can never provide the final answer. In the last analysis, a value judgment will have to be made by the individual in order for him to
↓    state what is "better."

6    A judgment to which facts may contribute, but which must be decided in the end by weighing values, is a rough definition of an ethical question. There was, in fact, an ethical decision hidden under the surgeon's clinical judgment. If we had disagreed with the surgeon's decision, chances are that we would have been unable to state our grounds for disagreement, other than to say, "I would have done otherwise." But once the hidden ethical assumptions are brought out in the open, we have a much better opportunity to find the root of our disagreement — or to reconsider our own ideas
↓    and conclude that the surgeon was right after all.

7    And the business of making concealed ethical decisions is not restricted to this particular kind of case. We can generalize all medical decisions to arrive at two conclusions, based on the fact that medicine is an applied art — science of persons, applied by persons:

   1. *Every medical decision involves human beings both as the decision makers and as those who have to live with the consequences.*
   2. *Every medical decision involves a choice between different outcomes, and human beings are likely to place different values on the different*
↓    *outcomes.*

Since both of the listed characteristics are characteristics of ethical ques-     **8**
tions (a more precise definition of ethics must wait until Chapter 2), an obvious conclusion is that *all medical decisions are ethical decisions, or at
least that they involve an ethical component in addition to the scientific or
clinical aspects of the problem.* If most medical decisions are made without
the ethical dimension ever being considered, it is because the ethical issues
involved are of a common variety about which there is almost universal
agreement. If the ethical question were to be raised as such, most people
would solve it easily.     ↓

Periodically, however, the physician is faced with a dilemma which forces     **9**
him to recognize the ethical dimension — an unmarried girl requesting an
abortion, or a terminally ill patient who requests that the doctor help hasten the end. These cases demand a particularly careful answering of the
ethical questions involved. But, if the physician has been in the habit of
ignoring the ethical component of his day-to-day decisions, he will find
himself at a distinct disadvantage when he faces this large-scale problem.
Like anything else, ethical decision making improves with practice. The
physician's entire training since high school has been directed at the techniques needed to make scientific and clinical decisions, but most likely he
has never had any formal training in making ethical decisions.     ↓

So what then does the physician do? He may choose to follow whatever the     **10**
current custom of his profession or community happens to be, he may do
what he emotionally "feels" is right at the time, or he may follow the dictates of his religion if they apply. In each of these cases he will take an
action. It may be the "right" action according to a subsequent rational analysis. If it is the "wrong" action, chances are that the consequences will be
much less dramatic than those of the surgeon whose scalpel slips and
severs a nerve, or of the internist who miscalculates the dose of a potent
drug. Physicians may lose hospital privileges for technical incompetence, or
for violations of professional etiquette (such as advertising); but they seldom are reprimanded in any formal way for wrong ethical decisions of this
nature.     ↓

In the last decade, however, the health professions have moved to correct     **11**
these deficiencies. Medical, nursing, and other health students are now
more likely to have medical ethics included as part of their formal training;
and many national conferences and articles in medical journals have shed
new light on troublesome ethical dilemmas. Once denigrated as merely applied ethics by philosophers studying ethical theory, medical ethics has
now also captured the attention of philosophers; and these philosophers,
often working in tandem with health professionals, have contributed to
teaching and research in this field.     ↓

**12**   Generations of medical students have been warned, "You may be the most humane and compassionate person imaginable, but if you can't correctly diagnose and treat disease, you are a danger to your patients." Recently, sensitive physicians such as Reiser (1978) and Pellegrino (1979) have called attention to the other side of that coin: The physician may be in the Nobel Prize category as far as his technical competence goes, but he is unable to be of real service to his patients unless he listens to them in an open-minded way and deals competently with the human values issues that he uncovers. Health care is just as much applied humanities as it is applied science. A new awareness of the role of the humanities disciplines in medicine — not just ethics and philosophy, but also history, religious studies, literature, and art — and the social and behavioral sciences has reminded us of this dimension of medicine that narrow focus on the biological sciences
↓   has tended to obscure.

**13**   So why study medical ethics in general, or this book in particular? We make two assumptions: (1) that the physician-to-be would rather be ethical than not; and (2) that ethical decisions, like clinical decisions, will be made better if they are made according to a rational methodology rather than haphazardly.

The idea of a rational methodology for ethical decision making may be a new idea. Popular conceptions of "ethics" often picture it either as the following of a set of commandments laid down by the Bible, the AMA, or some other authority; or else as a way in which some mysterious feelings deep within our souls magically transmute themselves into some kind of "force of will," "will to be," or some such thing. Chapter 2 will go into greater detail about the nature of ethics in order to show an ethical decision-making method that can be usefully applied to problems in medicine.

**14**   ↓   CH. 2

# A Method of 2
## Ethical Reasoning

Medical ethics is not a branch of medicine, but a branch of ethics. (The    **14**
question of the definition of ethics will be postponed for now.) Before
tackling the ethical issues that are peculiar to medical practice, it is best to
consider ethics in general, and to ask whether there is some general
method of problem solving that can be applied to any ethical question. This
method could then be applied to the ethical issues that arise in medicine. ↓

To begin with, one must be able to recognize an ethical, or moral, problem    **15**
when it arises. We can list two essential ingredients of an ethical problem.
The first is the existence of a real choice between possible courses of action. It makes no sense, for example, to make ethical statements about
whether or not a surgeon should perform a brain transplant — such action is
impossible now, and there are good reasons to believe that it will not be
possible in the near future, so the choice of whether or not to do a brain
transplant does not really exist.
WHAT ABOUT FUTURE POSSIBILITIES? * 17    ↓

The second major ingredient of an ethical problem is that the person in-    **16**
volved must place a significantly different value upon each possible action,
or upon the consequences of that action. For example, the question of
whether to use silk suture or nylon suture to sew a laceration is, for all practical purposes, not an ethical question; the choice can be made on purely
technical grounds. On the other hand, the question of whether to treat a
disease by drugs or by surgery has a definite ethical component, since both
doctor and patient may place a very different value upon taking medication
as opposed to undergoing surgery.    ↓ **18**

---

* Does this requirement mean that it is not worthwhile to make ethical    **17**
statements about those types of genetic engineering, such as cloning,
which are not now possible? But these technologies might well be developed in future years. In such cases where the implications may have great
social import, it makes good sense to get a headstart by thinking of future
ethical difficulties right now instead of waiting for the actuality and being
caught unprepared.    ↑ **16**

**18** In order to communicate about ethical problems and moral judgments, we must use moral statements. (At this point, we are using "ethical" and "moral" as approximately interchangeable terms; a distinction will be made later.) A formula for a moral statement is:

In situation X, person Y ought to do thing Z.

Note three ingredients to a moral statement:

1. <u>What</u> is to be done (Z).
2. <u>Who</u> is to do it (Y).
3. The <u>conditions</u> under which the statement is applicable (X).

While moral statements such as "stealing is wrong" do not fit this formula, they can generally be restated in accordance with the formula by filling in the obvious missing elements: "Under no conditions should any person
↓ steal."

**19** Before discussing how to use ethical statements in problem solving, we will compare ethical statements with various other types of statements. Failure to be absolutely clear about some of these distinctions is a primary cause of
**21** ↓ errors in ethical reasoning and of misunderstandings in ethical discussions.
WHY STATEMENTS? * 20

---

**20** * You might wonder why we are starting out with statements, which are, after all, only abstract representations of ideas, instead of the ethical judgments themselves. First, we are becoming more aware of the fact that language has a strong influence on the way we think, and that cultural patterns of thinking are reflected in language. (That is why, in order to learn Chinese, a Westerner has to learn not only vocabulary and syntax but also a whole new way of looking at the world.) Second, we find analysis of statements useful for making some important distinctions. Take the difference between our thoughts and our feelings, which can be very important in ethics. In our own minds we are both thinking and feeling together all the time, and it is hard to sort out the two. But by analyzing statements about thoughts and statements about feelings, we might gain some new insight
↓ into these actual mental processes.

A very common type of statement is the "empirical" statement, which as-     **21**
serts that a certain state of affairs does or does not exist. It is likely to cause
trouble when it occurs in a form closely resembling that of the ethical statement, such as:

In situation X, person Y often does thing Z.

The key difference is the absence of the word "ought." The ethical statement, by the use of "ought," both recommends action and suggests that
that action is better (has a higher value) than the alternatives. The empirical
statement is merely descriptive; it makes no value judgments and requires
that no action be taken.                                                     ↓

Empirical statements have the property of being either <u>true</u> or <u>false</u>. While     **22**
we sometimes hear these terms used also to apply to ethical statements, it
does not seem that a recommendation for action can be true or false in the
same sense that a description can. Rather, we would prefer to speak of ethi-
cal statements as <u>right</u> or <u>wrong</u>, or, even better, <u>valid</u> and <u>invalid</u>, to remind us that the method we must use to determine an ethical question is
fundamentally different from the method of settling an empirical question.
  *People trained in the sciences, who are most comfortable with empirical*
*statements, are especially prone to make the mistake of trying to solve ethi-*
*cal problems simply by accumulating data, while ignoring the need to make*
*value judgments. In theory, if we accumulate enough data, we can thereby*
*solve any empirical question. With an ethical dilemma, we can have all the*
*data in the world, and we still cannot arrive at an answer until we come to*
*grips with our values and make some value judgments.*                        ↓
  UNCLEAR * 24

Other statements, besides ethical statements, may be said to share the     **23**
property of being neither true nor false. One is the "aesthetic" statement,
such as, "I like to do thing Z" or "Thing Z is beautiful." However, these
should not be confused with ethical statements because, like empirical
statements, they contain no requirement of action. It is generally understood that "I like to do thing Z" does not necessarily suggest that "I ought
to do thing Z."                                                             ↓ **25**

---

* The reason truth and falsity apply to empirical statements and not to ethi-     **24**
cal statements is that in order to apply those concepts, we need a principle
of verification. We understand how to tell if a statement is true by
definition. Likewise, we know how to compare a statement with our observations of the real world in order to tell if an empirical statement is true.
However, the way we judge the validity of an ethical statement, which will
be shown in the problem-solving method below, is different from the
verification process: it involves the weighing of values. There is no "real
world" of what "ought to be" available for us to make comparisons — at
least, not one that has any degree of universal agreement.                  ↑ **23**

**25** Another neither-true-nor-false type of statement is the "command," such as, "Do thing Z." Since a command requires action, the difference between it and an ethical statement is not always so easy to grasp. The main difference is that a command is meant to apply only to the particular listener at that particular time. The drill sergeant who calls out, "Left face!" may call out, "Right face!" a minute later, and no one would accuse him of contradicting himself.

An ethical statement, on the other hand, implies by its "ought" that in theory it applies to all people in similar circumstances. The ethical statement, "The physician ought to provide contraceptives to sexually active minors regardless of whether parental consent is given," implies that all physicians should provide contraceptives to any sexually active minor who might request them. It is this principle of "universalizability" that distinguishes ethical statements from commands and gives ethical statements their particular force. As we shall see, it also provides a key way of testing the validity of ethical positions.

**26** For a summary of the above, we can construct the following table:

| Type of Statement | True/False? | Action? | Universalizable? |
|---|---|---|---|
| Empirical | Yes | No | No |
| Aesthetic | No | No | No |
| Command | No | Yes | No |
| Ethical | No | Yes | Yes |

**27** Now that the nature of ethical statements is clear, we may briefly consider the types of moral conflict that can arise. In general terms, these types of conflict differ according to the values that we place upon the choices available.

**28** The simplest ethical decision is made when one choice is considered to be "good" and the other to be "evil." Because this choice is so easy, it is a common human trait to view ethical issues in terms of good and evil, even when a closer analysis would reveal this to be an oversimplification. In actuality very few ethical problems are genuinely choices of unquestionable good versus unquestionable evil.

**29** Another type of ethical conflict arises when one choice is "better" and the other is "worse." This type of decision becomes progressively harder to make as the determination of which is better and which is worse becomes more indistinct. This is especially true where the units of value are very different: Is a job that pays $30,000 and entails considerable aggravation better or worse than one that pays $15,000 and offers peace of mind? Most ethical conflicts fit into this category.

A third type of conflict occurs when one must choose between two    **30**
"goods" that are mutually exclusive. An example in medical ethics is the
question of allowing a suffering and terminally ill individual to die; here the
two good actions of prolonging life and relieving suffering are in conflict. In
other cases, the conflict may arise between the doctor's role as a good physician and as a good citizen of the state, such as when it would seem to
serve the public good to violate his promise to keep the patient's information confidential. The problem with these conflicts is that we tend to view
the failure to do a good thing as "bad," and so we are forced into doing a
bad thing no matter which alternative we choose. While these conflicts
may not arise often in such clear form, they provide ethics with many of its
thorniest dilemmas.    ↓

The last type of ethical conflict calls attention to a more general point: the    **31**
principle of "you can't have your cake and eat it too." When there are alternative courses of action open, the decision to do one is also a decision
not to do the others. Thus, in ethics, it is easy to make a decision in this way
without realizing it — a decision one may come to regret later. Farther on in
this book, the question of the allocation of scarce resources will be considered as a separate issue in medical ethics. *For now, however, it is important
to note that any ethical decision involves the allocation and expenditure of
resources of which there is only a finite amount, such as time. And, of
course, the decision to allocate a resource in one place is simultaneously a
decision not to allocate it somewhere else.*    ↓

With all these introductory issues understood, we can progress to the major    **32**
business of outlining and explaining a general method of ethical decision
making. The method is diagrammed in Figure 1 and is explained in the
frames to follow.    ↓

The first step, obviously, is to perceive that a moral problem exists. As was    **33**
shown in Chapter 1, it is not always easy to sort out the ethical components
from the many other types of problems that face us in our daily lives.    ↓

Next, a list is made of the alternative courses of action that are open to deal    **34**
with the problem. An error that is commonly made at this step, and which
in fact was (deliberately) made above in the discussion of types of moral
conflict, is to assume that there must be two and only two alternatives and
then proceed to weigh one against the other, possibly ignoring completely
the existence of a third course of action that is much more desirable. The
human mind prefers "either–or" thinking to the complexities of juggling
three or more alternatives, so this error is often made unconsciously. Thus,
before proceeding to the next step, it is important to check to make sure
the list of alternatives is exhaustive.    ↓

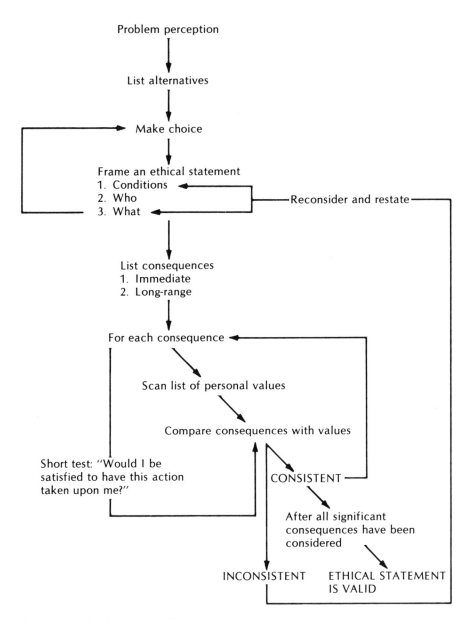

**Figure 1.** *Method for ethical decision making.*

Having listed alternatives, we next choose one of them as the appropriate       **35**
course of action. It may seem strange that the choice is made here instead
of as the last step of the decision-making process. All that is being done
here, however, is a recognition of how human beings actually function.
Faced with an ethical choice, in most cases, we immediately <u>want</u> to do one
thing, based on some gut-level reaction. There is nothing <u>wrong</u> with this,
so long as the initial reaction is then analyzed by some rational process, and
is rejected if it fails the test. That is the role of the rest of the decision-
making process.                                                                 ↓

The choice that has been made must next be framed in the form of an ethi-      **36**
cal statement, with all the ingredients described above: what is to be done,
who is to do it, and the conditions under which the statement is to apply.
Since the choice has been made, drawing up a detailed statement may
seem an unnecessary formality — in fact, in most ethical discussions, it is
never done. The value of this step lies in making explicit the element of
universalizability that is inherent in the ethical "ought."

"I have decided to do thing Z" carries no ethical weight; possibly later,
under essentially the same circumstances, I might instead decide to do
thing W. When cast in the form of an ethical statement, the implication is
far broader: "I have decided to do thing Z, <u>and</u> anyone like me, under the
same circumstances, <u>ought</u> to do thing Z also." The question then arises: If
everyone in fact did do thing Z, what would be the consequences? Would
these consequences be desirable or not? In these questions we have the
tools for a rational analysis to determine the validity of the ethical decision. ↓ **38**

"WHAT IF EVERYONE DID THAT?" * 37

---

* It has been objected that the question, "What if everyone did that?" is not     **37**
a valid way of judging ethical validity. For example, suppose a medical student is searching for a speciality field, and he learns that there is a shortage
of family physicians. He decides he wants to be a family physician. But then
he asks, "What if everyone became a family physician? There would be no
surgeons, obstetricians, and so on. Those consequences are bad; therefore,
I cannot be a family physician."

This difficulty is gotten rid of simply by stating the more general ethical
principle that is to be followed. In the case above, it is something like, "In
choosing a speciality, the new doctor ought to choose a field that is presently in need of more practitioners." If everyone did that, there would be
no problems.                                                                   ↓

**38**    The next step is, in fact, to determine the consequences if the proposed ethical statement were to be accepted. While the first thing that comes to mind are the immediate consequences of one's own act, it pays to devote some mental effort to predict the long-range consequences of one's own act in relation to the acts of others. The present interest in ecology is teaching us to be particularly sensitive to the aggregate consequences: The consequences of my throwing my beer can beside the road may be nil, but the consequences of everyone doing the same may be disastrous.

    Clearly it is impossible to list all the possible consequences, even if we could predict them — just as, in the scientific method, it is impossible to list all the variables that must be controlled in a particular experiment. Nor can we spend so much time listing possible consequences that we let the time for the action itself slip past. *This means, in the end, that we must always take action on the basis of some degree of uncertainty. The goal is to reduce that uncertainty to manageable proportions, and to ensure that we have at least considered all the major consequences that we are able to predict with our current level of understanding of the world.*

**39**    It should be noted here that this method of testing an ethical act by its consequences (or "consequentialist" ethics) is one type of ethical theory. By no means do all ethical philosophers adhere to this view, and several alternative methodologies exist. For simplicity, one ethical method is described in this book and is used as a basis for all further discussion. Some of the more common alternative forms of ethical decision-making processes are described in Appendix I.

**40**    How does one predict what consequences will follow from a certain action? In simple cases, we know from personal experience; in other cases, we can apply known empirical data, or we can make predictions using scientific methods. The statements about which consequences may or will follow from an action are empirical statements. Thus we see that while ethical and empirical statements are two different species of animal, they are closely related in the ethical decision-making process. Clearly, if the statements we now make about the consequences of our act turn out to be false statements, the remainder of our decision-making effort will be wasted.

**41**    The next step is to compare each of the consequences with one's own set of values. Since values are often only tacitly understood, this part of the process is less open to scrutiny than the rest. Essentially what is going on is that one asks, for each consequence, "Could I live with this?" If consideration of a consequence causes one some emotional discomfort, one may ask, "Why does this bother me?" and eventually arrive at a statement of the specific value that is inconsistent with the consequence.

This last set of instructions needs some clarification. First, obviously we do **42** not all go around with a list of values in our pockets ready to be pulled out and consulted as soon as an ethical question jumps out of the underbrush. But just as obviously, we do all value some things more than others, and if someone came to us with a long questionnaire that asked us to compare various things, we could, by our answers, make our values explicit.    ↓

Second, one might say that we have already made a choice by what we **43** "want" to do in this case, on a gut-level basis. Since our values are nothing more than gut-level intuitions, are we not doing the same thing here that we did before, when we stated that we just wanted to do one thing and not the other? If that were the case, our ethical method would just boil down to "Do what you want, and then use this fancy method to make it seem rational."

But that is not the case. If values are gut-level in their normal state, they are no longer gut-level once we have transformed them into language by stating them explicitly. Furthermore, at the beginning, when we "wanted" to do one thing, we had not yet predicted the consequences of doing so. Now we have both clearly stated values and clearly stated consequences to compare them to; we are no longer dealing with vague desires, even though we are still acting on a subjective level.    ↓

*In sum, what this ethical method really boils down to is the injunction that* **44** *we ought to make our values explicit so that we can judge acts by their consequences. We have just seen two steps to this process: (1) stating values and consequences in plain language; and (2) placing values and consequences in close juxtaposition, so that we can make direct comparisons and decide our preferences.*

In our ordinary activities, we do not do these things. We allow our values to govern our desires on a subconscious level, without examining the process by which this occurs. In these important respects, then, the ethical method put forth here is a distinct improvement over our "normal" way of acting.    ↓

A kind of short cut may often be useful in place of an exhaustive consider- **45** ation of lists of values. If the proposed action affects some other person besides the decision maker, he may ask, "If I were in that person's situation, and I were like him in morally relevant ways, would I be satisfied with having this done to me?" If the answer is "yes," it may be assumed that the action is consistent with the decision maker's own set of values, assuming he has been honest and thoughtful in his answer.

**45**
cont.  The successful application of this technique requires the decision maker to put himself in the shoes of the other party, and this requires in particular the ability to <u>imagine</u>. In some cases this may be very difficult — for example, in a case in which the other party is mentally retarded.

**46**  Once all the consequences have been compared to one's values, and no inconsistencies have been revealed, it may be concluded that the proposed course of action is ethically valid. It should, of course, be borne in mind that possibly all the significant consequences have not been considered, and that new knowledge in the future may cast doubt upon the decision in retrospect. There is no escape from this uncertainty, since all actions have consequences — including the decision not to take action.

**47**  Much more likely, some inconsistency will be found between one of the consequences and the set of values. When this occurs, the method calls for a reconsideration of the original ethical statement, and a restatement to remove the offending portion. The first thing to try is a modification of the <u>conditions</u> of the ethical statement.

For example, in order to rationalize why a physician should not perform an abortion, one comes up with the ethical statement, "Medical treatment should not be given to a person unless organic illness is present." This suits the purpose, since pregnancy is not considered an illness. However, one consequence of this statement is that a physician cannot perform elective plastic surgery. This is inconsistent with one's values, because one has sympathy with people who suffer emotional anguish due to unattractive features. One might therefore modify the original statement to, "Medical treatment should not be given to a person unless organic illness is present, <u>except</u> where the danger to life or health is negligible compared to the expected benefits." (What are some consequences of this new statement?)

**48**  In many cases, changing the conditions will suffice to bring the statement into accord with one's values. However, it may be necessary to change instead the <u>what</u> part of the statement — that is, the proposed action itself is realized to be inconsistent with one's values. This entails making a different choice, and in turn framing a new ethical statement.

Whatever the case, the modified, or the new, ethical statement must then be examined for consequences, and the process repeated, as shown by the circular arrows in Figure 1, until consistency wins out in the end.

If one is being really exhaustive, however, the process does not end here. **49** One should investigate the other choices as well; it may be that one or more of them are also ethically valid, as in the "good vs. good" type of conflict mentioned above. One then has a particularly hard decision to make. One must determine which of his set of values are most directly applicable to each of the alternatives. He then must weigh the values to see which he values most highly, and choose accordingly. In the euthanasia example mentioned already, a doctor who would oppose giving a terminally ill cancer patient an overdose of morphine may be saying that he values the principle of preserving life over the principle of alleviating suffering. A physician who decides to give the overdose may be making the opposite valuation.

Note that if one were being thorough in listing the consequences, "Not being able to do the other actions" would have been listed as a consequence of the choice that was made. One could have weighed this against one's set of values, without having to go through the whole process for each separate alternative.

So far we have been talking as if each time we applied the decision-making **50** method to an ethical question, we obtained one and only one ethically valid answer. This would be very nice if it were the case, but it is not. In many of the "hard" cases, both because of uncertainties in predicting consequences and because of confusions in how we rank our own values, it will be impossible to show that one alternative is clearly superior to the others. Several alternatives will be shown to be equally good, or more likely, equally bad, within the framework of the decision-making method; and we are still stuck with making a choice. We will run across several such cases in later chapters. (Note, in Appendix I, that alternative ethical methods share this problem of sometimes failing to come up with a "right" answer for each case.)

When these hard cases come up, however, we can learn something from **51** them. If we see that they tend to occur more frequently in certain circumstances, we can try to change those circumstances. For instance, if a physician who sees 60 patients a day in his office is always having to make difficult decisions about how to allocate his attention among patients with equally pressing problems, he might decide eventually to try to attract a partner to help with his practice. But in many cases we have no real choice about whether we are to go out on the ethical limb or not; or the consequences of changing the circumstances might be even worse ethical problems than we have now.

**52**  Now that we have gone through the entire method, we must go back and say a few more things about the so-called set of values. We have gotten around one objection by making our values explicit instead of allowing them to influence behavior on the subconscious level. We still have the objection that some values, even when rendered explicit, are still objectionable to others. According to the method as it stands, Attila the Hun could show up, placing a high value on murder, rape, and pillage, and so long as he made those values explicit, he could claim that his actions were ethically justified.

**53**  Does this mean that we are stuck with whatever set of values we find ourselves with, and there is no way to separate the good values from the objectionable ones? One preliminary way of testing values is provided in the ethical method. While we have described it mainly as a way of testing consequences, it can just as easily be used as a way of testing values. Explicate a value, take some sample cases, and determine how that value would lead you to act in each case. If a certain value tends to lead you to act in ways that are generally disapproved of, you would begin to give serious thought to changing that value, or at least giving it significantly lower priority.

**54**  If you do no more than accept values that are generally approved of and reject those that are not, you are adhering to "common-sense morality." This may be a useful guide in most simple cases, but it can be a source of inconsistency and irrationality in complex situations. We prefer a firmer basis for judging our values.

Many people feel at this point that the answer lies in religion. One adopts a religious outlook and judges values by how closely they agree with the doctrines of that religion. We will not be looking explicitly to religion for our ethical values in our later discussion; but this does not mean that we are rejecting religious values or that religion does not constitute an important source of ethical insight. (For more discussion on the role of religion in ethical decision making, see Appendix II.)

**55**  We are going to propose that there is a better basis for judging which values are best suited to meet the objective needs of human beings, and we will describe this basis in a preliminary way in Chapter 18. However, this basis is not yet so thoroughly worked out as to provide specific guidance on specific values; and even if it were, many ethicists would not agree with the results.

For the time being, therefore, we will accept the reality that different people have different values, and we will leave the ethical method open-ended to accommodate these differences. We will have to deal with Attila the Hun later.

In order to see how this whole process works, it will be illustrated by work-   **56**
ing through a sample case. Before doing this, however, a few more important points about ethical reasoning ought to be made.    ↓

*Rigor.* First, discussion of the decision-making process has hopefully dis-   **57**
pensed with the common view that ethics is a "soft" discipline, as opposed
to the sciences where conclusions are reached by rigorous application of a
specific method. While the ethical method certainly differs from the
scientific method, it should be clear that the process outlined is an arduous
one, which requires every bit as much sustained and disciplined thought as
any common scientific problem.    ↓

*Pluralism.* Second, it will have been noted that since individuals have dif-   **58**
ferent sets and scales of values, two people, each applying the decision-
making method faithfully, may reach two different ethical conclusions. This
may bother a reader who has been led to expect that it is the role of ethics
to provide unmistakable rules of correct conduct. Actually, such a
definition of "ethics" touches only on its very narrowest aspects (if you are
still unclear, review the "Objectives" and the "Not Objectives" at the beginning of the book).
   A common misconception is that, if we deny the possibility of a system
of ethics that clearly tells what is the right thing to do under any circumstances, past, present, and future, then the only alternative we are left with
is a totally vague ethics where any one person's opinion is just as good as
any other's. In technical terms, this is the conflict between "moral absolutism" and "moral relativism."    ↓

The absolutism vs. relativism way of phrasing the problem, however, falls   **59**
into the error already mentioned — assuming that there are only two alternatives. *The decision-making process outlined here in fact seeks a comfortable middle ground, which we may call moral pluralism. It allows for
differences in personal values and for change in ethical judgments over
time, as new knowledge about possible consequences is acquired. At the
same time, it prevents a moral free-for-all by insisting that no one can claim
ethical validity for his statements until he has subjected them to rigorous
and rational analysis. In this way, there may not be one "correct" answer.
There will, however, be no more than a few good answers, since the inconsistent or poorly thought out positions will have been eliminated along the
way. In any case, it would seem that a statement derived from the decision-
making process will prove to be a better guide to action, in important matters, than either one's initial gut reaction or blind adherence to preexisting
rules.*    ↓

**60** Still, to the ethical philosopher, absolutism and relativism are mutually exclusive categories; so since our pluralistic ethics are not absolutist, they must formally be listed as a type of relativistic ethics. We might also note that an ethical relativist may be saying two different things: either there really is no way finally to resolve a value conflict; or that ideally such a way exists but that in real life it is impractical to insist upon it. Frankena, in his book on ethics, discusses this matter more fully. Here the main thing is to see why a pluralistic ethic is not necessarily the same as "do your own thing."

**61** *Levels.* Since, as was noted in Chapter 1, there are potential ethical problems in all aspects of our daily lives (let alone in the practice of medicine), does this mean that we have to stop each time and apply the decision-making method just described in its entirety? Naturally people in practice do not do so. Even "ethical" individuals practice different levels of problem-solving behavior in accordance with the importance of the matter at hand, or in accordance with the novelty of the situation. One useful scheme for categorizing levels of moral activity has been proposed by Henry Aiken.

**62** Aiken (1962) suggests four levels of moral discourse, each of which is illustrated below by a sample statement on abortion made at that level.

| *Level* | *Statement* |
|---|---|
| Expressive Level | "I hate abortion" |
| Level of Moral Rules | "Do not perform abortions" |
| Level of Ethical Principles | "The right of the fetus to life is more important than the mother's right to the privacy of her own body" |
| Postethical Level | "It is important to respect the rights of others, else human life is not truly 'human' " |

**63** Notice that most daily decisions are made on the first two of Aiken's levels. In simple instances we allow our likes and dislikes to rule; in more complex cases we apply rules that we have come to follow. Every so often, we are faced with a more complicated problem and have to go through some kind of formal ethical reasoning process. (Note that in this scheme, a person can be moral, or acting in accordance with rules of "right" conduct, without being ethical, or having gone through a formal reasoning process to decide upon his behavior. In this sense, moral and ethical are no longer interchangeable terms but refer to different levels of activity.)

Any ethical statement raises another potential question: Why bother to do **64**
what is "right" anyway? Why bother to be ethical? Aiken's postethical level
deals with attempts to justify the need for ethical reasoning and ethical
conduct. Since this book is designed to be on the third level, the postethical
level is beyond our scope. Our basic assumption is that the physician wants
to be ethical and simply wishes to be told how to do it.

Aiken's levels raise two important points, which clarify the objectives of **65**
this book. First, it is often the case that conflict on one level requires re-
course to the next higher level to resolve the conflict. Thus, we can com-
fortably operate on the level of moral rules only so long as there is general
agreement. If someone questions our decision, or if two of our own rules
conflict, we have to either throw up our hands in despair, or else adopt an
ethical problem-solving approach to determine what is valid. The goal of
this book is not to make the reader use the decision-making process for
each moral question, but rather to provide the process as a tool that can be
brought into use when required. The ethical person does not use the process continually, but he is prepared to use it at any time whenever one of his
decisions requires formal justification.

The corresponding point is that, once a new situation has been dealt with **66**
on one level, recurrences of essentially similar situations can be handled
conveniently on a lower level. The physician faced with his first patient
who requests an abortion may have to go through a complex problem-
solving process. By the time he reaches his fifteenth patient, he has adopted
a set of "rules" as a shorthand for his previous thinking, and can reach the
decision much quicker. However, when the patient presents a novel aspect,
for example, an unmarried woman where all his previous rules had dealt
with married women, the physician may have to repeat the decision-
making process.

*Codes.* The distinction between moral and ethical levels of sophistication **67**
hopefully explains another point that may have puzzled the reader: why we
have begun a discussion of medical ethics without any mention of the various "codes of ethics" that already exist in medicine. There have been numerous such codes in the history of the profession, starting with listing of
fees and malpractice penalties in the Code of Hammurabi, to the famous
Oath of the Hippocratic school, to Thomas Percival's very detailed code
(1804), which formed the basis for the first Code of Ethics of the American
Medical Association (1847).

**68**     The limitations of such codes are the limitations of the "moral rule" level as opposed to the "ethical" level — they can apply only to situations stated in the code, not to any new situations that may arise later; and, if too detailed, different rules in the code are likely to conflict with each other. In fact, most of the codes mentioned above deal with the really hard ethical questions by ignoring them. Instead they concentrate on the matters that have come to be called "professional etiquette," such as whether a physician should advertise. Note that the entire first half of the famous Hippocratic Oath deals with how a physician should act toward other members of his profession (at that time, a religious cult); the admonitions about service to ↓ the patient and about respect for the patient's right to privacy come later.

**69**     *Law.* Many of the problems with codes also apply to those who would look to the law as a guide to ethical behavior. In that view, medical ethics can be reduced to one statement, "The physician should obey the laws of the area in which he practices," and all else will follow. One problem with that statement is that even the most patriotic physician will envision a few instances in which he would find it ethical to violate a particular law. A possible example occurred in the 1960s in Connecticut, where an archaic law from the Colonial era, never repealed, prevented physicians from giving any kind of contraceptive information. Civil disobedience by some physicians ↓ led to a landmark Supreme Court ruling, which overturned the law.

**70**     A more basic point is that the law and ethics, as Ladd (1979) points out, serve different purposes altogether. The law is primarily concerned with adjudicating conflicts in a way that preserves the basic social order. Ethics has a much broader range of concerns: our relationships with others, and how our values and character traits ought best to be expressed in action. It would be foolish to expect the law to do such a job, especially one for which it is poorly equipped.

   In practice, this will often mean that legal dictates are quite permissive with regard to medical practice. For example, right now the laws of most states permit a physician to do most abortions, and also to refuse to do any abortions. The physician seeking individual guidance on the ethics of doing ↓ abortions in certain cases will get no help from the law.

**71**     In this book we will address legal issues for two main purposes. First, we will point out important legal doctrines that limit the physician's behavior. Violating a law would be a major consequence to be considered in deciding whether to act in a certain way, and so knowing the law is important in such cases.

   Second, we will mention specific court decisions for the purposes of dissecting the ethical arguments that support the decisions. We may, on critical analysis, find that the courts have reached invalid ethical conclusions; but generally major court decisions contain ethical insights that are worthy ↓ of study.

*Rights.* You may have noticed that in describing our ethical method, we     **72**
have made no mention of "rights." But rights play a major role in medical
ethical debates — we hear often of the right to life, the right to privacy, the
right to health care. We must look, then, at what rights are and what arguments may arise about them.

First, we should be alert to a misuse of rights. It is easy to move from "I
want X" to "I have a right to X." But in doing so, one has advanced no ethical reasons to show that one's claim to X is a valid one, which others should
be obliged to honor. Talk of "the right to own a pet," "the right to eat in a
tobacco-free environment," and other such marginal rights merely
cheapens the notion. Also, if one party in a dispute advances a dubious
rights claim, the other party is liable to do likewise. When anti-abortionists
claim a right to life for the fetus, and pro-abortionists reply with the right of
a woman to control her own body, we can be sure that no ethical enlight-
enment is likely to emerge.                                                    ↓

One way to get rid of such nonserviceable uses of rights is to avoid claiming     **73**
any rights at all. For example, by our ethical decision-making procedure,
why not leave out all talk of a "right to life" and just say that life is of very
great value when one weighs the consequences of actions?

But getting rid of all rights talk may be likened to throwing out the baby
with the bath water. There are some things that seem fundamental to our
concept of a just society, so that the mere claiming of them gives rise to
very strong obligations on the parts of others to honor that claim — and the
others cannot use convenience, expense, or other ethical values as an excuse not to honor the claim. Except for calling these things "rights," there
seems to be no language that adequately expresses how basic these claims
are and how strong are the obligations arising from them. We may be thinking here of such basic constitutional or common-law rights as the right of
free speech and religion, the right to vote, and the right to a jury trial.     ↓

Generally, to say that "X has a right to A" entails an obligation toward X on     **74**
the part of others. If I have a right to life, you have an obligation not to kill
me. What we may call <u>perfect</u> rights entail <u>negative</u> obligations — obligations not to kill, not to prevent my speaking freely, and so on. These obligations apply to everyone equally. <u>Imperfect</u> rights — the right to health care
would be one — entail <u>positive</u> obligations (in this case to provide or to pay
for health care) and may not fall on everyone equally. For example, one
who is not a health professional, or who has very little money, may not be
obligated to pay for or provide my health care, even if we agreed that I had
a right to it.                                                                   ↓

**75** Because it's harder to allocate positive obligations fairly throughout society, and to make them stick, some argue that imperfect rights are therefore automatically harder to justify than perfect rights. Indeed, many of the marginal, rhetorical rights we condemned above are imperfect rights. But there are also many well-accepted imperfect rights — for instance, the right to vote clearly gives rise to positive obligations, since it is a great expense and inconvenience to the community to hold elections and set up polling places. Thus, just because a right such as the "right to health care" is an imperfect right, we cannot reject it on those grounds alone. (We shall have ↓ more to say about the right to health care in Chapter 16.)

**76** The connection between rights and obligations is often misunderstood. It is frequently said, "Your right to free speech means that you have the obligation to exercise that right in a responsible manner." And, indeed, people who speak irresponsibly are often justifiably condemned on ethical grounds. But that way of connecting a right and an obligation is <u>exactly what we do not mean</u> when we talk about how rights entail obligations. If you say, for instance, that a Nazi does not have the right to free speech because his views are appropriately despised by correct-thinking members of the community, you might as well say that free speech is a privilege to be accorded to those whose views you agree with — and that is to say that there is no right of free speech at all. *By talking about rights in the first place, we are pointing to claims that are so basic to our concept of justice that we are obligated to honor them, even when it is very cumbersome,* ↓ *difficult, or downright distasteful to do so.*

**77** Still, there are circumstances in which X, who has a right to A, does not get A, and yet we would still not say that X's right to A has been <u>violated</u>. First (taking A to be free speech, for example), X may simply have decided he doesn't want to speak freely, and this may be a voluntary choice. In this case, we say X has <u>waived</u> his right to free speech. (This means, in turn, that a right to do A is at the same time a right not to do A, if one so chooses.) Second, we may prevent X from shouting "fire" in a crowded theater, without violating his right of free speech. The rights of all members of the community to a minimal insurance of their safety <u>overrides</u> X's right to speak freely in this case. Generally, the only thing that is strong enough to override a right is an equal or more basic right of another, where the two rights are in direct conflict. X's right to life may be overridden by your right to life ↓ if X is the aggressor and you kill him in self-defense.

That a right may be waived or overridden is a further refinement on what     **78**
we mean by speaking of "rights," and does not count against their existence. It is sometimes argued that euthanasia cannot be ethical because it
would necessarily violate the right to life. But in some cases, individuals of
their own free will ask for death to end their suffering. We can reasonably
say that such an individual has voluntarily waived his right to life. In this
case, there is no contradiction between a right to life and the practice of
voluntary euthanasia.

Certainly it would be a mistake to reduce all ethical dilemmas to conflicts
of so-called rights. But when rights claims are raised in ethical debate, we
must know enough about rights to evaluate the claim critically, and to see
what the claim does and does not entail.     ↓

*Respect and Autonomy.* Consider this chestnut from Philosophy 101: We     **79**
are at a crucial decision point and have to choose what to do. There is one
action that allows us to promote the most values for the greatest number of
people; no other action provides for the same degree of value optimization.
But this action involves causing the suffering and death of a few people. Is
it right in such a case to sacrifice these few on the altar of the greater good
of the many? (It is dodging the question to reply that no such case is likely
to arise.)     ↓

By our ethical decision-making method, the proposed action would be     **80**
right. But many philosophers would use this as grounds to reject our ethical
system, as well as any other consequentialist ethics. They argue that it could
never be moral to commit an injustice to a few for the greater good. Any
truly ethical system, this argument goes, is based on respect for the dignity
and worth of the individual — in Kant's famous phrase, treat the individual
as an ends and not as a means only. Thus a system such as consequential-
ism, which would allow sacrifice of the individual for some greater good or
value, is fundamentally flawed.     ↓

To most health professionals, who ought to have as much if not more re-     **81**
spect for the worth of individuals than the average person, this argument
should carry great weight. For many, it will mean rejecting consequential-
ism altogether in favor of a deontological ethical theory (see Appendix I).  ↓

**82**    Still, there are many advantages to a consequentialist decision-making procedure; and we are allowed a great deal of flexibility in choosing the values
we will plug into the decision process. When values come into conflict, we
also have to decide which will have the higher priority. It seems, then, that
we can incorporate some of the strong points of deontological ethical theory into our own system if we stipulate that respect for individuals must be
regarded as a very basic value, to be given very high priority in our decision
making. And we may remember that many of the worst injustices are committed when short-sighted individuals place other values, such as the supposed good of the state, over respect for individuals. Thus, we will look
with great suspicion on any ethical argument that seems to give inadequate
emphasis to this important value. (Of course, adopting any ethical rule
which entails denying respect for individuals would also entail denying re-
↓  spect to ourselves, and thus would fail our "short-cut" test.)

**83**    What is involved in showing respect for individuals? To a large extent it
means treating others as our moral equals. We think of ourselves as free
agents, making our own choices. We are aware of sometimes being forced,
deluded, or subconsciously motivated into making choices; but we tend to
deny that choices made in those ways are "our own" choices or are
reflective of our true selves. We pride ourselves on the ability to make free
choices, even when we don't exercise that ability. Regarding others as our
moral equals, then, means respecting their ability for free choice equally to
↓  our own.

**84**    Respect for individuals thus involves respect for the autonomy of others.
We will try to promote circumstances that enhance the opportunities for
others to make free, rather than coerced, choices. Once those choices are
made, we will honor them as expressions of the other individual's autonomy, even when we disagree with the choice or think the choice is not in
the individual's best interests. Further, if we can do so without violating
other ethical rules, we will permit those choices to be translated into action. We will, in short, treat others as we would have them treat us, since
there is nothing more destructive to our self-respect than to have our autonomous choices belittled and thwarted by others who think they know
↓  better.

**85**    We have now reached the conclusion of our discussion about ethics without ever having defined "ethics." As a self-test, which of the definitions
below is the best summary of the points which have been attributed to
"ethics" so far? Check your answer . . .

1. Ethics is the study of right conduct.                                              ↓ 90
2. Ethics is the study of rational processes for determining the
   best course of action in the face of conflicting choices.                 ↓ 86

3. Ethics is a set of guidelines that, if followed, will always lead to
   correct behavior.                                                      ↓ 91
4. Ethics is the study of how people act in the face of difficult
   choices.                                                               ↓ 95

By choosing the second definition, you have summarized the major points    **86**
of the preceding discussion. Now go on to the sample case which illustrates
the application of the problem-solving process.                            ↓

---

We will now illustrate the problem-solving method by working through a     **87**
sample case. If you feel that you understand the method thoroughly without any illustration, go on to Chapter 3.                                  ↓

CH. 3 ↓ **115**

---

## CASE 1

You are a pediatrician in private practice. A mother and father bring in their    **88**
4-year-old daughter, who has been complaining for 3 days of slight fever,
runny nose, and irritability. Some of the irritability has rubbed off on the
parents and they demand rather abruptly that you prescribe an antibiotic
for the child.

According to your diagnosis, the child, with high probability, has a viral
infection. At any rate, the infection seems to be self-limiting and you feel
that no medication is required. You know that antibiotics can do no good
in viral conditions, and that the indiscriminate use of antibiotics is considered poor medical practice. Your first inclination is to explain that to the
parents and prescribe no medication, while encouraging them to call back
if the child gets worse. However, you see that the parents have a hostile
attitude, and you are aware that it is standard practice among many pediatricians to prescribe antibiotics just to save themselves the explanation and
to "make the parents happy." You are certainly not looking forward to taking the time to give the parents a full explanation, and even so they might
call another doctor or go to an emergency room.

What should you do?                                                        ↓

---

The ethical problem has been identified for you. The next step is to list the    **89**
alternative courses of action open. What are they, and how many are there?
Answer this for yourself before proceeding to the next frame.             ↓ **92**

**90** By choosing the first definition, you have selected what may be right by dictionary standards but which says very little about ethics. What is "right" conduct? How is it to be determined? Is the same conduct always right? Go **85** ↑ back to the list and try again.

---

**91** By choosing the third definition, you have shown that you are confused about the distinction that was made between "moral" and "ethical," or about the objectives of this book, or both. Review the sections on levels of moral activity, codes, and the original objectives; then return to the list of **85** ↑ definitions and make another choice.

---

**92** Technically, there are almost an infinite number of choices, since one of the questions is what to tell the parents, and there are innumerable ways of phrasing the exact words. For example, it may be a different matter ethically to tell them, "I will not give her any medication," as opposed to, "I will not give her any medication, because she has a viral cold and antibiotics are no good for that." As to alternatives that are both generally stated and realistic, we can at least identify these:

1. Prescribe a mild antibiotic; no explanation.
2. Try to explain why an antibiotic would not be indicated, without committing yourself to any action. If, after a few minutes, it seems that the parents do not understand or are still dissatisfied, give up and prescribe a mild antibiotic.
3. Explain to the parents the pros and cons of prescribing an antibiotic, ask them what they want, and follow their wish.
4. Same as above, but in addition to giving the pros and cons, add that you strongly recommend against prescribing. However, you will do it if they desire.
5. State, "I am not going to give your daughter an antibiotic because . . ." and then explain, taking as long as required to answer all the parents' questions.
6. State, "I am not going to give your daughter an antibiotic because in my professional judgment it can't do any good and may do some harm." Answer a few questions, but if they are dissatisfied after you have spent a few minutes with them, end the conversation by saying that if they don't ↓ like it they can see another doctor.

**93** Which of the positions listed would you choose? Or would it be a different one? Write out for yourself a formal statement of your ethical decision for future reference. Now you have to list the consequences of your action. Try to spend some time thinking of the long-range consequences as well as the ↓ immediate ones before going on to the next frame.

**Table 1.** *Partial List of Consequences for Case 1*

| Prescribing | Not Prescribing |
|---|---|
| 1. The parents will be satisfied with your action. | A. The parents will be dissatisfied with your action. (high) |
| 2. Parents will expect you to give a drug each time in the future when they bring child, will be dissatisfied if you don't. (high) | B. You will have the personal satisfaction of following your principles. |
| 3. Parents will be dissatisfied later if they find out that antibiotics are not indicated for viral disease. (low) | C. Parents may take child to an emergency room to get the drug, depriving child of the better follow-up care a private physician can give. (?) |
| 4. If your diagnosis was wrong, the patient may be cured. (low) | D. There will be no chance of the child developing an allergic reaction to the drug. |
| 5. Patient may develop an allergic reaction to the drug, possibly a serious or fatal one. (low) | E. By avoiding indiscriminate use of antibiotics, you are helping to avoid the emergence of new, more resistant strains of bacteria. (high) |
| 6. The child may become sensitized to the drug and suffer allergic reaction upon a subsequent exposure to it. (low–medium) | F. The parents will be saved the price of the drug. |
| 7. Use of the drug may aid in the natural selection of new strains of bacteria that are resistant to the antibiotic. (low) | G. If parents decide to seek another doctor, you will lose their fees in the future. |
| 8. You will be personally dissatisfied by having abandoned your principles. | H. If parents complain about you in the community, your reputation may suffer. (?) |
| 9. The parents will have to pay for the drug. | I. You will have made a contribution to the education of the parents on the appropriate use of drugs. (high–medium) |
| 10. You will reinforce the parents' erroneous notions about proper use of drugs. | J. If your diagnosis was wrong, the patient may get worse. (low) |
| 11. The patient may develop a side effect from the drug. (low–medium) | |

We can't list all the significant consequences of all the choices listed, especially since choices that are combinations of actions will have consequences for each part. For the sake of simplicity, a list of some of the more obvious consequences of prescribing an antibiotic and of not prescribing are listed in Table 1. If the consequences have different probabilities of occurring, these are indicated in the table as "high," "low," and so on.    94

↓ 96

By choosing the fourth definition, you have indicated that you may not be clear on the distinction between empirical and ethical statements. Statements about how people actually act are empirical statements, and are the subject matter of the behavioral and social sciences, not of ethics. Ethics is instead the study of how people <u>ought</u> to act. Go back to the list of definitions and make another choice.    95

↑ 85

**96** The next step is to compare the list of consequences with the individual's set of values. Of course, you can do this for yourself privately. However, since the purpose of this book is to make explicit things that we usually do without thinking about them, try this exercise instead. Suppose you adhere to the following list of values, that is, you value those things in the list below very highly. Which of the consequences listed in Table 1 are consistent with these values? Which are inconsistent? Are there any value conflicts that must be resolved by assigning relative weights to different values?

> Therapeutic conservatism (i.e., giving only treatment that is necessary and no more)
> Education of patients toward correct health habits
> ↓ Having other people like you

**97** Consulting Table 1, we see that for the value of therapeutic conservatism, 4, D, E, and F appear to be consistent with it while 2, 5, 6, 7, 9, 11, C, and J are inconsistent. For patient education, I is consistent while 2 and 10 are inconsistent. For having others like you, 1 and 4 are consistent while 2, 3, 5, 11, A, H, and J are all inconsistent. There are no specific value conflicts, that is, consequences that are consistent with one value and inconsistent with another. Note, however, that if the high-probability consequences are given greater weight, the value of having other people like you would tend to guide you toward prescribing the drug, while the value of therapeutic conservatism would lead to not prescribing. In the total decision-making picture, the primary conflict might be between these two values.

(Is having other people like you a good value to have? Is it particularly
↓ likely to conflict with other values?)

**98** Please note that there is one way not to reach a decision: by counting up the number of "consistents" and "inconsistents" and deciding by the majority. This is both because some consequences are more important than others, and because of the different probabilities. Is a favorable consequence of low probability more or less important than an unfavorable consequence of high probability?

This problem is a fatal error in all "arithmetic" approaches to ethics so far proposed, such as the situation-ethics rule of taking the number of people to be helped by an action minus the number of people hurt. A mathematical approach to the manipulation of values may yet be devised, but it will
↓ have to be more sophisticated than this.

By now you should be able to see whether the choice you made is consist-    **99**
ent or inconsistent with your values. Recall, however, that so far we have
only been talking about the consequences of this one case. Your formal
ethical statement, which you wrote out, must apply also to all similar cases.
You cannot accept this statement as a valid guide to behavior unless you
think of some of the other cases that it would apply to, and satisfy yourself
that the consequences in those cases would also be acceptable.

For instance, suppose you had decided not to prescribe the drug, and had
phrased your statement, "A physician should never prescribe a drug that is
medically contraindicated merely because the patient would be made happier by it." You might then envision a case in which a mentally ill patient is
requesting a harmless therapy, and threatens suicide or some other bodily
harm unless it is given. It might well be in accordance with your values to
give the patient a placebo for a while to buy time for the treatment of the
underlying mental illness. You might then change the statement to, "A physician should never prescribe a drug that is medically contraindicated
merely because the patient would be made happier, unless the patient may
suffer grave consequences as a result of a mental condition." Can you further refine this statement by thinking of new cases that would be similar? ↓

In complex issues, you might end up with an ethical statement that has so    **100**
many conditions tacked on that it would take up several pages. In such
cases, you might well conclude that a general ethical principle will not apply, and that each case presents so many unique features that it must be
decided on its own merits. The ethical statement may then be shortened to
simply list the basic criteria that you will apply to each unique case in order
to guide your decision.                                                      ↓

Without giving any right answer, we have outlined an approach by which    **101**
the ethical decision-making process can be used for a rational analysis of
Case 1. Before concluding this chapter, we will go into one other point that
might have been raised by the application of the ethical method to this
case.                                                                        ↓

*Rational Decision Theory.* As you went through Case 1, you may have been    **102**
dissatisfied with the rough way in which the consequences were compared
according to their consistency with values and also according to their high
or low probability. It may have occurred to you that there ought to be a
mathematical way of comparing these factors in order to obtain a more
quantitative answer. There is such a method, the basis of which is called
Bayesian decision theory, which can be very useful in some instances. A full
description of this theory and its modifications is given by Jeffrey (1965),
but we shall outline it here by giving one example.                          ↓

**103**  Let's suppose that we are trying to decide whether it is better to treat a certain patient by surgery or with medication. For simplicity let's also assume that we can list just three consequences that may follow each action, and that these consequences are mutually exclusive; we can call these the "good," "bad," and "very bad" consequences for each. In the case of surgery, say that the patient might have a complete cure, or he may suffer side effects from the surgical procedure, or he may die from the surgery. In the case of medication, the best he can hope for is a partial cure; and he also might have side effects, or might die from the drugs. Let's assume also that the side effects of the drug (unless they are fatal) are treatable with other ↓ means, but that the side effects of surgery are untreatable and permanent.

**104**  Now we construct a table, listing at the front of each row the various actions we might take, and at the head of each column, the possible contingencies that might arise outside of our control. Such a table for the case ↓ cited is shown in Figure 2A.

|  | Good | Bad | Very Bad |
|---|---|---|---|
| Drug Therapy | Partial cure | Treatable side effects | Death |
| Surgical Therapy | Complete cure | Untreatable side effects | Death |

A

|  | Good | Bad | Very Bad |
|---|---|---|---|
| Drug | .70 | .28 | .02 |
| Surgery | .50 | .40 | .10 |

B

|  | Good | Bad | Very Bad |
|---|---|---|---|
| Drug | .7 | .5 | 0 |
| Surgery | 1.0 | .2 | 0 |

C

|  | Good | Bad | Very Bad | Sum |
|---|---|---|---|---|
| Drug | (.70) (.7)= .49 | (.28) (.5)= .14 | (.02) (0)=0 | .63 |
| Surgery | (.50) (1)= .50 | (.40) (.2)= .08 | (.10) (0)=0 | .58 |

D

**Figure 2.** (A) Summary of case. (B) Probability table. (C) Desirability table. (D) Table of weighted desirabilities.

Now we have to determine the probability of each of these possible conse-    **105**
quences. We can assume that we have the data to do this. Using the convention of 1.0 = complete certainty and 0 = impossibility, we can state
that with drugs, there is a .70 chance of a good outcome, a .28 chance of
nonfatal side effects, and a .02 chance of side effects causing death. Say that
the surgery is of a relatively dangerous sort: there is only a .50 chance of a
good outcome, with .40 of the cases having a bad result, and .10 directly
resulting in fatality.

  We can substitute these values to obtain the table of probabilities shown
in Figure 2B.    ↓

We also need a term to represent the value, or desirability, placed on each    **106**
of the outcomes. Presumably we would have to obtain this from the patient
by asking some carefully designed questions. Let's say that we get the following results, also on a 0 to 1 scale: complete cure is highly desirable, at
1.0; a partial cure is worth .7; treatable side effects are .5; untreatable side
effects are .2; and death is at the bottom of the list with 0. (We could adopt
any other scale, calling death 0 and complete cure 100, for instance; so long
as the relative spacing between items and their rank ordering are the same,
the final results will be the same.)

  These desirability values are entered in the table in Figure 2C.    ↓

As we saw in Case 1, we want to weight the consequences differently, de-    **107**
pending on their relative probabilities. In mathematical terms, we do this
by multiplying the probability value in each square of the table by the corresponding desirability value; the product is called the weighted desirability. This is shown in Figure 2D.

  Since the events shown by the column headings are outside of our control, any of them may occur. Therefore, to decide what to do, we have to
add the weighted desirabilities for all the columns in each row. As Figure
2D shows, this gives us a sum of .63 for drug therapy, and a sum of .58 for
surgical therapy. We conclude, then, that drug therapy is superior to surgical therapy. Another way of saying this is that drugs come before surgery in
this patient's preference ranking.    ↓

Now we know what we want to do in this hypothetical case. To show the    **108**
other possible applications of the Bayesian system, let's take it one step further. Suppose you are a surgeon who wants to improve the surgical technique for this disease, so that it will be superior to the existing drug therapy.
Assume that for some reason the .10 mortality rate is relatively fixed, but
that you can possibly alter the surgical technique so that you lower the rate
of side effects and increase the rate of complete cure by a corresponding
amount. Question: How much do you have to increase the probability of
cure to make the surgery preferable to drug therapy?    ↓

**109**   We solve this problem by noting that the sum of the probabilities right now for complete cure and for side effects together is .90. Then, if we raise the probability for cure to some new rate x, the probability for side effects will be .90 − x. We also know that to make the preference ranking of surgery and drugs exactly even, we want the sum of all the weighted desirabilities in the "surgery" row to be .63. Keeping the same desirability values, the new row in the weighted desirability table would be:

$$(x) (1) + (.90 - x) (.2) + (.10) (0) = .63$$
$$\text{Solving,} \quad x + .18 - .2x = .63$$
$$.8x = .45$$
$$x = .56$$

**110**   These calculations tell us that the enterprising surgeon must aim at making the chance of complete cure greater than .56 before his surgical therapy will be preferable to drug therapy.

**111**   We have indicated that Bayesian decision theory has a number of advantages. Why do we not adopt it as the central ethical method?

First, remember all the simplifying assumptions that we had to make in order to get our sample case to fit into a simple matrix of six squares. In a real case, we might have five or six possible actions and each could have ten or twelve contingent consequences; we would have to go to a computer to solve the problem. (With increasing uses of computers in medicine this may in fact occur; indeed decision-theory programs might be added on to computer-diagnosis programs. How would you view such a development?)

**112**   But a more basic problem is deriving the desirability values. Once these are given, the calculations are easy. But do we always know what desirability values we place on things? We might know that we would prefer some degree of disability to death, but can we say just how much more we prefer it? If we can't, then our assignment of desirability values is nothing more than pulling numbers out of the air. There are several strategies to get around this, but none of them dispenses with the element of subjectivity.

**113**   Because of this problem with desirability values, we are often no better off using the supposedly quantitative Bayesian system than we would be using the qualitative method described above. In that case, we would prefer to use the qualitative method, to avoid giving our decision an appearance of "objectivity," which it does not deserve.

We can conclude that we ought to keep the Bayesian rational decision theory in mind as a useful strategy to apply when values of probabilities and desirabilities are readily obtainable, but that this system cannot replace a more general, qualitative ethical decision-making method.

This completes our discussion of the ethical decision-making method. This **114** method will be used in most of the case discussions in the following chapters. Space will not permit us to go into each case in as much depth as we did in Case 1; instead we will pick out the most interesting or the most controversial facets of each case. However, you will gain practice in the method by applying it to subsequent cases and using it to fill in the gaps in the discussion. Refer back to this chapter whenever you are unclear on how to apply the method.

Since our treatment of ethical theory has necessarily been rather brief, you may wish to supplement your knowledge by referring to the works listed in the References under the heading "Ethics, General." The works listed under the heading "Medical Ethics, General" are not only good survey works on medical ethics, but also contain useful analyses of different modes of ethical reasoning.

CH. 3 ↓ **115**

# Fundamentals 3
## of Medical Ethics

We will devote much of the remainder of this book to the particular types of ethical problems that arise in medicine and health care, and in doing so, we will spend a lot of time discussing specific cases. Medical ethics, after all, is supposed to be a guide to action; and our high-sounding ethical theories and methods will look very unimpressive if they do not, in the end, offer practical guidance in the sometimes confusing world of medicine. (Practical guidance, of course, need not mean an unmistakable, yes-or-no answer; but, at the very least, we should be able to use our ethical tools to see a puzzling issue more clearly and to have a better grasp of our alternatives.) **115**

↓

On the other hand, an ethical approach that proceeds merely on a case-by-case basis is also bound to be unsatisfactory. Medical situations differ in many respects, but also reveal striking similarities. *Unless we can pull out some general, fundamental principles as we go along, we will never be able to apply to new cases what we have learned from the previous ones.* The search for basic principles — which, when properly qualified, can fill the role of ethical rules in our decision-making method — is therefore as important as dealing with different cases. **116**

↓

Recall from our discussion in the last chapter that the very nature of ethical statements demands that they be both action-oriented and universalizable. Trying our ethical rules out on particular cases is one way of making sure they are properly action-oriented. Searching for basic, general principles is one way of making sure that our ethical rules are universalizable and are not simply ad hoc choices made for the convenience of the moment. **117**

↓

Four key issues emerge from the many issues that make up contemporary ethical concerns, and suggest themselves as especially important sources for basic principles in medical ethics. The next four chapters of this book will look at these issues. We will then proceed to a number of more specific issues, using as a guide the principles that we have learned from the first four. **118**

↓

The doctor–patient relationship (which serves as a model for nonphysician health professionals as well) leads us to ask what special ethical rules govern the way doctors and patients interact. Two subsidiary issues that arise directly from these questions are truth-telling and confidentiality. Chapter 4 will look at these matters. **119**

↓

**120**   Informed consent is another issue that arises directly from the doctor–patient relationship, since virtually every health care action is based on the assumption of either explicit or implied consent of the patient. However, the concept of informed consent is a complicated one, and hence is frequently misunderstood. We will try to achieve a proper understanding of it ↓ in Chapter 5.

**121**   Terminal care decisions are among the most difficult that health professionals must face; even if one has a good understanding of the doctor–patient relationship, it may not be clear what that relationship demands when the patient is dying. Most of the terminal care decisions must be made based on some assessment of quality of life, which is itself a problematic concept in many ways. These tough issues will be the subject of Chapter 6.

**122**   In many terminal care cases, either the patient himself is unable to participate in the decision, or other members of the family demand an equal voice. Such cases therefore remind us that participation in ethical decision making is a fundamental problem arising in many medical contexts, especially those dealing with children and the mentally incompetent. Participation will be discussed in Chapter 7.

**123** ↓  CH. 4

# The Doctor–Patient 4
# Relationship

A good place to start with medical ethics is to examine the human context **123**
out of which the ethical questions arise — the doctor–patient relationship.
Any relationship between two parties carries with it a set of mutual expectations. The special nature of the expectations in the doctor–patient relationship give rise to a number of problems, as well as a few solutions. ↓

To start with the obvious, we might state that the doctor–patient relation- **124**
ship is one of a human being toward another human being. While that does
not seem to tell us much, it is an important beginning and serves to alert us
to some of the more extreme misconceptions about the medical context.
For example, the statement, "The physician ought to have no emotional
involvement with his patients," becomes highly suspicious when the human nature of the doctor–patient relationship is considered. ↓

Obviously, however, the doctor–patient relationship entails a number of **125**
features that other human relationships do not share. A man carving on the
body of another person in a dark alley is a despicable criminal, while someone doing the same thing under the lights of an operating room in sterile
garb is a respected savior. The exact nature of these unique features, however, is not always clear, and different authorities hold up different factors
as being the most crucial to the doctor–patient relationship. A quick
beginner's guide to this territory has been provided by Robert Veatch
(1972), who has cited several idealized models of the doctor–patient relationship. ↓

In Veatch's "engineering model," the physician acts as a scientist who be- **126**
lieves that he must deal only with facts, and must divorce himself from all
questions of value in order to remain "pure." His role is to present all the
facts to the patient, let the patient make up his mind, and then carry out
those wishes. Morally, he is no more than the plumber called in to clean out
the drain. A Roman Catholic physician, who in his private life believes abortion to be an act of murder, will, in this model, perform abortions upon the
request of his patients in his role as "applied scientist." ↓

**127**  In the "priestly model," on the other hand, the physician plays a role that is frankly paternalistic. The patient (who, we might say, has somehow "sinned" by getting sick) comes for treatment, counsel, and comfort. The decision making is placed in the physician's hands, and the patient who does not follow the doctor's orders is adding an even greater "sin" on top of his illness. According to Veatch, a chief sign of this model is the "Speaking-as-a" syndrome: "Speaking as your doctor, I feel that it is definitely time for you to undergo surgical sterilization." The decision here is a moral, not a medical one; but the priest-doctor is presumed to have
↓ competence in both areas by virtue of his M.D. degree.

**128**  Each of these two models has features that most doctors and patients would consider undesirable. Each also has some desirable aspects. In many cases, it is well for the doctor to view himself as the agent responsible for carrying out the patient's desires. In many cases, it is also well for the doctor to feel that he has a responsibility to provide emotional support and comfort to the patient. As a result, most real doctor–patient relationships are a mixture of aspects of both models, depending on the immediate needs of
↓ both doctor and patient.

**129**  How might we go about deciding on an ideal model for the doctor–patient relationship? One way is through a sort of thought experiment: Imagine two people who have been removed from their daily lives, meeting together to draw up some guidelines for the doctor–patient relationship. These two know some general facts, but they are in ignorance about some particular facts. They know, for instance, about the sorts of values that most people have; about the nature of health care, illness, and death; about the way that medical and ethical decisions are made; and about how both illness and medical treatment can interfere with one's life. They also know that, when they return to their real lives, one of them will be the doctor, and one will be the patient; and that the guidelines they choose will be binding on them later. The one thing they don't know is which of them will be the doctor and which will be the patient; and whether the patient will turn out to be healthy, to have a minor illness, or to have a serious or ter-
↓ minal disease.

**130**  Put yourself into that thought experiment and consider what thoughts would pass through your mind. You would probably reject the engineering model — that would be just fine if you end up being the patient, but could be uncomfortable or even intolerable if you end up being the doctor. You would probably also reject the priestly model — if you are the doctor, you would probably feel secure in your ability to make the right choice for the patient, but if you are the patient, you might be unwilling to trust life-or-death decisions to someone who may not share your basic value outlook.
So what model would you choose? We think the best candidate is what
↓ Veatch calls the "contractual model."

*In the contractual model, the contract between doctor and patient is a non-*    **131**
*legalistic statement of general obligations and benefits for both parties. This*
*calls for a sharing of the decision-making responsibility. The physician ac-*
*knowledges that the patient ought to have control over his own life when-*
*ever significant decisions are to be made. Once the important, value-laden*
*aspects are dealt with, however, the patient recognizes that the physician*
*has the requisite skill to make the technical decisions needed to implement*
*the general goal that the patient has agreed to. The patient expects that the*
*physician will take no major action without allowing the patient to make*
*the decision, but does not expect to be consulted on all the technical de-*
*tails. The physician also retains the right not to enter into the contract, or to*
*end the contract, if the implementation of the patient's wishes would force*
*him to perform an act that he, the physician, finds abhorrent by his own*
*moral values.*    ↓

Before we discuss the positive aspects of the contractual model, we need to    **132**
clear up some possible misunderstandings. First, it does not claim or assume that the doctor ought to draw up a written contract with each patient.
The "contract" refers, instead, to a set of unspoken mutual expectations
that are, or ought to be, taken for granted by both parties.    ↓

Second, even though the word contract often implies financial consider-    **133**
ations, we are not here referring to how the doctor is to be paid. We will
assume that the doctor and the patient have a set of mutual expectations,
which are independent (or which ought to be independent) of whether the
patient has private insurance or Medicaid, or whether the physician is paid
on a fee-for-service basis or is on salary. (In Chapter 16 we will look at
whether certain social schemes of payment for health care might hinder the
establishment of an ethical doctor–patient relationship.)    ↓

Third, think now of a contract between two business people for the deliv-    **134**
ery of some goods. If the contract specifies that some of the goods are to be
stolen, any court would immediately void the contract, because it includes
an illegal act. And if one business person lies to the other, we would consider him unethical, and he could not use the fact that there was nothing in
the contract that explicitly prohibits lying as an excuse.

The doctor–patient contract, like a business contract, assumes the existence of other social, ethical, and legal obligations that are binding on both
parties as a background condition. The doctor–patient contract augments
these other obligations, and does not overturn or replace them.    ↓

**135**  Recall our discussion in Chapter 2 of the values of autonomy and respect for persons. We agreed that these values needed to be given special emphasis in our ethical decision-making method. And it would seem that the contractual model comes closer than either of the two alternative models to maximizing these values. (In fact, the very nature of our thought experiment was chosen so as to maximize these values. While we might be willing to sacrifice someone else's autonomy and respect if we are sure we will never be in his place, we are much less likely to do so when we could also turn out to be the victims.)

**136**  You can see why we referred to this model as "idealized"; obviously very few doctor–patient relationships fit this description. Very often the doctor makes no inquiries into the patient's wishes until a crisis occurs; and then there may be no time for inquiry, or the patient may be unable to communicate.

However, we can contend that if doctors and patients at least made an attempt to aim at this ideal model, the resulting relationship would be one that would provide a better atmosphere in which to act ethically, with a greater likelihood of long-term satisfaction for the patient.

**137**  We will accept the contractual model as the best single statement of the ideal doctor–patient relationship, and illustrate its applications in the cases that follow. Before doing so, however, we must provide some justification for this acceptance. The model itself has eliminated the possibility, which most physicians would find hopelessly impractical, that the patient ought to have a say in <u>all</u> medical decisions. The question, then, is whether the patient is to have input into <u>any</u> medical decisions; and if so, how those decisions he ought to be involved in can be distinguished from those in which the doctor has the final say.

**138**  Most people would agree that the patient has some rights to participation in the major decisions affecting his own life and body. At least, if it were to be widely known that doctors everywhere had adopted a totally paternalistic model, very few patients would go to doctors. Also, to return for a minute to the legal realm, the courts have consistently recognized the legal right of the patient to make decisions affecting his control over his body. The trend in recent court decisions has been indeed to broaden the area to which this legal right applies, as we shall see in the discussion of informed consent. Therefore, a physician who makes it a habit to exclude patients from decision making, whatever his moral justification or lack of it may be, may eventually find himself in legal trouble.

The question still open, then, is how to distinguish the morally significant decisions from the purely technical ones. The model itself does not provide much guidance; we can only attempt to point out some general principles by means of case illustrations.

*What we are saying in the contractual model is that the patient has the right*    **139**
*of participation in medical decisions that are morally significant to his life.*
We must immediately qualify this statement to apply to the conscious, rational patient who has passed the "age of understanding" (usually taken to be about 14 years of age).

In Chapter 7, when we discuss "Rights of Ethical Participation," we shall take the right of the patient for granted. We shall consider instead when others in addition to the patient have the right of participation, and who can assume this role for a patient who is irrational, unconscious, or a minor. ↓

---

## CASE 2

You are a partner in a urology practice. Your associate, Dr. X, tells you of a    **140**
patient who came in yesterday requesting a vasectomy. M.Q., apparently an intelligent and well-read man of age 32, has two children, aged 7 and 4, which he considers to be the ideal family size. His wife has a condition contraindicating the use of oral contraceptives and has expelled several IUDs. They are presently using the condom for birth control, and both find it unsatisfactory. M.Q. states that he and his wife are agreed that it would be best for him to undergo vasectomy.

M.Q. further states to Dr. X that he realizes that the operation must be considered irreversible. He has read in the papers of a case in which a sterilized man lost his wife and children in an auto accident, remarried, and then regretted not being able to father more children of his own. M.Q. says that he has pondered such possibilities, but upon weighing all the factors he has decided to undergo sterilization and accept any possible consequences.

Dr. X says he does not want to perform the operation. Before joining you in partnership, he had a case where the tragedy alluded to by M.Q. did indeed occur. The other man, who had cheerfully consented at the time of surgery, later bitterly attacked Dr. X for performing the sterilization. Dr. X feels that M.Q.'s present statement is worthless, since no one can predict how one would actually feel in the face of such a tragedy until it has occurred. For all these reasons, Dr. X has made it a personal rule never to do vasectomies on patients of M.Q.'s age, who still have many potential child-conceiving years ahead of them. However, he wants your views before making a final decision.

Would you perform the vasectomy?    Yes ↓ 141
No ↓ 142

**141**  By agreeing to perform the vasectomy, you have shown accord with the contractual model. By just about any standards, the choice of sterilization is a morally significant one for the patient and thus earns his right of participation in the decision. As a physician, you have the duty to make sure M.Q. knows all the important facts about vasectomies and their consequences, since, as we saw in Chapter 2, ethical judgments made on the basis of inaccurate data are worthless as practical guides to behavior. Since vasectomies have been the subject of much attention in the popular press, and since M.Q. has illustrated a grasp of the most relevant points, you seem justified in engaging him in a minimum of questioning and explanation before ↓ agreeing to do the operation.

**142**  If you refuse to do the vasectomy, you are apparently putting decisive weight on the arguments raised by Dr. X. Let's examine them. First, what is the actual probability of the hypothetical auto accident actually occurring? How does this compare to the number of men who were quite satisfied with the results? If the probability is sufficiently low, is it correct to give that consequence so much weight in the final decision?

While all negative consequences must be considered, it is in general an ethical "error" to allow a bad consequence of very low probability to decide the question by itself. An example of this error from another medical issue is to refuse to allow a terminally ill cancer patient to die, "because who knows, tomorrow they might discover a new miracle drug that would have cured him." In this case it is a good consequence instead of a bad one, ↓ but still of very low probability.

**143**  But more important than this is the difference of opinion between Dr. X and M.Q. Dr. X's statement that no one can really predict how he would act in a hypothetical situation he has not experienced is factually true. But it does not follow logically from that that Dr. X ought not perform the vasectomy — <u>unless</u> one makes the assumption that Dr. X knows <u>better than</u> M.Q. how M.Q. would act in that hypothetical situation. This is the element of paternalism that we found fault with in the priestly model, and which we specifically excluded from the contractual model.

This is not to say that in some cases Dr. X might not know the patient's true mind better than the patient. But then it is incumbent on Dr. X to demonstrate by the patient's words or behavior that the patient knows his mind poorly. On the other hand, M.Q. appeared to be a uniquely rational and ↓ thoughtful individual, so these proofs would be hard to come by in his case.

As this case illustrates, it is easier to remove paternalism from one's ideal    **144**
model of medical practice than it is to avoid slipping into it unconsciously
in one's actual activity. This is because the priestly model has traditionally
been very powerful in medicine and has shaped patients' expectations of
their doctors' behavior. Also, the paternalistic role fits in well with the average physician's own emotional needs.

While many patients allow their doctors to act paternalistically by de-
fault, because the patient is unaware of any alternative, some patients genuinely want this relationship, due to their own inability to, or fear of,
making important decisions. If, early on in the relationship, the patient says
something like, "You're the doctor, so just do what you think is best and
don't bother me with the gory details," he has made his own moral decision as called for by the contractual model, and the physician may then be
justified in making subsequent major decisions on his own.    ↓

---

## CASE 3

The population of a very small country in Asia is doubling every 21 years.    **145**
This growth is negating economic gains and hindering meaningful economic development. The country's Family Planning Council, after a massive study, concludes that continued rapid growth jeopardizes the very
existence of the country and the health and welfare of its citizens.

They have recommended drastic action: that every citizen who voluntarily agrees to accept sterilization be given coupons redeemable for 100 kadis
($20 U.S.) worth of food. Any individual who voluntarily requests steriliza-
tion after no more than two children will get an additional 100-kadi coupon. And to increase recruiting, a similar coupon would be provided for
persons bringing to a government clinic anyone who subsequently accepts
sterilization.

In defense of its proposal, the Council argues: "No one will be penalized
for having children; no one will be forced to refrain from having children;
no one will suffer. In accord with the U.N. Declaration of Human Rights,
every citizen should have available to him those means of controlling family size which are consistent with his own values and religious beliefs."

The traditional religious beliefs of the country apparently offer some resistance to limitation of family size on the grounds that such matters should
be in the hands of God. However, studies have suggested, in past population programs in that country, that in practice, the religious objection was
limited to a very small minority of the population.

You are a high official of the World Health Organization (WHO), charged
with recommending whether WHO will provide assistance to this program.
Since WHO money is vital to equipping the sterilization clinics, you have
considerable leverage over the provisions of the plan.

**145**
**cont.** Do you recommend WHO participation? If not, what changes, if any, would you require in the proposal in order for it to get your approval?

↓ (Adapted from R. M. Veatch, "Case 59." In *Case Studies in Medical Ethics.* Cambridge, Mass.: Harvard University Press, 1977.)

---

**146** Case 3 was included to remind you that paternalism can exist on the social level as well as in individual relationships, and this will become increasingly important as social policy in medical areas becomes more widespread. While there are a number of pros and cons on either side, one question we could ask here is: Does the Council know what is good for the people of Kadi-land better than the people? (How does the fact that they are poor, uneducated Asian peasants influence your decision?) If the program is really good for the people, why is it necessary to "bribe" them to participate? Especially, why is it necessary to pay some of them to recruit others?

This case is well worth discussion in a small group — especially since, within your professional lifetime, you may be called in to judge a similar ↓ proposal for some community in the United States.

---

## CASE 4

**147** You are the family physician of Mr. R., a rather likable 33-year-old man with a wife and two children, who works in an electronics factory and is covered by that company's health-insurance policy. Lately he has had some acute anxiety attacks, brought on by some crises in his personal life; you have treated him with some antianxiety medication and with frequent, lengthy sessions of office counseling.

On today's visit, Mr. R. happily reports that his symptoms have abated and that he feels past the need for more medication or further counseling. However, he is concerned about the bills for his many office visits, which now total several hundred dollars. He points out that his health insurance policy does not reimburse for psychotherapy or counseling. He requests that you fill out his insurance papers, substituting some organic diagnosis instead of his real problem. Otherwise he will be stuck with the bill, causing some hardship for himself and his family.

↓ What do you write on the papers?

If one looked at Case 4 from the narrow perspective of the doctor–patient    **148**
relationship only, probably no conflict would arise. Mr. R. has asked for
your help, and you are eager to help him if you have the power. You do not
want to see his family suffer financially if some outside source of payment
is available.

The conflict arises between your desire to help your patient and your
duty to tell the truth to others. As we noted, the doctor–patient contract
does not override your other pressing social and ethical obligations.    ↓

We might imagine the physician in Case 4 using any of the following argu-    **149**
ments. Each one is only partially satisfactory. Either the argument deals
with some consequences of the proposed action while ignoring other important consequences; or the argument looks at the consequences of this
one action and fails to look at the consequences if that action were to be
made into a general rule of conduct. Can you find a flaw in each argument?

1. "Putting down the wrong diagnosis would be a lie, and lying is always
   wrong, however much I'd like to help the guy."
2. "If I get Mr. R. off the hook this way, and if other physicians did likewise,
   the insurance company would pass along the increased costs to all their
   policyholders, and it wouldn't be fair to others."
3. "Let's see — I think with one of his anxiety attacks Mr. R. complained of
   nausea. If I put down the diagnosis of 'Nausea, rule out peptic ulcer and
   gastritis,' then I'm not really telling a lie."
4. "My job as a physician is to help my patient. If I have to bend my conscience a little to do it, that's just part of my job."
5. "People can be just as sick and disabled from emotional complaints as
   from physical ones. If the insurance company had any sense they'd recognize that. Since the policy as it stands is stupid and unfair, I can be
   excused if I lie about the diagnosis."

Remember from Chapter 2 that one of the cardinal ethical mistakes is to act
as if you have only two alternatives when more exist. Did you consider as
one alternative refusing to lie on the form, but setting up a payment sched-
ule of a few dollars a month to allow Mr. R. to pay his bill without undue
hardship?    ↓

### Truth-Telling

**150**  Let's now examine some of the consequences of the contractual model. *If the patient has a right to participate in decisions that are morally significant for him, and if a correct ethical decision depends on the accuracy of the relevant data, it follows that as a general rule, the patient must at all times be told the truth about his medical condition.* This brings up the issue of what to tell the patient, especially one who is dying or who has a potentially fatal illness. This is a problem on both the ethical and emotional level — even after making an ethical judgment about what we should divulge, we may not have the nerve to actually face the patient and say it. While this applies to every communication with the patient, consideration of the more dramatic cases highlights the crucial issues.

---

### CASE 5

**151**  As a new intern in a large city hospital, you take the initial history and physical of Mrs. P., a 54-year-old, postmenopausal Jamaican-born woman who comes in complaining of severe pain and a mass in the right lower quadrant of the abdomen. After the interview and after establishing some initial rapport with the patient, you elicit from Mrs. P. the fear that she has cancer. You reassure her that she will get a complete workup with laboratory tests. She replies sadly, "I know if it was cancer you doctors wouldn't tell me." You end the conversation by saying that you and the other doctors will know much more after the initial lab tests are done.

A tentative diagnosis of degenerating fibroid was made and the patient underwent surgery. Later, the pathology report showed that in fact Mrs. P. had Stage IV cervical cancer. While the surgeons had removed all the tumor they could see, the spread was such that distant metastases were very likely, and the most they could do would be to try radiation and chemotherapy. The 5-year survival rate of Stage IV cervical cancer is 0 to 20 percent.

Your first response is to want to go to Mrs. P. and explain to her that she has cancer and that she has a limited time to live, although every possible effort will be made to prolong her life. You want to try to help ease her grief and offer continued moral support. Since you are new, however, you want to first ask your chief resident how to proceed.

The chief resident says that you should "never use the word 'cancer' to a patient or they lose all hope; it's best to use a lot of medical jargon to soften it." You reply that somehow or other you feel that Mrs. P. has to be told her survival chances. After an increasingly angry interchange, the resident exclaims, "Look, how would you like it if you told her she had incurable cancer, and she walked over to the window and jumped out? Just let me handle this on rounds."

Later the resident tells you shortly that he has informed Mrs. P. that she had a malignant process and the surgeons had removed it.

**151**
cont.

Are you satisfied with this? If not, what do you do now?

(Adapted from R. M. Veatch, "Case 43." In *Case Studies in Medical Ethics*. Cambridge, Mass.: Harvard University Press, 1977.)

↓

---

Case 5 illustrates that the problem of what to tell the patient is one where general rules are least likely to be of benefit. The resident's rule, never tell a patient they have cancer, clearly saves him a lot of hard thinking, but it displays a singular disregard for the individual emotional states and emotional needs of patients.

**152**

↓

The argument that a patient, if told the truth, might "jump out of the window" has gained widespread currency. However, it may be an example of basing an ethical conclusion on an unproved, and highly suspicious, empirical claim. Reich and Kelly (1976) studied all suicide attempts by patients at a major teaching hospital over a 7-year period. Less than one-quarter occurred in patients with serious or terminal illness, and all of the latter attempts were triggered by some other sort of psychologic stress, not depression over being told their diagnosis. Veatch (1976) also reported that directors of suicide prevention centers have observed no increased suicide risk in people who have just received word of a terminal diagnosis.

**153**

It appears that the "out the window" excuse reflects our own irrational fears about confronting patients, rather than a likely outcome.

↓

It is tempting to use the empirical approach to lend support to the obligation to disclose a true diagnosis. Oken (1961), in a classic paper, showed that while about 90 percent of physicians avoided telling cancer patients the truth, 90 percent of patients would prefer to be told. While such percentages have been debated by McIntosh (1976), most other investigators have confirmed Oken's findings on patient desires.

**154**

↓

But data such as these do not settle the ethical question. Even if 90 percent of patients want to be told, you don't know if the patient in front of you is one of the 90 percent or one of the 10 percent.

**155**

To tell patients unpleasant news in a compassionate and helpful way, we need to be skilled at the science of human behavior as well as medical ethics. We need to be aware of what the patient already knows or suspects, what he wants to hear, and what he is most concerned about, before we can decide what to tell him. We need first of all to be sensitive listeners before we can decide what to tell the patient, and how to do it in the most humane manner.

↓

**156** Case 5 has another point worth pondering. Consider the statement of Mrs. P.: "If it was cancer you doctors wouldn't tell me." Mrs. P. did not make up this idea out of thin air; she has been exposed to instances in the past, her own experience or that of friends, in which the doctor withheld information that was later found out. This shows that we cannot decide whether to tell the truth or not on an ad hoc basis, without considering the future consequences both for our relationship with that patient and for the trust placed by all patients in the doctor–patient relationship in general. Any decision made with an eye toward getting us out of a temporarily sticky situation may come back to haunt us in several forms later on.

Some of the unanticipated consequences of medical deception are
↓ nicely illustrated in Case 6.

---

## CASE 6

**157** The prize fighter J. J. Corbett had died of cancer, and *The New York Times* ran the story with this headline: "Ex-Champion Succumbs Here to Cancer. He Believed He Had Heart Disease." Such was the conscientious lie with which Gentleman Jim's doctors had let him live out his last days. However, other doctors soon began to violently protest the open publication of the deception in a news story, one physician complaining to the editor that several of his own patients with heart diseases were wild with fear that they too had cancer of the liver.

↓ (Joseph Fletcher, *Morals and Medicine*. Boston: Beacon Press, 1960.)

---

**158** Case 6 illustrates the medical attitudes prevalent at the turn of the century. It is revealing, in this light, that in books on medical ethics, this issue is usually titled "truth-telling." In most other walks of life, "lying" is seen as being the thing that needs justifying; why is it that in medicine, telling the truth is seen to be in need of defense? This reflects the extent to which physicians have come to see themselves as immune from considerations
↓ that affect other people.

**159** These attitudes, however, are changing rapidly. Oken, in 1961, found almost 90 percent of physicians opposed to telling the truth about a cancer diagnosis; but today, as Novack (1980) shows, the figure would be much lower. There are several reasons for this. Investigators of the dying process have revealed that most terminally ill patients already know or suspect their diagnosis. Also, cancer has become more treatable with advances in technology, and the diagnosis is no longer the equivalent of a death sentence in most people's minds. On a more pragmatic level, informed consent is needed for any life-prolonging surgery or chemotherapy in cancer, and in-
↓ formed consent requires that the patient know the true diagnosis.

*The contractual model would seem to suggest the following ethical rule:*   **160**
*"The physician should tell the patient the truth about his condition, in lan-*
*guage he can understand, unless the physician has reason to believe that a*
*degree of harm, more serious than merely a temporary emotional depres-*
*sion, would follow as a result."*

This means that the burden of justification of not telling the whole truth
rests on the physician; and that, in order to avoid slavish adherence to
truth-telling as a rule, he must be alert to any signs or "messages" from the
patient that would indicate that the patient would be better off not having
the entire truth thrust upon him at once. In particular, the physician dare
not take "Tell it to me straight, Doc, I can take it" at face value.   ↓

---

## CASE 7

A hospitalized man has had a biopsy taken of an enlarged cervical lymph   **161**
node, and you are awaiting the results of the pathology report. The patient
appears to be rather agitated by these proceedings. He finally states that if
the biopsy showed cancer he wouldn't want to live; and if the report came
back negative, he would be convinced that you were lying to him in order
to spare him the shock.

The biopsy report indicates a malignant lymphoma. Furthermore, a more
thorough physical exam has turned up a mass in the patient's abdomen,
and all indications point to its being of lymphatic origin and also malignant.
Lymphomas of this type, in general, respond fairly well to chemotherapy;
but it is difficult to predict the outcome of any individual case before a
course of therapy is attempted.

What do you tell your patient?

(From a case report by B. C. Meyer. In E. F. Torrey (Ed.), *Ethical Issues in Medicine.*
Boston: Little, Brown, 1968.)   ↓

---

If you tell the patient he has cancer, you are either adopting the general rule   **162**
of always telling the truth, or you are assuming that his statements do not
reflect his true mental status. Possibly he might really want to know and
would be happier knowing. Possibly if he really did not want to know, he
would simply deny the truth when it is told to him ("they must have gotten
my specimen mixed up with someone else's in the lab") and no harm
would have been done, except possibly for some anger at you.   ↓

**163**     If you elect not to tell, either you have adopted the general rule of not telling patients they have cancer, or you are taking at face value the fact that revealing the true diagnosis would send the patient into a significant depression. Or possibly you wish to avoid an emotion-laden confrontation.

In the actual case, the physician did neither of the above. Instead, he adopted a procedure that ought to be used much more in medicine. Sensing his own inadequacy to evaluate the patient's possible emotional reaction, he called in a psychiatrist to advise him as to how to proceed.

**164**     Meyer reports that after evaluating the situation, the psychiatrist advised the physician to tell the patient that the biopsy of the cervical node showed cancer; that he also had a growth in the abdomen which was very likely cancer; that the type of cancer involved tends to respond well to chemotherapy; that if chemotherapy, in turn, were to cause him any discomfort, he could receive medication for its relief; and that the doctors were very hopeful of a successful outcome. The physician, a surgical resident, was "both appalled and distressed" when he learned what he was to do, but he steeled himself and spoke the required formula with conviction.

**165**     While happy endings are not reliable indicators that the original ethical decision was correct, this case ended happily. Says Meyer:

> The patient, who, it will be recalled, had declared he wouldn't want to live if the doctors found cancer, was obviously gratified. Immediately he telephoned members of his family to tell them the news . . . That night he slept well for the first time since entering the hospital . . . Just before leaving he confessed that he had known all along about the existence of the abdominal mass, but that he had concealed his knowledge to see what the doctors would tell him. Upon arriving home he wrote a warm letter of thanks and admiration to the resident surgeon.*

**166**     Several points about this case deserve comment. First, it provides an excellent example of how empirical findings can be "fed in" to the ethical decision-making process without making the error of assuming that the ethical question is an empirical one. The resident realized the ethical question at stake, but also saw that information about the patient's emotional state, with predictions about his reactions, were essential empirical data upon which the ethical question was based. Accordingly, he called in a specialist who was best suited to supply the missing empirical data.

* B. C. Meyer, Truth and the Physician. In E. F. Torrey (Ed.), *Ethical Issues in Medicine.* Boston: Little, Brown, 1968.

The second point is that telling a patient something takes place over a span     **167**
of time, and is not a one-shot affair. Thus, the shading of the phrases used, whether the truth is delivered all at once or in small doses, and the kind of follow-up are all important parts of the ethical decision, as well as "tell" or "don't tell." A decision to reveal a grave prognosis, which may be ethical in itself, may become unethical if the physician tells the patient bluntly and then withdraws, without offering any emotional support to help the patient resolve his feelings. In fact, the assurance that the physician plans to see it through along with the patient, and that he will always make himself available to offer any comfort possible, may be more important than the bad news itself. In many of the "sour cases" that are offered as justification for withholding the truth, it may well be the absence of this transmission of compassion, rather than the telling of the truth, that produced the unfortunate result.

↓

All the truth-telling cases we have considered so far deal with terminal ill-     **168**
ness. But there are many, more mundane areas of medicine where telling "white lies" seems to be either convenient or in the best interests of the patient. Think of the medical student who introduces himself to the patient as "Doctor Smith," or the nurse who tells the child before she gives a shot, "Now this won't hurt a bit."
Case 8 depicts a fairly common example of medical deception.     ↓

---

## CASE 8

Your instructors in nursing school would have primly referred to Mr. C. as a     **169**
"difficult" patient, but, as you work on the medical ward, you are inclined to use more blunt and colorful language to describe him. He has end-stage kidney failure and is having his waste chemicals removed by flushing fluids through his abdominal cavity (peritoneal dialysis), while awaiting surgery on the blood vessels in his arm that will allow him to be hooked to a kidney machine. He has an infantile personality and is continually whining and complaining in order to get the staff's attention. You know that beneath all of that, he's probably scared stiff and can't admit it; but none of the nursing or medical staff have been able to establish any rapport with him.

His complaints are of vague pains for which he has been receiving high doses of narcotics every 4 hours. He claims marked relief with every shot, but is then asking for another one 2 hours later. The physicians are convinced that the pains are of psychologic origin.

Today, when Mr. C. again starts complaining of pain, the intern caring for him goes into the room and gives him a shot. Coming to the nursing station, the intern says, "I just gave him a shot of sterile water. I'm sick of giving that

**169**
**cont.** SOB narcotics when the pain is all in his head anyway. If it works, change his medicine to sterile water every 4 hours. Let him think he's still getting the narcotic."

Half an hour later you hear Mr. C. say that that new pain medicine worked better than any he's had before.

↓ What do you do about the intern's order?

---

**170** A treatment that is pharmacologically inactive but is given under the guise of active medicine is called a "placebo." As Case 8 illustrates, placebos often work to relieve pain and other symptoms. But, contrary to what the intern apparently believes, placebos work just as well on symptoms caused by "real organic disease" as they do on symptoms that we believe to be
↓ psychologic or hypochondriacal.

**171** Many physicians would argue that Case 8 does not present any truth-telling dilemma. Nothing in the intern's order requires that the nurse lie outright to the patient. "If the patient chooses to believe that the water is really narcotic, he's deceiving himself; you're not deceiving him."

But patients expect, legitimately, that a medicine given to them by physicians or nurses will be "real" medicine. (Think how hard it would be to treat patients if they routinely suspected that medicines were really something different from what you said they were.) When you give something that outwardly appears as a medicine, you are creating a false impression if the medicine is a placebo, even if the words you use do not constitute a barefaced lie. The crucial test is: If the patient later learns what the medicine is, would he feel deceived, or would he simply agree that he had made an erroneous conclusion? If he would feel deceived, you have been guilty
↓ of causing the deception.

**172** Still, deception may be justified in some cases. Physicians have defended placebo use when it is for the good of the patient (such as substituting water for a potent medicine much more likely to cause addiction and side effects).

Unfortunately, surveys reveal that it is precisely the least likable patient, like Mr. C., who ends up being given the placebo. Perhaps Mr. C.'s need to keep others at a distance through his infantile behavior is so strong that no one could have established a good relationship with him regardless; but at any rate the placebo is being used as a cheap substitute for that relationship — and one, in addition, that would overturn the relationship altogether if the deception is later discovered by the patient.

Placebos, then, violate our general rule about telling the truth to patients, and should be avoided unless particularly strong justification exists in a cer-
↓ tain case.

## Confidentiality

What are some of the other consequences of the contractual model? We    **173**
might consider also one of the terms of the implied contract — that the
information gained by the physician in the course of the relationship will
be kept confidential. While many patients may not be aware of any right to
be told the truth, or to avoid a paternalistic physician, the "right to privacy"
is very well known because of its existence as one of the most ancient traditions in medicine. As the Hippocratic Oath held, what the physician hears
"which ought not to be noised abroad" will be kept in confidence. Of
course, the Oath offers no clarification as to <u>what</u> ought not to be noised
abroad. The corresponding statement in the AMA code is qualified: "unless
the law requires it or if necessary to protect the welfare of individuals or the
community." It is in deciding when these loopholes apply that many of the
ethical dilemmas related to confidentiality arise.    ↓

---

## CASE 9

You are the family doctor of 26-year-old A.T., and just now you're very an-    **174**
gry with him. Some friends of his called you from a local movie theater to
say that A.T. was having a seizure, and you are now with him in the emergency room. You know A.T. has been on antiseizure medications since he
had brain surgery in his youth, and that he had a seizure 2 years ago caused
by neglecting to take his medicine. He now meekly admits that he has been
slipping up on taking his medicines again; and, worse, that he had another
seizure last year (again while off medicines) while alone, which he never
told you about.

   A.T., as you know, is in a car pool and drives to work and back one week
out of every four; and he makes two 25-mile trips each month to visit his
elderly mother. In your area, there is no public transportation and new jobs
are very scarce.

   A.T. pleads with you not to notify the State Motor Vehicle authorities
about the seizure, lest he lose his driver's license. He admits to having been
lax about medicines before but insists he has learned his lesson and will not
forget to take his pills in the future.

Do you notify the authorities?    Yes  ↓ 175
                                  No   ↓ 179

(Adapted from an unpublished case by George Agich and Theodore LeBlang.)

**175** If you choose to notify the authorities, you are judging that A.T.'s diagnosis is "fit to be noised abroad." There is both legal and ethical justification for this judgment — the former because of licensing laws requiring reports of such illnesses, the latter because of possible harm to others if A.T. has a seizure while driving. Of course, another reason you might report A.T. is simply because you are angry with him, but that hardly counts as ethical justification.

Suppose you really believed that A.T. would, in the future, take his medicine. In that case, the probability of another seizure would presumably be ↓ quite low. Would that factor make you less likely to turn him in?

---

**176** A major feature of Case 9 is that if you choose to respect confidentiality, the benefit will accrue to A.T., whom you know and are concerned about; the risk will be borne by the general public, most of whom are unknown to you and to whom you have no explicit relationship of trust. This makes it easier to decide not to report him. In Case 10 the danger is directed more specifi- ↓ cally at one individual.

---

## CASE 10

**177** You are a psychiatrist for the student health service at a large university. One of your patients is a foreign graduate student who has been extremely depressed since his affections were rejected by his former girlfriend, who lives in the city with her parents. Today, expressing his anger to you over the way the girl treated him, he announces his intention of killing her when she returns from a trip out of the country.

You know that the business of predicting violent behavior is not as clear-cut as some would like to think; nevertheless you feel that your patient is seriously disturbed and that there is a fair probability that his threat will be carried out.

What should you do with your knowledge?

↓ (Adapted from *Tarasoff* v. *Regents of the University of California*, 551 P. 2nd 334, 1976.)

---

**178** The direct danger to the life of another is precisely the sort of justification that clearly overrides the duty of maintaining confidentiality. (A similar concern is expressed in the laws that require physicians to report cases of contagious diseases, so as to prevent possible epidemics.) There can be lit- tle question in this case that the psychiatrist is duty bound to protect the girl. He may feel obligated to tell his patient that he plans to do so, in order to try to maintain the patient's trust; but in this case a person's life counts **180** ↓ for more than the doctor–patient relationship.

Not notifying the license board is probably the easy thing to do — A.T. will **179** be pleased with you, and no one will be likely to find out. On the other hand, if he has a seizure while driving and runs into a school bus full of kindergarten children, you might have cause to regret your choice later on. And again, recall that a proper ethical choice must be translatable into a universal rule — so that it would be acceptable to you if all the other drivers on the road turned out to be people with uncontrolled epilepsy whose doctors had refused to notify the authorities.

↑ **176**

---

However, this decision ought to bother us at least a little. Presumably one **180** of the reasons people with psychiatric disorders are willing to seek help is the trust that psychiatrists will respect confidentiality. If the duty to disclose confidential psychiatric information were to be broadened, a point might be reached where patients would be unwilling to speak openly. We might then have destructive and homicidal persons roaming the streets instead of seeking psychiatric help, which would not be much of an improvement in public safety.

The negative consequences of violating confidentiality are not compelling enough to cause us to want to maintain confidentiality in Case 10; but they should give us pause if further inroads into confidentiality rights are suggested.

↓

The actual outcome of Case 10 created a medico-legal quandary. The psy- **181** chiatrist notified the campus police, who detained the foreign student, judged him to be rational and not dangerous, and let him go with a warning — and with no warning to the girl or her family. Two months later the student went to the girl's house and killed her when she would not talk to him. The girl's family sued the university health service and the police.

The California Supreme Court ruled that the psychiatrist had had a duty not only to warn the police, but also to warn the girl herself, and therefore could be liable for damages. Psychiatrists and lawyers have quarreled with this ruling, saying that the duty should have been only to notify the police, not to second-guess them and take over their job. (The ethical conclusion, that the girl's danger overrides the patient's right to confidentiality, holds up whether you agree or disagree with the Court.)

↓

In both Cases 9 and 10, the danger if confidentiality is maintained affects **182** other parties. In Case 11, respecting the confidence will harm no one except the patient.

↓

## CASE 11

**183**    Your hospital's open-heart surgery team uses a psychologic evaluation as part of its presurgery workup. Research has shown that patients who go into open-heart surgery with severe depression, or who are hopeless regarding their future outcome, have a much higher incidence of death during and immediately after surgery. You are the psychiatric social worker who conducts the interviews, looking for these psychologic risk factors.

You are talking to a 44-year-old man who has already had a one-vessel coronary artery bypass operation following a heart attack 6 years ago. He later had a second heart attack, and severe heart failure has made him an invalid, able only to take care of his immediate physical needs and unable to work or leave the house. He hated this sort of life and felt that his family resented him as a burden.

After being very reticent, he asks if he can speak to you in confidence. When you agree, he admits that he thinks he has nothing left to live for, and has been planning his own funeral and writing his own obituary. He had agreed to surgery because he saw in it a way "to die like a man," and was sure that he would in fact die. Naturally he had not revealed any of this to the surgeons, and he repeats that he is telling you this in the strictest confidence.

Should you inform the surgeons of this conversation? Under these circumstances, should the operation proceed or not?

↓  (Adapted from an unpublished case, used by courtesy of Sumer Verma, M.D.)

---

**184**    Case 11 is a grotesque example of a patient manipulating the doctor–patient relationship for his own purposes, while concealing those purposes from the physicians. We might observe that it was unwise of the social worker to agree to keep the confidence in the first place. It would be better to have said at the start that any information divulged that was of importance for the operation would have to be shared with the surgeons. Of course, had you said this, the man might never have revealed his purposes; so the dilemma of what to do now remains.

**185**    In the real case, the mental-health worker explained to the patient that he was there representing the entire surgical team, and was, in effect, not a free agent; he asked that the patient voluntarily release him from the pledge of confidentiality. After some discussion the patient reluctantly agreed. The surgeons, however, on being told, decided to proceed anyway, as the operation (a three-vessel bypass) was felt to be the man's only hope of survival, since his heart function continued to deteriorate.

The man survived the operation. On awakening in the recovery room, and    **186**
being told he was alive, he began to sob uncontrollably, then became de-
lirious and lapsed into a coma. Five days later, while still comatose, he
suffered a new, massive heart attack and died.    ↓

Case 11 is an interesting test of the contractual model. Once the man's pur-    **187**
pose is known, the surgeons' responsibilities are unclear. One could say
that no doctor–patient contract exists, since the surgery was initially agreed
to under false pretenses. At any rate, if being possible accessories to the
man's suicide is repugnant to the surgeons' personal values, the contractual
model recognizes their right to refuse to proceed. The engineering model,
by contrast, would dictate that they must operate.    ↓

We can summarize our discussion of confidentiality. *Confidentiality is a*    **188**
*traditionally recognized and highly desirable right of the patient under the*
*terms of the contractual model. However, the right is not absolute and may*
*be overridden by clear and present danger to other persons or to the public*
*welfare. Those who would overturn confidentiality in any particular case*
*must bear the burden of demonstrating that some real and specific danger*
*exists.*    ↓

One final comment on the doctor–patient relationship is necessary. You    **189**
may have been disturbed that in all the sample cases cited in this chapter,
the social context was that of one doctor in private practice seeing one
patient. A number of developments are now occurring in the field of
health-care delivery that make it likely that, inside of 20 years, such a social
relationship will be in a minority status within the health-care field. Which
of the ethical principles that are valid for the one-on-one relationship will
still be applicable in, say, a health-care delivery team concept is an open
question, which will have to be worked out as these future developments
take a clearer shape. For example, experimental use of computer storage
and recall of patients' medical records have already raised significant questions about the future of the right to privacy.

For an example of a problem that could arise within a health-care team
setting, see Case 27 in Chapter 7.

CH. 5 ↓ **190**

# Informed Consent 5

The contractual model of the doctor–patient relationship requires that the **190** patient be involved in any major medical decision. To be involved meaningfully, the patient must first be given any information he requires about the risks and benefits of the medical treatment and whether any alternative treatments exist. Next, the patient must be allowed to make a voluntary choice to accept the treatment or not. These two features make up <u>informed consent</u>. ↓

REVIEW CONTRACTUAL MODEL ↑ 131

In the past, physicians have generally avoided giving full information about **191** treatment to the patient — especially about the risks of treatment. They chose what they thought was best for the patient, and patients generally accepted that. When the American Hospital Association proposed its Patients' Bill of Rights in 1972 (see Appendix III), informed consent was listed prominently as a right — an indication of the extent to which it had been neglected in the past. ↓

Today, informed consent is taken much more seriously by health profes- **192** sionals. Unfortunately, this is due not to any heightened ethical awareness on the part of physicians, but to highly publicized lawsuits in which physicians who did not obtain informed consent, and whose patients subsequently suffered from the risks of treatment, collected damages. Physicians are now very careful to obtain the patient's informed consent, generally in writing, and to document consent carefully in the medical records. ↓

But this new emphasis on informed consent does not mean that informed **193** consent is well understood by physicians. We have the advantage of tying informed consent to our contractual model, which, as we saw, has as one of its basic features the preservation of the patient's autonomy. Respect for autonomy requires that we honor a person's free choices, even when we think those choices may be ill-advised. If we overrule a person's autonomous choice because we think that we, as health professionals, "know best," we have fallen back into the priestly model of paternalistic medicine. ↓

REVIEW AUTONOMY ↑ 79–84

The medical journals, however, are full of articles on informed consent that **194** fail utterly to see its connection with patient autonomy and respect for persons. In one, Coleman (1974) says flatly that informed consent is a "law" designed to protect physicians from lawsuits. Nothing is said about protecting patients from physicians. ↓

**195**  Possibly the most bizarre misunderstanding of informed consent appeared in a letter to a medical journal. Kaplan and his colleagues (1977) described two cases in which patients with no known heart disease suffered heart attack or irregular heart rhythm about 12 hours after "informed consent" had been obtained for unrelated surgery. They suggested, first, that the informed consent procedure may have caused the heart problems; and second, that because of such a risk, the whole idea of informed consent was medically unsound.

Had a physician written to a medical journal to report two patients who had had heart attacks 12 hours after drinking a glass of milk, under the title, "Does milk cause heart attacks?", he would have been laughed out of the profession. The fact that the Kaplan letter even saw print reflects the widespread ignorance about informed consent.

**196**  A fanciful way to explain why so many physicians fail to grasp what is essentially a common-sense notion (as we saw when discussing the contractual model) is to hypothesize that there must be some other doctrine floating around that really is ridiculous, and that physicians have mistaken for the doctrine of informed consent. We might label our hypothetical doctrine the "doctrine of omniscient decree."

**197**  The doctrine of omniscient decree might go as follows:

1. The patient must be given complete information about all facts that could possibly be relevant to his case.
2. The patient must use those facts in a logical reasoning process to make his choice.
3. The patient must be emotionally stable and free of any psychologic pressure that could affect his decision.
4. The physician must be completely neutral and must not sway the patient toward any alternative.
5. After the treatment is given, the patient must be able to look back on his choice and agree in retrospect that it was for the best.

**198**  It is not difficult to see that the doctrine of omniscient decree really does place ridiculous demands on both doctor and patient. Several arguments are evident that reveal its flaws (arguments which physicians have raised against the doctrine of informed consent).

**199**  First, knowing all the facts is an impossible requirement, even if each patient were forced to go to medical school for 4 years before submitting to treatment. Often the physician himself does not know the facts, and indeed the facts are often unknown to medical science. Medicine is always practiced under the limitations of a great deal of uncertainty.

Second, physicians fear that if patients are told every conceivable risk of every procedure, patients would be so scared that they would refuse even simple procedures. (Coleman makes much of this argument, and Kaplan felt duty bound to tell the patient every horrifying detail whether or not the patient wanted to know.) **200**

Third, a number of studies have shown that patients often make up their minds independent of the facts presented to them. Fellner and Marshall (1970) found that prospective kidney donors generally made up their minds firmly before ever being told about risks. Robinson (1976) found patients unable to recall what they had been told some time after the informed consent interview; some even denied having had the interview. **201**

Fourth, a patient who is ill and needs treatment is hardly in the ideal emotional state to make a dispassionate choice. The more crucial the medical decision is, the more likely the patient is to be emotionally distressed at the time the decision must be made. **202**

Fifth, the physician, try as hard as he may, can never remain strictly neutral. Generally he will think one alternative to be superior and will want the patient to know that. Even if he tries to conceal his bias, he is liable to betray it by subtle changes in voice or phraseology. **203**

All these arguments suffice to overturn the doctrine of omniscient decree, were anyone to propose it as part of medical practice. Of course, no one has. But many have assumed that the doctrine of omniscient decree is what the doctrine of informed consent would entail, if it were carried to its logical conclusion. Thus, Laforet (1976) felt obliged to speak of the " 'fiction' of informed consent." And some authors on ethics (including this one, in the first edition of this book) have added to this misunderstanding by suggesting that "there is no such thing as 'fully' informed consent in the strict sense." **204**

Our discussion so far has provided a sort of backdoor way of getting at what the doctrine of informed consent really is. If the doctrine of omniscient decree is ridiculous, while the doctrine of informed consent is common-sensical and pragmatic, then it must follow that the latter differs from the former on all major points. **205**

To see what it means to give adequately informed consent, it may help to turn away from health care for a minute and to look at examples from everyday life. (While we could obviously come to erroneous ethical conclusions in medicine if we fail to see that medicine deals with problems not found anywhere else, we could also be led astray if we jump to the conclusion that medicine is completely different from the rest of human existence.) **206**

62

**207** Consider the problem of buying a car. There is certainly a lot of technical information available about the different models (some of which is unknown, such as which ones will have to be recalled in the future), and you generally make your choice based on a small fraction of all the technical information. A lot of your information comes from salespeople, who are clearly biased in favor of their product. (You assume, however, that they are not telling you any outright lies.) You are yourself not free of emotional pressures to decide one way or the other; cars, after all, are very important in our society. Finally, after you have bought the car, you may look back with regret and wish you had chosen another.

**208** Notice that the car-buying example fulfills none of the requirements listed under the doctrine of omniscient decree. Still, you are willing to accept your choice of a car as your own free choice, not something that is forced upon you. You accept it as a choice made based on the information you had available at the time. The fact that you did not have more information also reflects your own choice, as you could have read some more auto magazines or test-driven some more models. In short, buying the car fulfills all the necessary criteria for informed consent.

**209** Consider one more nonmedical example: You are at a fancy restaurant, and the wine waiter comes for your order. You tell him what dinner you're ordering, and about how much you want to spend, and ask him to choose a wine for you.

In this case, you do not make your own choice at all, but you voluntarily place the choice in the hands of someone who knows the situation better than you do. Maybe the wine waiter has very different tastes from yours; or maybe he has been looking for a sucker to unload a bottle that no one else wants. But those are risks that you assume voluntarily, with your eyes open. This choice, too, fulfills the requirements for informed consent.

**210** The wine example reveals why Coleman and Kaplan have misread the requirements of informed consent. Informed consent may be viewed as a right, and rights can be voluntarily waived. If the patient knows he may ask questions and make up his own mind, but says instead, "Gee, Doc, I'd rather you spare me the gory details" or "You're the doctor, you know what's best for me," he has voluntarily waived his right to informed consent. The doctor then has no obligation whatever to tie the patient to the chair and tell him about every possible side effect.
REVIEW RIGHTS ↑ 77–78

Having used these nonmedical examples, we need to remember that there 211 are still some features of the medical case that are not strictly analogous, especially to the car example.

First, the car salesman has a duty not to defraud you or to lie about the car; but he has no obligation to look out for your best interests. If he sees you about to buy a car much more expensive than the one you really need, he has no duty to point this out. The physician, on the other hand, is expected under the contractual model to be an advocate for the patient's interests (in legal terms, the doctor–patient relationship is a <u>fiduciary</u> one); so the doctor's responsibility will be judged according to much stricter standards. ↓

A second nonanalogy is the degree of emotional impact that illness has on 212 the patient. Serious illness may influence one's judgment directly, by toxic effects on the brain, or indirectly, by causing depression or other psychopathology. In such cases a patient's decision may reflect his disordered judgment rather than his autonomous choice. (A choice made because of mental upset or delirium is, in a sense, a coerced choice and not an autonomous one — the sort of choice that one, looking back later, will describe as "I wasn't really myself when I did that.") ↓

The physician, aware of the impact of illness on reasoning, must therefore 213 walk a narrow line (as some of our cases will illustrate). On one hand, he must be alert for signs that the patient's choice is not truly autonomous. On the other hand, he must not imagine these signs when they do not exist, lest the impact of illness be used as a handy excuse to revert to the priestly model and to rob the patient of autonomy altogether. ↓
REVIEW PRIESTLY MODEL ↑ 127

So far we have seen what is required ethically under the doctrine of in- 214 formed consent. The most recent legal decisions generally support this ethical analysis. The value of patient autonomy has been upheld widely in the courts, going back at least as far as Justice Cardozo's often-quoted decision in *Schloendorff* v. *New York Hospital,* 1914: "Every human being of adult years and sound mind has a right to determine what shall be done with his own body." ↓

Having established patient autonomy, the courts have been primarily in- 215 terested in the physician's duty that corresponds to the right of informed consent — the duty to disclose. Until recently the duty to disclose was judged according to the standards of community practice among physicians. This was clearly inadequate by our ethical analysis — if physicians in general chose to disclose too little information to allow patients to make reasoned choices, no one physician could be held liable for concurring with that community practice. ↓

**216** In 1972, however, two major court decisions rejected the community-standard rule in informed consent. In the District of Columbia, the *Canterbury* v. *Spence* decision ruled that the test should be whether that particular patient, his own needs being taken into account, received enough information to make a reasoned choice. In California, the *Cobbs* v. *Grant* decision ruled that the physician should disclose whatever information was necessary for a prudent person to make a decision.

Our ethical analysis would cause us to favor the *Canterbury* formula. Our object should be determined by the individual patient and his real needs, not the hypothetical needs of the "reasonable man."

**217** Courts have also recognized two exceptions to the informed-consent doctrine. The first is emergency situations where consent cannot be obtained and where the patient's life would be jeopardized by waiting for consent. In such cases the physicians proceed under <u>implied consent</u>.

The second exception is when the physician has reason to believe that full disclosure would lead to severe emotional trauma. We might add that the physician should have clear evidence that this will occur, not just a vague suspicion, lest this turn into a loophole to justify a general policy of nondisclosure.

**218** Incidentally, the argument that full disclosure will scare patients away from needed procedures is an empirical question and is susceptible to research. Several studies, such as one by Alfidi (1971, 1975), have showed that patients are not generally scared away by full lists of all possible risks of the procedure (although, if given the option, they often choose not to hear all the risks).

---

## CASE 12

**219** A 14-year-old girl is referred to you, a general surgeon, with a complaint of severe abdominal pain of one week's duration. Based on a thorough workup, you narrow your differential diagnosis to several conditions, all of which require surgery, and you decide that the best course is exploratory laparotomy as soon as possible.

Of the several diagnostic possibilities you are considering, the most likely one can be corrected only by a procedure that carries with it a 50 percent or greater risk of subsequent sterility, as a result of compromising the ovaries and uterus. The results of mortality and serious complications are otherwise those of any surgical entry into the abdominal cavity.

The girl's father is deceased and her legal guardian is her mother.

What will be your procedure for obtaining informed consent for the surgery you propose? Will you direct this procedure at:

| | |
|---|---|
| The girl only? | ↓ 220 |
| The mother only? | ↓ 222 |
| The girl and mother, in separate interviews?. | ↓ 220 |
| The girl and mother, both in the same interview? | ↓ 220 |

**219 cont.**

---

Your primary question as to how to proceed is: Who is the patient? That is not as silly as it may sound. The girl will have her belly cut open and will have to live with whatever consequences arise. However, since it is the mother, as a fellow adult, that the physician is most comfortable communicating with, and since it is the mother who pays the bills or who will withhold payment if not satisfied, there is a natural inclination to treat the mother as the real patient and to relegate the girl to secondary status when it comes to explaining risks.

**220**

↓

Ethically speaking, the girl has reached the "age of comprehension" — a 14-year-old girl is capable of understanding information about risks and benefits and applying them to her own present needs and future desires. Legally speaking, she has not reached the "age of majority," so her mother must sign the consent form for surgery. This means that the mother must have the final say, but that the girl ought to be a part of the decision-making process nonetheless. It might be best to describe the risks and benefits of the surgery to both of them at once, and then later have separate interviews to see if either has questions they were unwilling to raise in front of the other.

**221**

↓ 223

---

You obtain consent from the mother only and do the surgery.

**222**

With the girl convalescing well and ready for discharge the following day, you consult with the girl's mother in your office to discuss your follow-up management plan. You explain that while the girl has not been informed of her chances of sterility — you did, as it turned out, have to do that procedure — you feel that her well-being can best be safeguarded by telling her as soon as possible. Thus she will have been able to assimilate this fact gradually by the time she reaches the age of wanting a family.

You are surprised to learn that the mother regards your plan as cruel and that she feels that it would expose her daughter to constant emotional anguish; that it would destroy any of the "joy of youth" she might experience in her adolescence. The mother feels that she would be clearly deficient in her maternal role were she to allow you to tell the daughter.

Upon further prodding by you, the mother agrees that it might be unjust to allow the girl to enter into marriage later in ignorance of her condition. She says that she would just attempt in subtle ways to discourage her

**222**
**cont.** daughter from marrying. If, however, the girl did become engaged, the mother states that she would tell the girl after the wedding had taken place.

Since you note that the mother is stating her views calmly with an appearance of having thought through the situation, you try, as gently as possible, to dissuade her from her proposed action. As you proceed, however, she becomes hostile and expresses her fear that you will upset her plans by telling the girl without her consent. She forbids you to say anything and threatens legal reprisals if you ignore her injunction.

**220** ↑ What do you do now?

---

### CASE 13

**223** A woman comes to your surgical practice with a lump in her right breast that, to manual palpation, strongly suggests malignancy. You explain that you would like to take a surgical biopsy, and, if it is positive, you feel that only removal of the entire breast will give a hope of cure. The middle-aged woman states that she wants you to do the biopsy, but that she will not have her breast removed and will only give permission for removal of the lump. You decide that this is another of those women who are so emotionally confused about their breasts that they would rather die of cancer than lose one. You determine to cater to her present whims without giving up your option to do what is in her long-term best interests once she is under anesthesia.

On the day of surgery, you note in the chart a consent form for the operation of mastectomy, duly signed by the patient. As you see her just before surgery, she again repeats her desire that you are to remove only the lump and not the breast.

↓ Do you have consent to perform right mastectomy when the biopsy comes back positive?

---

**224** In this case, you have a lot of evidence that the woman does not want her breast removed. The only evidence you have to the contrary is a piece of paper that says "consent" at the top and has her signature at the bottom. For all you know, she signed the paper not knowing what was in it; or she ↓ did not know that "mastectomy" means having a breast removed.

Case 13 illustrates a danger from misunderstanding informed consent as    **225**
legal red tape, rather than something arising from the ethics of the doctor–
patient relationship. It is easy to come to think that informed consent
means getting a signature on a piece of paper, not sitting down with the
patient and engaging in a human exchange. Obtaining informed consent
was often a task relegated to the nurse, as one more preoperative chore.

In Case 13, if you did do the mastectomy and the patient sued for damages, and the patient could prove in court the facts as described, the piece
of paper would be no protection against your being found liable for damages.    ↓

It is also conceivable, though unlikely, that the patient did knowingly and    **226**
willingly sign a form to have her breast removed; but then, just before surgery, changed her mind again and decided she wanted only the lump taken
out. Respect for the patient's autonomy requires that we respect the
patient's right to change her mind, too. Therefore, informed consent may
be withdrawn at any time prior to the actual start of the procedure. (Case 14
deals also with withdrawal of consent.)    ↓

Since we know that the right of informed consent is grounded in auton-    **227**
omy, we conclude that informed consent does not apply when autonomy
is impossible. This occurs in the case of children below the age of comprehension, and in adults who are mentally retarded, or else so mentally compromised that they cannot comprehend reality and make rational judgments. These classes of patients are considered <u>incompetent</u>, and others
must make decisions for them — a problem we will consider at length in
Chapter 7.    ↓

---

## CASE 14

You are a psychiatrist. Mrs. R.L., a 56-year-old widow, voluntarily hospital-    **228**
izes herself to be treated by you for psychotic depression. You explain to
her that a condition such as hers often responds best to a series of electroshock treatments, and after explaining the procedure, you obtain her verbal
and written consent. Mrs. R.L., however, finds the first treatment a very
frightening experience. When the attendants come to get her for second
shock, she refuses to go.

You can have the attendants forcibly take Mrs. R.L. to the treatment room
and administer the shock. Do you zap her or not?

1. Zap — because she is, after all, psychotic, so you can't place much weight
   on her expressed wishes.    ↓ 230

68

**228**
**cont.** 2. Don't zap, yet. Get a court order to have her committed as mentally incompetent, then proceed with treatment.                                    ↓ 231
3. Don't zap. Talk to her, get at the basis of her fears, remind her that such
an experience is not abnormal with shock, and explain again the possible
benefits. Try to get her to agree voluntarily again.                       ↓ 234
4. Don't zap. Mrs. R.L. has withdrawn her consent for the therapy. She has a
right to do this, so you might as well send her home.                      ↓ 235

(Adapted from R. M. Veatch, "Case 99." In *Case Studies in Medical Ethics.* Cambridge, Mass.: Harvard University Press, 1977.)

---

**229**      Regarding the option of having Mrs. R.L. legally committed, this task would
not necessarily be an easy one. Most states have now adopted laws protecting the rights of the mentally ill, demanding proof that the person is a danger to himself or others, or totally incapable of taking care of his most basic
needs, before a court can declare a person incompetent. It is not likely that
Mrs. R.L. could be made to fit into these categories unless she were actively
**232** ↓  suicidal.

---

**230**      If Mrs. R.L. is psychotic and therefore she cannot give true informed consent, what right did you have to start treatment at all? She is no more incompetent now than when she came in; since she had one treatment, she
should actually be a little better.

Or you may have reasoned that since she has refused beneficial therapy,
she is now incompetent and can be ignored when she refuses to cooperate.
The practical consequences of this view are twofold. First, you are in effect
denying the right of any psychiatric patient to refuse treatment. Second,
you are saying that the psychiatrist always selects the best possible therapy
and is never mistaken.

Is mental illness, of any sort, an automatic indication that a patient cannot make a rational judgment for informed consent? Go back and choose
**228** ↑  another alternative.

---

**231**      What is the practical and ethical difference between this alternative and
the first one, even though there is a great legal difference? You are still administering shock to Mrs. R.L. against her will. Therefore, you must be willing to accept all the ethical implications of the first choice if you go this
route. Either go back and read the frame for the first choice, or make an-
**228** ↑  other choice.

## CASE 15

As a family nurse practitioner, you believe strongly in the right of patients    **232**
to make their own decisions and the desirability of patients' being responsible for their own actions. Thus you are very frustrated with Mr. B. This
44-year-old man is about 75 pounds overweight, has borderline hypertension, and a family history of diabetes and heart disease. Your supervising
physician has emphasized how important it is for him to lose weight.

You know from experience that different approaches to diet and exercise
work better for different people; and that weight loss is almost impossible
unless the patient can take responsibility for altering his own habits.

Mr. B. affirms that he knows he absolutely must lose weight. However,
when you try to present different weight-loss approaches to him so that he
can help you select the one best suited to his life-style, he keeps putting off
the information you are trying to convey: "Just pick the one you think is
best and tell me what to do, and I'll do it." You reply that you can't decide
which approach is best for him without his thoughtful consideration of the
alternatives. "You're the expert," he replies. "I want to lose weight. You tell
me what to do." You want to scream.

What do you do with this patient?    ↓

---

What Case 15 probably boils down to is that Mr. B., despite his protesta-    **233**
tions, doesn't want to lose weight and doesn't intend to do so. For our purposes, however, think of this as an attempt to have the patient give his informed consent to one of several alternative treatments, while the patient
is exercising his prerogative to waive his right to be informed. (We need to
remember that the concept of informed consent applies to all encounters
between patients and health professionals, not just to surgery and other
dramatic procedures.)    ↓ 236

---

You seem to have chosen the most acceptable ethical course of action.    **234**
However, to a certain extent, you are postponing your decision. What if
Mrs. R.L. still continues to refuse?    ↑ 229

235     By choosing this course you seem to be saying, in effect, that by refusing her treatment, Mrs. R.L. has rejected you, so now you will get even and reject her.

Mrs. R.L. has refused to undergo this treatment, but she did come in voluntarily to be treated. Possibly if you explain matters further to her she will change her mind. If not, there are some alternative forms of treatment for depression that might, while not as satisfactory as electroshock, still be better than nothing.

Is it ethically valid, where genuine treatment options exist, for a doctor to insist that the patient agree to the doctor's choice or else go elsewhere for
228 ↑     care?

---

236     Clearly Mr. B. is refusing to accept the responsibility for his own actions, and is practically begging you to respond paternalistically as in the priestly model. But this is his choice — and probably a true reflection of his personality. The doctor–patient contract requires only that the patient be given the <u>opportunity</u> to act autonomously and make his own value choices. Ironically, to force a patient to act more responsibly, because you think that is how patients ought to act, would also be to revert to the
↓     priestly model.

237     The hooker here is your judgment that in this particular illness, the priestly model just won't work — that accepting responsibility is an <u>essential</u> feature of the treatment of obesity.

You would seem, then, to have two viable alternatives. You could recant on your views, accept the paternalistic role that the patient is forcing on you, and rigidly prescribe a diet plan for him — reasoning that this is less than ideal treatment, but better than nothing. Or you could argue that Mr. B.'s attitude effectively precludes your treating him at all. You might then
↓     point this out to him and recommend that he seek another nurse or doctor.

---

### CASE 16

238     You are an American physician in the jungles of Nigeria, and you are there to try out a new vaccine for measles, a disease that is causing significant childhood mortality in the region. The vaccine that you will be using causes encephalitis on rare occasion. It also has the potential of sensitizing the child to proteins in the vaccine besides the measles material itself, so that the child might have an allergic reaction to a subsequent vaccination of a different type. The relation of such sensitization to various auto-immune diseases is not known at present.

The mothers are all uneducated and speak their tribal language, which   **238**
you do not. How do you go about getting informed consent, or do you   cont.
bother to do it at all? (This case is intended for thought and/or discussion.)

(Adapted from F. D. Moore. In J. Katz (Ed.), *Experimentation with Human Beings.*
New York: Russell Sage Foundation, 1972. Used by permission of the Russell Sage
Foundation.)   ↓

---

We can now summarize some of the major points we have made on the   **239**
doctrine of informed consent.

1. *The basic purpose of informed consent is to protect patient autonomy,
   not to have patients make the choice that we think is best for them.*
2. *As a right within the doctor–patient relationship, informed consent may
   be waived. The patient may choose not to be informed about some features of the treatment, or may choose to allow others to make the decision for him.*
3. *The physician's duty includes disclosing the information that that particular patient would ideally require in order to make a reasoned choice.
   This will depend in part on the patient's own values. Generally this will
   include mention of the risks and benefits of the proposed treatment, and
   the risks and benefits of any alternative treatments.*
4. *Informed consent, once given, may be withdrawn.*
5. *Emotional stress or mental illness does not by itself necessarily preclude
   the possibility of informed consent.*   ↓

A final point worth mentioning parallels our comment on telling the true   **240**
diagnosis to a terminal patient — "telling all" can be done either compas-
sionately or brutally, depending on how well one is tuned in to the
patient's state of mind. Similarly, if the patient desires to hear about the
remote but disastrous risks of a treatment procedure, you may frankly describe them; but you are also free to add that these risks are highly unlikely
and that you will do all in your power to prevent them. The ability to explain alternative treatments to a patient in a thorough yet sensitive manner
is a valuable clinical skill, which all health professionals ought to cultivate.

CH. 6 ↓ **241**

# Terminal Care and 6
# Quality of Life

## CASE 17

As head nurse of the hospital ward, you have gathered together the other
nurses to meet with the surgeon caring for Mr. T.S. Two years ago, at age 71,
Mr. T.S. underwent colostomy for colon cancer; and then underwent x-ray
therapy when the cancer recurred. Now, blood tests suggest metastasis of
the cancer to the liver. While often drowsy or obtunded, Mr. T.S. has nevertheless communicated to various nurses that he realizes he is approaching
the terminal state, is tired of medical procedures, and wishes they would
"just leave me alone." You have called a conference to deal with the nurses'
dissatisfaction over the surgeon's plan to treat Mr. T.S. aggressively with
palliative radiation and surgical procedures.

The surgeon, Dr. H., admits that the patient is terminal and that cure is
impossible, and that death will occur within several months even with aggressive therapy. Still, he argues, "If we take it upon ourselves to end his life
before then, we are playing God. Who gave us that right? And how would
we feel if the week after he died, somebody discovered the cure for cancer?
I've been brought up to believe that human life is sacred, and we ought to
do anything possible to preserve it."

What do you think of Dr. H.'s argument? Would you try to dissuade him?
Or would you try to convince the other nurses that their emotional reactions, while understandable, are ethically unsound?

---

Case 17, while presenting a common dilemma, still represents a type of
problem that constitutes only a small minority of all patient–health professional encounters. But because issues surrounding death lead to some of
the most perplexing ethical dilemmas — and because each patient and each
health professional must sooner or later face his or her own death — issues
of terminal care, including the notion of quality of life, deserve discussion
as part of the fundamentals of medical ethics.

Our main purpose in this chapter will be to divide cases of terminal-care
dilemmas into three general categories. In practice, terminal-care cases involving very different ethical features are often lumped together and
treated according to the same principles. While people with different
values will disagree about cases within each category, getting the categories straight will at least ensure that we are all arguing about the same thing
in each instance. And the disagreement should not surprise us; in this area
we should be especially wary of easy answers.

**244** Case 17 portrays Dr. H. giving examples of several overly easy answers. Before dealing with the three categories, then, we need to look more closely ↓ at some inadequate forms of argument about terminal care.

**245** First consider the accusation, "If you do so-and-so then you're playing God." This is heard with amazing frequency in ethical discussion, even though it is almost totally devoid of meaning. Such a statement makes sense only if we assume that God is one who takes an active interest in, and intervenes in, the daily lives of individual human beings. It then follows that either medicine is totally ineffective in accomplishing its goals — if God wanted Mr. T.S. to go on living, our stopping aggressive treatment would make no difference — or else physicians are "playing God" every time they intervene in the natural course of an illness. If you do not object to playing God by giving penicillin to treat a strep throat, you have to explain why it is ↓ wrong to play God in terminal-care decisions.

**246** A sympathetic interpretation of the playing God objection is that it warns physicians not to be too eager to make life-and-death choices for others as if we knew better than anyone else what is best for them. But we have already called attention to this problem by contrasting the priestly and the contractual models of the doctor–patient relationship.

   In short, if we agreed to outlaw the expression "playing God" from all medical-ethical discussion, the quality of such discussion would be signif-↓ icantly enhanced.
   REVIEW PRIESTLY MODEL ↑ 127

**247** Next, what do you think about the new-miracle-cure argument? Again, it is useful to compare the terminal-care case to the more usual medical circumstances, granted that the stakes are often much higher in terminal situations. And nowhere in medicine do we find responsible physicians relying on such remote possibilities as the appearance of a new miracle cure — even leaving aside the fact that today, new cures seldom burst unannounced onto the scene, but are used experimentally for years before they ↓ are released for general use.

**248** For example, when Mr. T.S. was first diagnosed with cancer, it was at least barely possible that he would have a miraculous spontaneous remission without treatment; and if such had occurred, he would have been saved the pain and the toxic effects of surgery and radiation. But his surgeon wisely based his therapeutic plans on the probable outcome, not the wildly improbable one. Now, if in fact a new cure was discovered the day after we had let Mr. T.S. die prematurely, we would regret our actions. But we should regret our actions even more if the something-may-turn-up argument condemned Mr. T.S. to months of additional, unnecessary suffering; ↓ and this is a much more probable outcome.

Presented with these arguments, Dr. H. might agree that his statements    **249**
about playing God and miraculous cure do not lend the support to his actions that he thought. But what about his insistence on the sanctity of human life? This line of argument holds special appeal to health professionals.
After all, it seems that our primary task, no matter what else we do, is to
preserve life. And, if the sanctity-of-life view is correct, we would never be
justified in taking action to end anyone's life; thus a lot of ethical problems, such as euthanasia, would be swept aside. Finally, the health professional might find that the sanctity of life view is supported by some of the
major religious ethical systems.    ↓

Since, so far, we have not paid much attention to religion as a source of    **250**
ethical principles, it is worth quoting at length from a particularly precise
statement of "sanctity of life" as viewed by an orthodox theologian — in
this case, Dr. Moshe Tendler, professor of Talmudic law at Yeshiva University, in a 1972 Symposium on Ethical Issues in Human Experimentation:

> As you know, the ethical foundation of our society of Western civilization is a
> biblical one. . . . There are certain indispensable foundations for an ethical system
> and one of them is the sanctity of human life. This concept has a corollary; that is
> that human life is of infinite value. This in turn means that a <u>piece</u> of infinity is also
> infinity and a person who has but a few moments to live is no less of value than a
> person who has 70 years to live.    ↓

> And likewise, a person who is handicapped and cannot serve the needs of society is    **251**
> no less a man and no less entitled to this same price tag — a price tag inscribed with
> an infinite price. A handicapped individual is a perfect specimen when viewed in an
> ethical context. This value is an absolute value. It is not relative to life expectancy, to
> state of health, or to usefulness to society. . . .
>   When does man become man is the real definition of the problem of the morality
> of abortion. When is man no longer man is similarly the real definition of the prob-
> lem of euthanasia, and all of it depends on your concepts of the rights of man. . . .
>   Another principle germane to the discussion is that the protection due your fel-
> low man is directly proportional to his helplessness. The more helpless he is, the
> more he must be protected. This is the key to the ethical principle of man imitating
> God, illustrated in biblical literature by the men who care for the orphans and
> widows, and for the helpless and defenseless. . . .    ↓

> It is not necessary in a system of ethics to which I adhere — a biblical system of    **252**
> ethics — to have informed consent if you know for sure, with the best of your
> scientific and ethical ability to evaluate, that the action is for the benefit of the pa-
> tient. Just as a man cannot commit suicide under our ethical system, he cannot re-
> frain from benefiting from medical advances and by doing so forfeit his life pas-
> sively. If indeed a procedure is looked upon as a proper medical procedure, it will
> be proper to institute it even without informed consent. It is only when there is a
> question of probability — odds on the chance of helping, or on the chance of hurt-
> ing — that we expect adults to be able to make a consensual decision. . . .    ↓

**253** What, now, can be said against the sanctity-of-life view? Its very comprehensiveness makes it suspect. If we take one thing and declare it to be of infinite value, so that we never have to examine any competing values in making ethical decisions, the decisions certainly come more easily — but the decisions are not necessarily better ones.

**254** A quick test of the sanctity-of-life view is the issue of rational suicide. Do you think that suicide is <u>ever</u> morally acceptable? Consider, for instance, extreme cases such as suicide by a captured secret agent who knows that if he does not kill himself, he will be mercilessly tortured and forced to divulge important national secrets, and then killed anyway by his captors. If you feel that such a suicide could ever be justified, then you do not hold a view consistent with the absolute sanctity of life.

**255** The basic question is: Do we feel that life is of infinite value? Or do we feel that life is of very great value, precisely because most of the other things we value cannot be realized without life? If we hold the latter view, we are bound to preserve life in almost all cases; but we have to consider the possibility that in a few cases, life does not further other major values and may indeed be of negative value. Case 17 may be an example of such a case.

**256** The sanctity-of-life advocate may fear that if we act to bring about an individual's death, we cannot respect the value of that individual; and we saw in Chapter 2 that respect for individuals is a basic feature of any acceptable ethical system. But theological ethicists such as McCormick (1978) have argued that, from the infinite value of the <u>individual</u>, we cannot conclude that the individual's <u>life</u> always has value; again, in Case 17, it is precisely our respect for Mr. T.S. as an individual that prompts us to accede to his requests. (Compare punishment, which is certainly a disvalue in itself; from the fact that we punish a child it does not follow that we do not value that child as an individual.)

For a more detailed discussion of the sanctity-of-life view, see Clouser (1973).

**257** The sanctity-of-life principle can, however, be restated in a consequentialist form more in keeping with the principles we have been using — that is, that one ought never kill an innocent human being because following such a course would have undesirable consequences. As emotionally stated by certain vocal proponents of sanctity-of-life views, the undesirable consequences are as follows: first you allow abortion, then you open the door to mercy killing, then you start shooting inmates of mental hospitals, and eventually, in short order, we will have resurrected Nazi Germany.

We can label this type of argument, which is often seen in ethical debates, a **258** "domino-theory" strategy of ethical argument. We need to be alert for two types of domino theory; the first is not a consequentialist argument while the latter is.

1. We are unsure about whether to accept action X. Morally speaking, action X is, in principle, indistinguishable from action Y; and action Y is morally unacceptable. Therefore, since accepting X is the same in principle as accepting Y, we ought to prohibit X.
2. We are unsure about whether to accept action X. If people in general did X, there is a high probability that they would also begin to do action Y; and Y is morally unacceptable. Thus, we should prohibit X, because it would lead to Y. ↓

A philosopher, Tooley (1972), used the first type of domino-theory argu- **259** ment in the case of abortion and infanticide. He argued that a fetus, morally speaking, is no different in its essential characteristics from a newborn baby; therefore, if it is all right to do abortions, it should be all right to kill infants. If we added the stipulation that infanticide is clearly immoral, we would have a domino-theory argument of the first type against abortion.

For our purposes it is important, not to agree or disagree with Tooley, but to see the type of argument used. For example, the argument that nowadays, in countries where abortion is widely practiced, infanticide is still condemned, would not count against this domino-theory position. It is an argument about what acts are similar or dissimilar in principle, not about the practical consequences of adopting a certain policy. ↓

The second type of domino theory is often seen in arguments against le- **260** galizing active euthanasia, which we will be discussing in Chapter 13. It may be argued that we will start off by using active euthanasia in clearcut cases, to eliminate suffering of terminal illness at the individual's own request; but as we become more used to the idea, abuses will inevitably occur. This argument is about the practical consequences of our policy decisions. It does not say that we cannot distinguish in principle between giving an overdose of morphine to a terminally ill cancer patient in excruciating pain, and giving an overdose of morphine to Aunt Sally in a nursing home to collect on her life-insurance policy. It argues instead that a policy allowing the first type of action will lead to increased incidence of the second. ↓

**261**   The two types of domino-theory arguments, then, demand different types of reply. To the first, we must show that we can distinguish between the two types of cases on the basis of ethically important characteristics. To the second, we must show that, based on studies of actual behavior, the first type of behavior is unlikely to lead to the second. Domino theorists like those who cry "Nazi" at any mention of euthanasia or allowing to die often overstate their case, claiming that the deleterious consequences are inevitable. Unfortunately, we can prove the issue for certain only by making the policy change; it is then too late to retreat if the domino theorists turn out to have been right. On the other hand, we could imagine deleterious consequences to any policy choice; so the domino theory, if accepted without close scrutiny, could become an argument against any change whatsoever.

**262**   If we reject the sanctity-of-life view, we have to judge individual terminal-care cases to see whether life should be preserved, or whether respect for individuals or other, overriding values require that we choose another course. We will now look at three major categories of cases in which such questions might arise.

## CASE 18

**263**   You are the neurosurgery resident assigned to take care of Johnnie Tibbs, a 10-year-old boy with severe head injuries from an auto accident that occurred the day before. After getting blood transfusions and being placed on a mechanical respirator, Johnnie was observed to have fixed and dilated pupils, no spontaneous attempts to breathe, and no reaction to stimuli such as pain. An electroencephalogram done at that time showed no electrical activity of the brain, and today's EEG shows the same result. Johnnie's heart is beating normally, but his status is unchanged.

You now have to speak to the Tibbses about Johnnie's further treatment. Your attending neurosurgeon says that you should ask them for permission to stop the respirator and allow Johnnie to die.

What do you say to the parents?

**264**   Johnnie Tibbs's sad case represents the first of our three categories of cases. Ten years ago, had such a case arisen, it would have been a straightforward question of allowing to die as opposed to continued heroic therapy.

Since then, however, the concept of brain death has become widely accepted in medicine, and has been enacted into law in 23 states as of 1980. According to the brain death criteria, there is no opportunity in Johnnie's case for you either to allow him to die or to continue treatment, since he is already dead.

*By brain-death criteria, a person is dead if he has suffered irreversible loss of*    **265**
*spontaneous function of the entire brain.* Several sets of clinical measurements have been suggested to determine the presence of brain death. Most
widely known are the Harvard Medical School ad hoc committee criteria:
(1) total unresponsiveness to external stimuli, (2) lack of spontaneous
movement or respiratory effort, and (3) no elicitable reflexes. A flat-line
EEG is of "great confirmatory value" but is not required. These findings
must be present over a 24-hour period, and do not apply in cases of hy-
pothermia (body temperature below 90°F) or barbiturate overdose, in
which brain recovery has been observed.

Other proposed criteria include absence of cerebral blood flow, as determined by radioisotope scan or angiography. Black (1978), reviewing the
different criteria proposed, concluded that all are free of false-positive results; that is, no recovery of brain function has been observed in anyone
declared brain dead by the careful use of any of these criteria, even where
the respirator and other care have been continued.    ↓

Brain death has often been seen as a radical departure from our traditional    **266**
idea of death, and in addition has been held to be highly suspect, since its
adoption has been motivated in large part by the desire to get healthy organs for use in transplantation. But it is possible to view brain death instead
as a conservative revision necessitated by our modern medical technology.    ↓

The reason heart and lung function became the legal and social standard to    **267**
determine the time of death, we might argue, is that when one either
stopped breathing or suffered cardiac arrest, irreversible loss of total brain
function invariably followed within minutes. Today, however, mechanical
devices have made it possible to maintain artificially heart and lung function even in the presence of brain death. If we have other tools, such as the
Harvard criteria, to tell us what is actually going on with the brain, we
should rely on those, and not the artificially maintained heart and lungs, to
determine death.    ↓

This argument assumes that heart and lung function are important, not for    **268**
themselves, but as signs of brain activity. And this assumption seems quite
plausible. When surgeons stop the heartbeat for an hour or more during
open-heart surgery, and a bypass pump is used to prevent any brain damage, we do not normally say that the person has died and then been reborn,
unless we are speaking metaphorically.    ↓

**269**   If we accept the notion of brain death, Case 18 is considerably clarified. The attending neurosurgeon is mistaken in suggesting that we allow Johnnie to die, or that we ask consent from the parents to unhook the respirator. We cannot allow a corpse to die, nor need we ask consent to unhook the respirator from a dead body.

On the other hand, were Johnnie's parents to consent to donating his kidneys, there would be nothing incorrect about continuing mechanical respiration until after the surgery to remove the kidneys, to guarantee their freshness. We would still be removing the kidneys from a corpse, and our removing the kidneys, or shutting off the respirator afterwards, would not be the cause of death.

**270**   If the resident in Case 18 tells Johnnie's parents that Johnnie is already dead, and that therefore the respirator should be turned off, they might be quite bewildered. Medical professionals currently have an awareness of brain death in advance of the views of most of the public. The Tibbses may reason that, since Johnnie's body is still warm and has a heartbeat, he cannot possibly be dead; and they might indignantly reject such an assertion.

**271**   Encountering such resistance, many physicians, even in states that have legalized brain-death criteria, would choose to avoid creating additional emotional turmoil for the parents (and perhaps a lawsuit for themselves, though such a suit would be destined to fail) by not discontinuing the respirator until the parents had accepted the fact that Johnnie would never recover, or until he suffered a cardiac arrest, which in the vast majority of brain-death cases occurs within a few days anyway. This course may avoid conflict, but risks leading to a confusion between brain-death cases and the next category of cases we will discuss below.

**272**   In Case 18, brain death simplifies matters considerably and allows us to avoid a number of sticky ethical questions — allowing to die, euthanasia, quality of life, extraordinary means, and so on. While few cases of terminal care fall under the brain-death category, the concept is still a highly useful one when it does apply.

The very simplicity of the brain-death notion has led to a misunderstanding — that we have replaced complex ethical dilemmas with simple, empirical measurements of death.

**273**   To understand brain death correctly, however, we have to sort out its empirical and ethical elements. Whether irreversible loss of spontaneous brain function has occurred when the Harvard criteria are present, and whether the criteria were present in Johnnie's case, are empirical questions. But whether irreversible loss of spontaneous brain function is to be equated with death is an ethical question, and one that requires ethical arguments of the type that we have just been reviewing.

Some ethical ramifications of revising criteria for death are illustrated in the next case.

## CASE 19

The year is 1988; Michigan's brain-death statute has been in effect for 15 **274** years, and a law to allow mercy killing in terminally ill patients at their request or at the request of the next of kin was passed by the legislature last session. None of this is of much help to you as you try to figure out what to do with Mr. L. Mr. L. has been in a coma and maintained on a respirator for 26 days, ever since the auto crash in which his wife was killed. For 3 weeks you still had some hope that the 58-year-old patient might be brought back to consciousness; now you have pretty much given up, but the state of his reflexes and movements are too equivocal to allow you to pronounce him dead by the Harvard criteria. You have told Mr. L.'s two grown children that it seems as if there is nothing to be gained, and if no dramatic change for the better occurs within 24 to 48 hours, you will disconnect the respirator.

This morning you have a visitor — a lawyer for the Great Atlantic and Pacific Life Insurance Company. He tells you that Mr. L. is protected by a six-figure insurance policy that pays double indemnity in cases of accidental death. However, to qualify under that clause of the policy, the death must take place within 30 days of the accident.

The lawyer says that his company has developed a fear that you are plotting in concert with Mr. L.'s children to turn off the respirator inside the magic 30-day limit, "despite the fact that he is obviously still alive." In order to guard itself against this course, the company has authorized the lawyer to inform you that you will be sued for the amount of the insurance policy should the respirator be turned off, in the absence of clear signs of death, within the 30-day period.

No sooner has this gentleman left than you are visited by the attorney newly retained by Mr. L.'s children. He reminds you that proper regard for the best interests of your patient's family would require that the respirator be turned off immediately, "since he is obviously already dead. Anyway, he should have a right to death with dignity, without all sorts of tubes stuck in him." In case you need encouragement to consider these interests more closely, the lawyer notes that should you cause the family to lose the double-indemnity sum, they plan to sue you for that amount.

After finishing the half-full bottle of bourbon in the bottom drawer of your desk, what do you do then? ↓

**275** We have no intention of offering an answer to this rather fanciful case. It is included to remind us that defining and pronouncing death are in no sense isolated medical functions. Death to the public at large means not only respirators, defibrillation, and autopsies, but also funerals, mourning, insurance policies, wills, and many other things. No medical approach to death can be viewed apart from its impact on these other social and legal considerations; and a new concept such as brain death must be judged for its impact on the entire social structure, not just on narrow medical grounds. All indications are that brain death will meet these tests well, so we are ↓ justified in adopting it.

**276** The concept of brain death, however, does not help us in the following ↓ case.

---

### CASE 20

**277** On April 15, 1975, 21-year-old Karen Ann Quinlan was taken to a New Jersey hospital in comatose condition, apparently having taken an overdose of drugs combined with alcohol while partying with friends. While meeting none of the Harvard brain death criteria, she remained in a coma for five months, supported with a respirator and tube feedings; her doctors felt that if she was removed from the respirator she would die, but held out no hope for recovery of consciousness. Karen's parents requested that the respirator be withdrawn, citing their view that this was in accordance with God's will and also what Karen herself would have wanted. The doctors refused to stop support on a patient who was not brain dead.

What should be done with Karen Quinlan?

↓ (Adapted from *In re Quinlan*, 355 A. 2nd 647 [N.J. 1976].)

---

**278** In this widely publicized and discussed case, a lower court first refused to grant the parents' request. On appeal, the New Jersey Supreme Court overturned this lower ruling, and appointed Karen's father her guardian for purposes of discontinuing the respirator. Basically, the court held that when a person has no chance of recovering a "cognitive, sapient state," the usual overriding interest that the state has in protecting life weakens. Instead, the individual's right of privacy, exercised through a guardian, may call for dis- ↓ continuance of burdensome life support.

While some newspapers, confusing this case with cases in the first category    **279**
we discussed, headlined the Quinlan decision as "a new definition of
death," no one in fact ever argued that Karen was dead. All agreed that the
question was whether she should be <u>allowed to die</u>. In fact, the physicians
were wrong, and after discontinuing the respirator Karen continued breathing on her own, and still does so at this writing 5 years later. She has never
recovered consciousness, however.    ↓

Unlike brain death, the *Quinlan* case presents a different set of ethical    **280**
questions. We might refer to this second category of cases as those involving a chronic vegetative state.
   The way we will approach the question of what should have been done
with Karen Quinlan is to ask whether Karen Quinlan is still a person, and
what personhood means in this context. To do this, we will have to deal
with some rather abstract philosophical points; but getting these clear will
help us to see the doctor–patient relationship in such cases in a more useful
way.    ↓

Much of the original debate about the *Quinlan* case was based on whether    **281**
Karen, who was not yet dead, had a right to life, or whether, since continued existence presumably could be of no benefit to her, she had instead a
right to die. We discussed the nature of rights briefly in Chapter 2; but here
we might ask a more basic question – *not whether a being has or doesn't
have some particular rights, but what sort of beings can be said to have
rights at all.* Clearly, human beings who are alive and conscious have rights,
while it would be absurd to speak of a rock or of a tiger lily having rights.
What is the essential difference?    ↓

Several philosophers, notably Feinberg (1974), have addressed the question    **282**
of what characteristics a being must have in order to be eligible as a bearer
of rights. In brief, one could construct the following argument:

1. To be eligible to have rights, X must be the sort of being that could be
   said to have interests. That is, some things must be good for X for X's own
   sake, and not merely because X is useful to somebody else.
2. To be said to have interests, X must have wants and purposes – it would
   seem absurd to say that X had an interest in, say, being fed, if X never
   wanted to be fed, and being fed furthered no purpose that X had in life.
3. At the very least, having wants and purposes requires memories, expectations, and beliefs – that is, a minimal level of cognitive awareness existing over time.
4. Therefore, if X does not have a minimal level of cognitive awareness, or
   has irreversibly lost all such awareness, then X cannot be said to be the
   bearer of rights.    ↓

**283**   It follows from this argument that Karen Quinlan cannot have a right to life — or, for that matter, a right to die. If, by a person, we mean a being who is eligible to have rights — to be a member of a moral community — then Karen Quinlan is no longer a person. This is not to say we can then do anything we please with Karen Quinlan. Johnnie in Case 18 was not a person either, being dead; but we could not remove his kidneys for transplant without his parents' consent. Other persons may have rights that dictate how we treat beings that are not persons; or there may be important moral ↓ values independent of rights.

**284**   It is very important to see what this argument does and does not claim. It is an argument not about what rights Karen Quinlan does or does not have, but about what sort of being Karen Quinlan is now. Before she became comatose, for example, Karen may have had a right to a college education at public expense, or she may not; this right is arguable, but at any rate it makes sense to speak of Karen, before she was comatose, having or not having such a right. After she became comatose, however, it makes no sense to talk of Karen having rights or not having rights, because in her chronic vegetative state she lacks the characteristics that make her eligible for right-bearing at all. (Maybe Reggie Jackson hit a home run today, or maybe he didn't; but at least he is the sort of being about which it makes sense to talk of him hitting home runs. By contrast, it makes no sense to talk ↓ about the Pythagorean Theorem hitting a home run.)
          CONSEQUENTIALIST? * 286

**285**   What does all this abstract philosophical rigmarole have to do with ethical decisions in medicine?
          We discussed in Chapter 2 the basic value of respect for individuals, and we then saw in Chapter 4 that the contractual model of the doctor–patient relationship best served this value. We now see that really what we mean by respect for individuals is respect for individual <u>persons</u>. Respect for individuals means respecting that individual's wants and purposes, and seeing that certain things are good for that individual for his or her own sake. But
**287** ↓  to have wants, purposes, and an "own sake," one must be a person.

---

**286**   * This argument about persons is not a consequentialist ethical argument such as we have previously discussed. It is a deontological argument (see Appendix I), based on a priori considerations. It does, however, suggest a related consequentialist argument. There are good consequences to be served by not keeping Karen Quinlan alive — her parents' desires, preserving expensive medical resources, and so on. The only bad consequences we might be worried about would be those that are bad for Karen, or for others in her class of individuals, those in a chronic vegetative state. But we saw that such individuals cannot be said to have interests, so nothing we do can run counter to their interests. Thus, in deciding the ethical course of action,
**285** ↑  we can essentially leave Karen herself out of the equation.

When a patient is in an irreversible vegetative state, he or she is no longer a **287** person. We can no longer, by treating or failing to treat, pursue the value of respect for persons regarding that individual. The only exception is that we can respect any promise that was made to the person, while still a person, about how they wished to be treated should such a vegetative state occur; or we can honor a document or "living will" left by the person giving those directions. (See Appendixes IV, V, VI, and VII for examples of living wills; they will be discussed further below and in Chapter 13).

Since the individual in a chronic vegetative state is not a person and has no conscious awareness, it can make no difference to him whether we respect our promise or not. The duty we have to do so is like the duty to respect the will made by a person who is now dead.  ↓

Suppose that Karen Quinlan had left a document requesting that she be **288** kept alive as long as possible even in a chronic vegetative state; or that her parents had requested this. We might then feel an obligation to carry out this wish, assuming that our society does not prohibit using medical resources for such an end — a prohibition that may be imposed someday due to rising health costs. The person argument does not prohibit treating Karen in this way; it merely reminds us that by doing so we should not assume that we are doing it for (the present) Karen's "own good" or in accordance with her (present) interests, as she cannot be said meaningfully to have either.  ↓

This argument based on personhood may be very upsetting to some peo- **289** ple. They will recall that societies in the past, when intent on carrying out some monstrous wrong against a minority group, frequently began the campaign by depicting the victims as less than fully human or as nonpersons. By a domino-theory argument, claiming that any class of patients are not persons in the full sense would be very dangerous and could open the door to all sorts of future inhumanity.  ↓

But this objection, based on historical analogy, fails to see that all we re- **290** quire for personhood is the most minimal level of cognitive awareness. Our personhood criterion, furthermore, meets the "what if it were me?" test. If we were Nazis persecuting the Jews, and if we imagined that we were to be changed into Jews overnight, we presumably would object to receiving similar treatment ourselves. But if we were to become irreversibly comatose, would it matter to us whether or not we had certain sorts of medical treatment, or if we lived for 5 minutes or 5 years? It might matter now to us thinking about it, and it might matter to our surviving families; but if we

**290**
cont.
↓
approach the question rationally, we would have to include that it would make no difference to us, at the time, given our inability for any sort of cognitive awareness.

HOW DO WE KNOW? * 294

**291** Our approach to chronic vegetative states based on the idea of personhood could be criticized from another point of view. One objection would be that in selecting a rock-bottom, minimal criterion for personhood we have been too conservative; and that one should define personhood in terms of optimal, rather than minimal, human qualities. One such attempt is Joseph Fletcher's list of indicators of personhood (see Appendix VIII).

If personhood is to be used in ethical decision making, however, the farther we get away from the very minimal criteria, the more objectionable our view is likely to become. When we start demanding higher levels of intelligence, imagination, and sensitivity, we run the risk of including criteria that reflect our own personal value biases, and thus are not universalizable to others holding different values. We might then be in a position of imposing those idiosyncratic value judgments on others, under the guise of separating persons from nonpersons. The Nazi analogy starts to sound
↓ more relevant once we adopt this posture.

**292** We must also remember that the person–nonperson distinction in no way parallels the save-or-don't-save distinction. From the fact that X is not a person, it does not follow that I may kill X if I so choose, or allow X to die if I could easily save him (suppose X were my neighbor's dog, for example, about to run into traffic). Similarly, from the fact that X is a person, it does not follow that I must not kill X (perhaps I may kill in self-defense, or perhaps in a case of justified active euthanasia) or that I must not allow X to die
↓ (as with Mr. T.S. in Case 17).

**293** Finally, we must keep in mind the rather technical definition that we used in defining "person" in this context — *a being that could meaningfully be said to be potentially the bearer of rights. (Or, put another way, a being who could meaningfully be said to be benefitted or harmed for that being's "own sake.")* In this technical usage of <u>person</u>, we do <u>not</u> mean: a human being, a "decent" human being, a "worthy" human being, a human being "leading a meaningful life," and so on. When we say that Karen Quinlan has lost her status as a person, we do not mean that we don't like her any more, or that we think that she has done something nasty and should be punished for it, or anything of that nature. We are saying here that Karen

---

**294** * Some might object here that perhaps Karen Quinlan has some sort of inner existence that we cannot know about and that neurophysiologists cannot detect. We cannot refute this with certainty, but it seems a very slim
**291** ↑ thread on which to hang an ethical argument.

Quinlan has irreversibly lost some basic capacities, and that those capaci-   **293**
ties are necessary conditions for us to be able to relate to Karen Quinlan as   cont.
an equal in our moral community and as a bearer of rights (as Kant would
say, "as an end and not as a means only").   ↓ **295**

---

Another argument is that we could accomplish our purpose more directly   **295**
by expanding our first category of cases, rather than creating a second category based on the concept of persons. That is, why not redefine death further so that all people in chronic vegetative states will be judged dead? One
might argue that the Harvard criteria are too conservative, since according
to them, someone with a functioning brain stem, who therefore has spontaneous respiration and some reflexes, is alive. But is merely having a functioning brain stem to be alive in any human sense of the word? From this
view has come the recommendation for a neocortical criterion for death: A
person would be considered dead if only the higher brain centers, and not
the entire brain, had irreversibly lost spontaneous function. Along these
lines, some have recommended that a flat EEG be taken as an adequate
criterion for death, even if the other Harvard criteria are not present.   ↓

There is a good deal to be said for this neocortical approach to death; and   **296**
perhaps in the future this concept will even be enacted into law, just as
brain death has been enacted.
   However, a number of objections have been lodged against it. For one
thing, it stretches our traditional concepts of death much farther than brain
death does. A body declared dead by brain criteria, once artificial life support is stopped, becomes dead by traditional criteria in a very few minutes,
since it cannot breathe and therefore cannot sustain a heartbeat. A body
with a flat EEG but with an intact brain stem may go on breathing
indefinitely, however. Many of us would find it hard to imagine declaring
such a body dead, holding a funeral, and lowering it into the grave, still
warm and breathing.   ↓

Also, instead of trying to answer all ethical questions regarding terminal   **297**
care by manipulating our definitions of death, we might make clearer and
more precise judgments if we recognized a category of human beings that
are alive and yet are not persons. Karen Quinlan in a coma fits into this
category. An anencephalic infant (one born without any brain apart from
the brain stem) would be another example. Depending on your views on
abortion (see Chapter 10), a living human fetus might be still another example.   ↓

**298** Finally, we should note that of all individuals in chronic vegetative states, many do not exhibit a flat EEG pattern — Karen Quinlan did not. Thus, even if we adopted a neocortical criterion for death, we would fail to deal with
↓ many Quinlan-type cases.

**299** We have now discussed two categories of terminal-care cases — those involving individuals who are brain dead, and those involving individuals who, because of chronic vegetative states, have irreversibly ceased to be persons by our definition. But these two categories together account for only a minority of all cases of terminally ill patients. The dilemma presented by Mr. T.S. in Case 17 is much more typical. Mr. T.S. is clearly not brain dead, and he also possesses the degree of cognitive awareness necessary to be regarded as a person. Thus, his case represents our third category of
↓ terminal-care cases, as does the case following.

---

## CASE 21

**300** Joseph Saikewicz had lived all of his 67 years in institutions for the severely mentally retarded. With an IQ of 10, he had the intellectual capacity of a 3-year-old child. On April 19, 1976, he was diagnosed as having acute myelogenous leukemia.

You are the physician called in by the institution to advise on Mr. Saikewicz's treatment. You know that this form of leukemia is incurable, but that with aggressive chemotherapy, the patient has a 30 to 50 percent chance of achieving a remission lasting from 2 to 13 months, after which the leukemia will recur. The chemotherapy involves several weeks of treatment with potent drugs, which entails severe discomfort and nausea, and could itself be fatal. Because of the patient's inability to understand or communicate other than by grunts and gestures, he could not cooperate in the therapy and would probably have to be physically restrained. Without treatment, he would live some weeks or months and would probably die of infection.

What course of treatment do you advise for Mr. Saikewicz?

(Adapted from *Superintendent of Belchertown State School* v. *Saikewicz*, 370 N.E.
↓ 2nd 417 [Mass. 1977].)

The superintendent of Joseph Saikewicz's institution appealed to the court    **301**
for guidance. At a hearing, two doctors testified against giving chemotherapy, and the court ruled that chemotherapy not be given; this decision was
appealed directly to the Massachusetts Supreme Judicial Court, which upheld the lower court ruling. Some months later, after Saikewicz had already
died of pneumonia, the Supreme Court issued its full opinion, which took
place alongside the New Jersey *Quinlan* decision as one of the most widely
discussed judicial pronouncements on terminal care.    ↓

As interpreted by Annas (1978), the Massachusetts court based its decision    **302**
on the finding that a competent adult has the right to refuse life-prolonging
treatment — a right fully consistent with our views of the doctor–patient
relationship and informed consent. Since Saikewicz was not competent,
however, the court allowed that it was possible for someone representing
his interests to look at the situation as nearly as possible from Saikewicz's
own point of view, and to make a decision of discontinuing treatment on
his behalf. But, to ensure that his best interests were really protected, the
court required that an adversary judicial hearing be held to decide such
cases — going against the reliance on doctors, families, and hospital committees proposed by the New Jersey Court in *Quinlan*.    ↓

The fine points of the *Quinlan* and *Saikewicz* rulings have been extensively    **303**
debated by authorities on medical jurisprudence, and physicians in Massachusetts and New Jersey will want to study these rulings to see what is required of them legally in those respective states. Recall, however, that the
law, even when nationwide in scope, cannot finally answer ethical questions. Therefore, we will have to supply the ethical reasons that might underlie a decision such as *Saikewicz*, and criticize the court's ruling if necessary.    ↓
REVIEW LAW ↑ 69–71

First, note that Saikewicz falls into our third category of cases. Unlike John-    **304**
nie Tibbs, Saikewicz was not brain dead, and unlike Karen Quinlan, he was
not in a chronic vegetative state. While not experiencing the sort of life any
of us would find gratifying, Saikewicz could experience human relationships, pleasure and pain, and probably had some sense of himself and of his
bodily integrity. Thus he was a person by the minimal criteria we proposed
for personhood. As a person, he had rights and interests that needed to be
protected when a decision was made regarding his care.
  In all these respects Saikewicz was like Mr. T.S. in Case 17. He was unlike
Mr. T.S., however, in that Mr. T.S. was considered competent to speak for
himself, while Saikewicz was not.    ↓

We saw in Mr. T.S.'s case that most of the arguments commonly raised    **305**
against ceasing aggressive treatment, when he requested the cessation himself, did not stand up to critical scrutiny. Furthermore, as would be implied
by our views on the doctor–patient relationship and informed consent, and

**305**
**cont.** our rejection of the sanctity-of-life view, Mr. T.S. has the <u>right</u> to refuse therapy, even when refusal leads to death. Furthermore, given the certainty of death, the discomfort of treatment, and, presumably, the absence of any unfinished business that Mr. T.S. desperately wants to complete before dying, it could be rationally in his best interests to be allowed to die. In this view the *Saikewicz* decision implied its concurrence. In fact, if a physician persisted in treating Mr. T.S. regardless of the latter's refusal to consent, he
↓ might legally be guilty of the tort of battery ("unconsented touching").

**306** Mr. T.S. would make this decision for himself on highly individualized and subjective grounds, comparing what life would be like for him if different, alternative plans of medical care were to be adopted. As a shorthand phrase for the many subjective factors the rational person would take into account in making such a judgment, we can refer to a decision based on <u>quality of</u>
↓ <u>life.</u>

**307** We need right away to scotch some confusions adhering to quality of life. This phrase has often been used in popular debate to justify allowing patients to die, and has been contrasted with a right to life approach. Some have thus come to fear that quality of life is yet another slippery slope, sounding innocent enough at first but leading inevitably into inhumane abuses. (Picture inmates of a nursing home being lined up and shot by storm troopers because their quality of life is felt to fall below some mini-
↓ mum level.)

**308** To rebut this domino-theory type of objection, we must note first that there is no conflict between the concepts rights to life and quality of life. Mr. T.S. is a person, and if persons have any rights at all, the right to life is one. But Mr. T.S., as a competent adult, may waive any of his rights, including this one, if he judges it in his best interests. Thus Mr. T.S., looking at the quality of life he would experience if kept alive by aggressive treatment, may waive
↓ his right to such treatment.
REVIEW RIGHTS ↑ 77–78

**309** Second, we have noted the sorts of considerations Mr. T.S. might take into account in making his quality-of-life decision. Notably absent are the sorts of reasons particularly open to abuse — reasons regarding his worth to the community, his economic contributions, the cost of his care. By quality of life we have in mind quality according to the perspective of the person himself, and his own value system — not the perspective of the community, the state, or of some value system imposed from outside.

This is why we insisted that the quality-of-life judgment must be highly subjective by its nature. Some, such as Ramsey (1978), see in this subjectivity a great danger for abuses. But consider instead the danger of abuse if we
↓ tried to impose an "objective" value scale on an individual's life.

Considered in this way, the quality-of-life approach is fully consistent with      **310**
the values of respect for individuals and respect for autonomy that we have
been speaking of all along. In fact, we might ask, if Mr. T.S. did <u>not</u> make his
decision on whether to continue treatment based on quality of life as we
have defined it, on what basis <u>could</u> he possibly make such a decision that
would make any sense at all?                                                          ↓

One alternative to quality of life decisions is the position taken by Roman       **311**
Catholic theologians — that one may ethically choose to forego "extraordinary means" of preserving life but is obligated always to continue "ordinary
means." A brief discussion of this alternative may be useful here.                   ↓
    MAY SKIP TO ↓ 319

------------------------------------------------

The modern statement of the Roman Catholic position on ordinary and ex-        **312**
traordinary means appears in the 1957 encyclical "Prolongation of Life" by
Pope Pius XII, which states that in prolonging the patient's life, "one is held
to use only ordinary means — according to circumstances of persons,
places, times, and culture — that is to say, means that do not involve any
grave burden to oneself or another," although one may choose to use
extraordinary means providing no other duties conflict. The ordinary–
extraordinary distinction is not confined to the Catholic position, however;
it has been adopted by the American Medical Association code of ethics,
for example.                                                                         ↓

Why might this approach be preferred to a decision made on the basis of        **313**
quality of life (assuming we are not, by our religious beliefs, committed to
following Papal dictates)? The main reason seems to be a hope that, by focusing on the means used to preserve life, one can ethically allow some
patients to die while still insisting upon the absolute value of life itself.        ↓

But how, then, is the ordinary–extraordinary distinction to be applied in      **314**
practice? Two ways have been demonstrated. One way — often used in
practice by physicians — has been to set up categories of treatment and to
label each treatment (by reference to criteria that are usually unspecified or
idiosyncratic) as ordinary or extraordinary. Thus, respirators and kidney machines might be seen as extraordinary while penicillin and tube feedings
might be ordinary.
    This method seems overly rigid, attempting to reduce major ethical di-
lemmas to a cookbook solution. It seems much more reasonable to hold
that a kidney machine would be extraordinary treatment for an 80-year-old
man in a coma with terminal cancer, and ordinary treatment for a 35-year-
old, otherwise healthy and active mother of three children.                          ↓

**315** The other approach, then, is recommended by sensitive theologians, such as Ashley and O'Rourke (1977). They reject any a priori classification that does not take into account the patient's situation, and quote Pius XII that "all . . . treatments . . . which offer a reasonable hope of benefit for the patient and which can be obtained without excessive expense, pain, or other inconvenience" is ordinary treatment. These theologians refuse to fall into the trap of assuming that because one is talking of types of treatment, then physicians are the appropriate experts to have the final say. The judgment on what means are ordinary or extraordinary is an ethical question, they insist, and must be made with the participation of the patient and
↓ family.

**316** But now consider some of the value terms in this construal of ordinary treatment: "reasonable" hope of "benefit," "excessive," "pain," "inconvenience." By what standards is the patient to judge these, or are we to judge for him if the patient is incompetent? Presumably, these are to be judged by looking subjectively at what life would be like for the patient if the treatment were, or were not, to be used, given that patient's particular values and interests. But that is precisely what we have designated as the quality-of-life approach to these decisions. We might thus conclude that anyone making the ordinary–extraordinary distinction in a sensitive way is really making a quality-of-life decision, but for some reason doesn't want to use
↓ those terms to describe it.

**317** Thus, one might say, "Treatment X would lead to an unacceptable quality of life (e.g., excessive pain with little reasonable hope of benefit), so it is extraordinary for this patient. Since X is extraordinary treatment, we may ethically dispense with it." Or one may say, "We may dispense with treatment X because it would lead to an unacceptable quality of life for this patient." The second way seems much more direct; so in practice we may avoid use of the ordinary–extraordinary distinction altogether.

There is also an advantage to avoiding use of this distinction. By phrasing the question in terms of ordinary or extraordinary means, this mode of reasoning may falsely suggest that what is at issue is a technical, empirical decision about medical treatment, and therefore one best made by the physician alone. We may then forget that a quality-of-life judgment is being
↓ made, which demands input from the patient or his family also.

**318** However, we cannot merely condemn the ordinary–extraordinary distinction. So long as they avoid the simplistic cookbook approach, health professionals deciding terminal-care cases in this manner will often make the
↓ same conclusions we would make using the quality-of-life approach.

- - - - - - - - - - - - - - - - - - - - - - - - - - - - - - - - - - - - - - - - - -

Even if the quality-of-life approach is fully appropriate in the case of Mr. **319**
T.S., however, its use may still be challenged in the case of Joseph Saikewicz. Ramsey (1978), for instance, would support such decisions in the case
of competent individuals but would disallow quality-of-life thinking in deciding on behalf of incompetents, lest we commit the fallacy of treating the
two categories as one. Ramsey points to the Massachusetts court's formulation, "The decision in such cases should be that which would be made by
the incompetent person, if that person were competent, but taking into account the present and future incompetency of the individual as one of the
factors which would necessarily enter into the decision-making process."
This labored rendition, he notes, illustrates the muddle in the court's thinking. According to Ramsey, the only way to be sure of protecting the rights
of incompetent patients is to use life-prolonging therapy unless the patient
would still be dying even if the therapy were given — that is, we are obligated to use all <u>effective</u> life-prolonging therapies on incompetent patients,
where effectiveness is measured by the ability to change an (imminently)
dying person to one who is no longer dying.                                      ↓

But surely Ramsey gives an unsympathetic account of the court's intent. **320**
Elsewhere, the court states,

> One would have to ask whether a majority of people would choose chemotherapy
> if they were told merely that something outside of their previous experience was
> going to be done to them, that this something would cause them pain and discom-
> fort, that they would be removed to strange surroundings and possibly restrained
> for extended periods of time, and that the advantages of this course of action were
> measured by concepts of time and mortality beyond their ability to comprehend.

Clearly the court is here trying to put itself in Saikewicz's shoes as closely as
sensitive imagination will allow — not to treat Saikewicz as if he were something different from what he was.                                               ↓

We might reformulate the court's instructions as to making decisions on **321**
behalf of incompetent patients as follows: Think what the patient would do
if competent — that is, if able to verbalize his own rights and best interests;
but in determining what those best interests would be, remember that the
incompetent person, because of his deficits, may see the world differently
than we do. (Saikewicz would have had much lower ability to tolerate
chemotherapy than would someone who could understand its end; but
he had also a much greater ability to get enjoyment and contentment from
an institutional life that would drive most of us crazy in a week.) Expressed
this way, there is no muddle.
    In the next chapter we will take up questions regarding making ethical
judgments on behalf of others. For now, we should just note that, unless we
have a mechanism for making quality-of-life judgments on behalf of incompetent patients, many such patients may be forced to endure types of treatment which, if competent, they would instantly and vigorously renounce.   ↓

**322** Before leaving *Saikewicz* we should note two points that are rather peripheral to medical ethics and of more interest to medical jurisprudence. First, the court decision explicitly rejected a quality-of-life evaluation of Saikewicz's cause in reaching its decision. But in doing so they appear not to be disagreeing with anything we have said above. Rather, they feared quality of life would be taken in this case to mean that Saikewicz, because retarded, was of less worth than a person of normal IQ. We, of course, have noted that Saikewicz is a person with rights and interests, and our use of quality of life takes this into account. For example, had the chemotherapy been painless and had it had a high probability of returning Saikewicz to the life he had known for an extended period, we would have no business

↓ using <u>our</u> distaste for that sort of life as a reason to withhold therapy.

SCARCE RESOURCES? * 324

**323** Another point from the *Saikewicz* decision has engendered the greatest amount of debate — the insistence that such cases must be brought before the court to be adjudicated, and cannot be decided by physician and family only. (The *Quinlan* decision, on the other hand, said the physician should consult a hospital ethics committee, but seemed confused on what the precise role of the committee should be.) It is still somewhat unclear which sorts of cases the court meant to include. The court apparently intended that some very clear cases, in which the treatment was not altering the terminal illness, could be decided by physicians and family without a court

**325** ↓ hearing. What sorts of cases do you think demand court hearings?

---

**324** * Clearly, in talking about Joseph Saikewicz's right to life-prolonging treatment, we are assuming that we have the resources to provide the treatment, and that, if resources are limited, there is no one else who has a greater right than he does. These assumptions are debatable, and will be the focus of Chapter 12. Our goal here is to get straight on what rights and interests someone like Saikewicz has, and what ethical obligations they entail. We must then later deal with complicating factors such as other, competing obligations from other sources. If we move immediately to the question of how to conserve scarce medical resources, we run the risk of forgetting the

**323** ↑ high value we placed on respect for individual persons.

## CASE 22

Mrs. E.W. is a 64-year-old woman being treated on your medical service for    **325**
acute myelogenous leukemia. Attempts to achieve remission with chemotherapy have failed; the attending hematologist has explained this to the
patient and her husband, and all have decided on a course of palliative
treatment only. Now, as the intern responsible for her care, you are worried
about Mrs. E.W.'s increasing shortness of breath, in addition to her general
wasting and loss of appetite. Unfortunately, x-rays and other tests lead you
to suspect that she probably has developed pulmonary aspergillosis — a
fungal lung infection that can be treated only with a highly toxic antibiotic,
which can make the patient ill, may lead to renal failure, and often fails to
cure the aspergillosis anyway. Discussing the matter with the hematologist,
you conclude that therapy with this antibiotic is inappropriate, given Mrs.
E.W.'s overall situation. You are aware, however, that not treating the infection may hasten her death.

Now the nurse approaches you with the hospital chart. She wants to
know what orders you want regarding Mrs. E.W.'s oxygen, pain medications, diet, and IV fluids.

What orders do you write in the chart?    ↓

---

In ethical debates, terminal-care decisions in cases such as Mrs. E.W.'s are    **326**
commonly labeled "treatment or nontreatment." But, as the nurse's questions remind us, treatment does not stop — at least it should not stop — just
because a particular treatment has been thought to be detrimental to the
patient's quality of life. (This applies to our third category of cases, of
course; "treatment" in the personal, caring sense is no longer possible with
the brain dead or those in chronic vegetative states.)

Having decided to withhold the antibiotic in Case 22, we still must decide whether to give Mrs. E.W. oxygen to relieve her shortness of breath,
intravenous feedings, and pain- and anxiety-relieving drugs. Some of these
treatments might shorten life; some might lengthen life and thus have the
capacity to increase her suffering before the inevitable death occurs. Sound
medical judgment is needed here as well as compassion and ethical insight.    ↓

Ramsey (1970) nicely summarizes our obligations in such cases by his chap-    **327**
ter title, "On (Only) Caring for the Dying." When curing is impossible, the
caring function goes on and indeed assumes supreme importance. Instead
of asking whether to treat or not to treat, we should ask which treatment is
most appropriate for this patient in these circumstances?

Techniques to approach both the physical and the emotional needs of
the terminally ill were the subject of Kubler-Ross's pioneer book, *On Death
and Dying* (1969), and have been developed by Saunders and others active
in the growing hospice movement.    ↓

**328** We must now deal with another problem in terminal-care decision making. Both the *Quinlan* and the *Saikewicz* decisions assumed that had the respective patients been conscious and competent, they could legally have refused life-prolonging therapy, with no court hearing being necessary. This follows from the idea of informed consent that we developed in the last chapter. But does this mean that any reasoning, no matter how idiosyncratic or irrational when viewed from the social perspective, can be used to justify the refusal of life-prolonging therapy?

---

### CASE 23

**329** As the hospital administrator of a New Jersey hospital, you are summoned by the surgeon treating Mrs. Heston, a 22-year-old woman injured in an automobile accident. The physician says that he has diagnosed a ruptured spleen; she will need surgery to correct it, and will certainly die without blood transfusions. The woman, however, is of the Jehovah's Witness faith and adamantly refuses the transfusions, calmly acknowledging that she may die as a result. The surgeon demands that you get a court order to allow him to proceed with treatment immediately.

What do you do?

(Adapted from *John F. Kennedy Memorial Hospital* v. *Heston,* 58 N.J. 576, 279 A. 2nd 670, 1971.)

---

**330** Jehovah's Witnesses interpret several passages from the Bible — Genesis 9:3,4, Leviticus 17:13,14, and Acts 15:28,29 — to mean that blood transfusions represent a contamination of the soul and thus are absolutely prohibited in one who hopes for final salvation. In such cases, does our value for human life outweigh the value of religious freedom and individual autonomy — especially in the case of a 22-year-old woman who would lead a normal life if she allowed the transfusions? Or would this be an unacceptable example of government interference?

**331** In the *Heston* case, the court decided to grant permission for the transfusion, on the grounds that refusal was tantamount to suicide, and suicide was a violation of the law. The woman had the operation and survived.

From an ethical, as opposed to a legal, standpoint, is this a valid argument — that refusal of treatment is wrong because it is suicide? This argument would assume that suicide is always morally wrong. On the other hand, some would argue that suicide is justifiable in some cases, and in the past those committing suicide in support of their religious beliefs have been praised. To try to settle a moral question simply by redefining a word begs the question, and is a commonly seen ethical "error" that should be avoided.

The legal status of Jehovah's Witness cases is somewhat confused, re-    **332**
flecting the genuine ethical dilemma. Three general trends have emerged.

1. In some cases, unlike *Heston,* the courts have allowed a competent adult
   to refuse therapy on religious grounds, even if death results. This is most
   likely to occur if the adult has no minor dependents. (In *Application of
   President and Directors of Georgetown College,* 118 U.S. App. D.C. 80,
   331 F.2nd 1000, 1964, refusal of treatment by a mother was held to be
   child desertion and therefore illegal.)
2. Courts have uniformly ordered transfusions for children of Jehovah's
   Witness parents, on the grounds that one's own religious freedom does
   not allow imposing one's views on another.
3. Occasionally a Jehovah's Witness patient will give mixed messages to
   the court, implying that he may be wavering in his beliefs. For example,
   the patient may say that he opposes transfusions but will submit if the
   court orders them. In such cases the court has often ordered the transfusions.    ↓

Consider this statement: "You are talking about these cases as if the patient    **333**
is clearly competent. But that's ridiculous. Anyone who would want to
commit suicide, which is exactly what refusing blood transfusions on religious grounds amounts to, is showing that they are mentally unbalanced.
So their refusal should be ignored."

Many people who want to commit suicide are subject to depression and
other mental illnesses that can be treated, and it would be a cardinal mistake to miss such a treatable illness and allow death to occur. But, assuming
that one has investigated and found no such illness, the mere desire not to
go on living cannot be used by itself as evidence for incompetence. (As we
saw, the view that it is always irrational to want to die is a disguised version
of the sanctity-of-life view.)    ↓

In many cases, however, the question of competence is not so clear-cut.    ↓ **334**

---

## CASE 24

You are treating an 80-year-old widow suffering from diabetes and ad-    **335**
vanced arteriosclerosis. She has been in a home for the aged for the past 2
years and has just recently been admitted to the hospital with diabetic gan-
grenous infection of one foot. You can solve the present problem by doing
an above-the-ankle amputation. You know, however, that this cannot be a
life-saving procedure; that there is no chance of the lady ever walking
again; and that, as often happens in diabetics, the same infection may recur
above the amputation site later. You might, by doing the operation, give the
woman another 1 or 2 years of life.

**335**
**cont.**     The patient, from an overall view of mental function, is probably mentally incompetent. However, she can communicate desires and is aware of
her body. She tells you that she wants to keep her body intact and is totally
opposed to amputation. She does not specifically state that she wants to
die — which might easily follow within a month or so if the gangrene is not
treated — and you cannot be perfectly certain that she perceives that this is
a consequence of refusing to have the surgery.

You speak with your patient's three sons. Two of them tell you that they
feel that everything should be done to prolong their mother's life, and are
willing to go to court, if necessary, to be appointed her legal guardians for
the specific purpose of consenting to the operation. The third son, himself a
physician, says that he is opposed to the surgery because he fears that the
anesthesia might prove a greater risk to a compromised circulatory and
respiratory system than the infection would.

You are also aware that if you do the surgery and the patient wakes up to
find her foot gone, she might either accept it or go into a depressed state,
which in itself might hasten her demise considerably. However, you are not
willing to predict her emotional state in that hypothetical event.

Do you do the amputation or not? (If you decide to do it, is the consent of
two sons sufficient, or do you have to go to court?)

(Adapted from *Petition of Nemser,* 51 Misc. 2nd 616, 273 N.Y.S. 2nd 624, Sup. Ct.
↓ 1966.)

---

**336**     We had another case previously where a psychiatrist called in as consultant
provided valuable input for the physician's ethical decision. Did you think
of a psychiatric consultant to evaluate this patient's status?

This case presents a number of uncertainties, which probably means that
it is closer to the usual reality than a number of the cases discussed so far.
For one thing, how competent does a person have to be to refuse consent
in a life-and-death situation? One argument might be that since this decision is so important, one must demand a very complete degree of mental
power, and reject any decision where mental competence can even be
called into question. Another would be that since whether one wants to
live or die is so basic a decision, a person should be able to express his true
wishes on that score even if his mind is unable to grapple with more sophisticated problems. In sum, it seems that this woman is making a quality-of-
life judgment that has to be given considerable weight in the final analysis.
↓ Exactly how much weight may be debatable.
    REVIEW PSYCHIATRIC CONSULT ↑ 163–164

**337**     In this case, the court refused to appoint guardians to order the amputation
over the woman's objections, but it did not directly address the issue of
↓ whether she should be allowed to die.

Case 24 points out the importance of the concept of the living will we have    **338**
referred to before. Were we making the decision in this case, we might
wish that the widow, back when she still had full use of her senses, had
written a document stating explicitly whether, under these circumstances,
she would rather die than have a leg amputated; or at least, that she had left
a document directing which of her sons, or which of her other acquaint-
ances, she wanted to speak on her behalf should the need arise.    ↓

Objections to the living will concept arise from the observation that when    **339**
in full health, we often think that we would never want to put up with
heroic medical therapy just to maintain a borderline existence; but, were
we actually to become terminally ill, we would quickly change our minds
and would beg for any chance for a little more life. And, indeed, if a person
who had signed such a document verbally repudiated it at the crucial moment, we would feel obligated to honor the repudiation and not the (supposedly more rational and thoughtful) decision contained in the document. When in doubt, we would always choose to go with life rather than
death.    ↓

On the other hand, if we truly value the autonomy of persons, then some    **340**
sort of living will device would seem to be the best way to assure the continued autonomy of those who are originally competent but have become
incompetent at the time a major decision must be made. (This does not
help us, incidentally, with severely handicapped newborns, who were
never competent to begin with.)

A living will respects autonomy in that the act of executing one is a
totally free choice. If you seriously worry that you might change your mind
when ill, the obvious answer is not to sign a living will.    ↓

However, a document of directions to the physician may not be the best    **341**
manifestation of the living will concept, since cases often will arise that do
not match the situation described in the document. One can never predict
in advance all the possible medical predicaments that may arise. Had our
widow in Case 24 signed the documents shown in Appendixes IV, V, or VII,
we would have no guidance regarding the question of amputation. On the
other hand, appointing an agent whose judgment will be called upon if one
is unable to choose for oneself, as provided for in Bok's proposal in Appendix VI, avoids this problem. Often the agent chosen might be a close friend
and not a relative. The current legal convention of turning to the next of
kin, by contrast, may allow the decision to be made by someone of a different generation and who perhaps knows the patient only slightly.    ↓

## CASE 25

**342**  Mr. and Mrs. H.D. are the parents of four healthy, normal children and one 2-year-old child who was discovered at birth to have the appearance characteristic of Down's syndrome or Trisomy 21; further chromosomal tests confirmed this diagnosis. The child was noted early to have a loud systolic heart murmur and now has progressive symptoms of heart failure. As the H.D.'s family physician, you refer the patient to a cardiologist, who reports that the child has a large ventricular septal defect and possibly other heart defects. Correction would require inserting a catheter into the heart through a vein in order to determine the precise extent of the anomaly, then cardiac surgery. This cardiologist is of the opinion that since the family already has four healthy children, and since this mentally retarded child can never be a functional or significant member of society, it would be a waste of funds and manpower to do either the catheterization or the surgery. In this case the child would most likely be progressively unable to tolerate exercise, be confined to bed, and die from a secondary infection within one year or so.

With the parents still uncertain, you refer to another cardiologist who confirms the first one's diagnosis and prognosis. However, he says that he would go ahead and correct the defect if possible. In fact, referring to the age-old medical dictum of <u>primum non nocere</u> ("first, do no harm") he states categorically that it would be unethical for you to do harm by allowing the child to die.

You again confer with the H.D.s. It is clear that they are thoroughly confused at this point and your injunctions that the decision is theirs to make have been to no avail. They are looking to you for the decision, and any preference you suggest one way or the other, no matter how many reservations you tack on to it, is probably going to sway them.

Incidentally, while the family is not destitute, they cannot afford such complicated surgery and the cost would have to be financed publicly through Michigan Crippled Children's funding.

↓  Do you favor cardiac catheterization or not?

---

**343**  Which of our categories does this case represent? This child is clearly not brain dead. Also, this child seems clearly to be a person — while, as we will see in Chapter 10, the case for fetuses and perhaps even newborn babies is questionable as to whether they have the minimal capacities for personhood, a 2-year-old child clearly has a sense of self, a memory, and pursuits that are his own. Thus, this child falls into the third category and can be assumed to have rights and interests that must be weighed in any decision made about his care. His quality of life both with and without the proposed medical procedures must be weighed. However, like Joseph Saikewicz, this child is incompetent to speak on his own behalf, so others must
↓  choose for him.

A few of the phrases encountered in Case 25 are worth looking into in more **344** detail. First, we find that the H.D.s are the parents of "four normal, healthy children" besides the infant with Down's syndrome. This phrase has a tendency to come up in case descriptions of genetic problems. Why? If all that is needed is data about how many other children the H.D.s must care for, in order to determine how much time and energy they have to take care of a mentally retarded and sickly youngster, it would be sufficient to say "four children." There is at least an implication here that since the H.D.s have other children who are well, they would be less likely to miss the "defective" one if you were to allow him to die. Not only is this not true empirically, but it reduces all the children to the status of pets — they are considered in terms of how good they make the parents feel, not as individuals with needs of their own.    ↓

Next we come to the first cardiologist who states that a mentally retarded **345** child "can never be a functional or significant member of society." Can one make a categorical statement about the entire field of mental retardation? Even within the one disease category of Down's syndrome (or "mongolism") one can find individuals who are of low-educable IQ, who can perform simple tasks and do routine work, and who are capable of giving and receiving love within their family units. We also find severely retarded individuals with multiple physical defects as well. We have no data here about where the H.D. child fits on this spectrum as far as mental competence goes, so it is premature to make judgments about his worth as an individual.

(If you are not familiar with Down's syndrome, and with the range of mental retardation in general, you might wish to read a little in standard genetics or pediatrics texts.)    ↓

Finally we encounter the second cardiologist who tells us what is moral and **346** immoral based on the age-old dictum of <u>primum non nocere</u>. This seems to be invoked as a supposed last word in ethical discussions about as often as the adage about playing God, and so we must subject it also to a similarly close inspection. First, assume that "harm" simply means "hurt." Who is to say that we would be hurting this child more by letting him die than by keeping him alive? Moreover, much of medicine involves doing a small amount of hurting in anticipation of a greater good to follow. Are we to interpret <u>primum non nocere</u> as prohibiting any sort of surgery, or prescribing a drug with a known side effect, or puncturing a vein to draw blood?    ↓

REVIEW PLAYING GOD ↑ 245–246

347 But a philosopher might object that strictly speaking, harm and hurt are not equivalent, and that harm means "wrongful hurt" or "hurt deliberately done without any accompanying benefit." By this definition, <u>primum non nocere</u> is the same as "don't hurt anyone unless the good consequences outweigh the bad consequences," which is really no more than a recommendation to use a consequentialist ethical method, such as we proposed in Chapter 2. But the ethical method is just the beginning, and gives no answers until we fill in the relevant data and values. Thus, <u>primum non nocere</u> can never be accepted by itself as the "last word" in an ethical argument; and, like playing God, we might decide that an agreement to ban it from ethical discussions would be an improvement and a clarification.

---

## CASE 26

348 As her family physician, you accompany Mrs. M.K. to the Regional Perinatal Center when, at the twenty-eighth week of her pregnancy, you discover during an office physical that she is in heart failure and that she has a rhythm disturbance (ventricular tachycardia). It is found that drug therapy is unable to convert her to normal rhythm, and because of the danger of the tachycardia progressing to fatal ventricular fibrillation, the specialist wants to convert the heart with DC current. You ask about the effect of the electric current on the baby's heart rate; no one seems to be sure, although healthy infants have been delivered after the mothers had DC cardioversion earlier in pregnancy.

You explain to Mr. and Mrs. M.K. both the danger to Mrs. M.K. and the potential hazard to the fetus, who, if born at this stage, might have some chance of survival. The parents are agreed that every effort should be made to ensure a viable baby, so an emergency unit for caesarean section is readied as you prepare for the DC cardioversion. At this point, as you are watching the monitor of Mrs. M.K.'s EKG, you see a ventricular fibrillation pattern develop.

1. Would you electrically defibrillate Mrs. M.K.?
2. Would you do an emergency caesarean section to remove the infant before extreme lack of oxygen has compromised its survival chances?

Think about these questions, then proceed with the rest of Case 26.

Before a decision is reached as to defibrillation, Mrs. M.K. spontaneously converts to her previous rhythm of atrial fibrillation. At this point, rather shaken up, you obtain further consultation from an obstetrician. He is of the opinion that a caesarean section could well be fatal for Mrs. M.K. because of the sudden load placed on the circulatory system, whereas a normal delivery, which spreads the stress out over a longer period, should be tolerated well.

Meanwhile, an obstetrical consultant has been administering test doses **348** of oxytocin (a hormone stimulating contraction of the uterus) and finds cont. that even a slight uterine contraction seems to produce significant slowing of heart rate and lowered blood pressure in the fetus. This obstetrician states that the infant will not survive a normal vaginal delivery; however, if the pregnancy is continued one more week, the infant would clearly sur- vive a caesarean section. You now have to decide whether to recommend a caesarean section which will most likely kill the mother, or await sponta- neous onset of normal labor and most likely lose the baby.

What is the most appropriate manner of reaching this decision? What would be your recommendation? ↓

---

In Case 26 you have a situation that is often talked about in medical-ethics **349** discussions, but which in real life seldom occurs in such pure form — a situ- ation in which you have to choose between the lives of two individuals. Quality-of-life criteria are hard to apply to the situation of comparing two individuals; and, in addition, data about either individual is hard to come by here.

Presumably you must talk this over with the parents. If Mrs. M.K. says that she wants to live, who is to speak for the baby's point of view? On the other hand, if Mrs. M.K. says that she wants the baby to live even if it is at the expense of her own life, is she expressing her real feelings or some idea of what society expects of a mother, that is, to be self-sacrificing for her child? And if Mr. M.K. says that he wants the baby, does he have the right to make a martyr of his wife? ↓

Case 26 is based on a real case. In the end, the physicians decided to await **350** spontaneous labor — apparently because it is more of an established medi- cal tradition to sacrifice the infant to save the mother, and also because the quality of life the infant would face growing up without its mother was judged to be low enough to justify this decision. As it turned out, this was another happy-ending case. The second obstetrician's prediction was wrong and the child survived. ↓

**351** In this chapter, we have covered a lot of very controversial ground. (We have also failed to develop a number of controversial issues, which will be taken up in the next chapter and in subsequent chapters on abortion, allocation of scarce resources, and euthanasia.) Some of our main conclusions can be summarized:

1. *The sanctity-of-life view, that life of whatever quality must be preserved at all costs, cannot be defended without committing major inconsistencies.*

2. *In deciding terminal-care issues, the three categories of cases must be clearly distinguished. Talking about withdrawing the respirator from a brain-dead individual to allow him to die, or talking of the right to life of an individual in a chronic vegetative state, betrays a failure to assign these cases to the proper categories.*

3. *The quality-of-life view, as we have defended it, implies an assessment based on the individual's own values and interests. To use quality of life to indicate the individual's worth to society, or his economic contributions, is to misuse the term and to tread on dangerous ethical ground.*

**352** ↓ CH. 7

# Determination 7
## of Ethical Participation

In Chapter 4, we concluded that so long as the contractual model is ac-    **352**
cepted, we must acknowledge the right of the patient to participate in ethical decisions that affect his life. This leaves unanswered two important
questions, which we shall take up now. First, in those cases where the patient is incompetent to assume this responsibility, who ought to participate
for him? Second, are there cases in which others besides the patient have so
much at stake that they have a right to participation also?                    ↓

This question of ethical participation is obviously an important one. Ironi-    **353**
cally, it can at times become too important. In ethics, we must be most
interested in the decision itself — the basis on which it is justified, and the
criteria by which it is to be applied. Being human, we often, without realizing it, search for some means to escape the responsibility of confronting the
decision directly. Too often, a handy way out is to start worrying about who
should decide instead of what decision should be made. If we worry first
about who should decide, we can then get into detailed considerations of
who should be consulted, when, how, in what order, and so on, and conveniently let our minds drift from the basic issues.                             ↓

The worst form of the preoccupation with "who" instead of "what" is the     **354**
"Let's form a committee" syndrome, which has been much too prevalent in
the areas of allocation of scarce resources and of human experimentation.
It is pleasant to discuss how many members the committee should have
and how they should be chosen in order to represent all the different interest groups. You then feel that you have done your duty, while the committee itself is stuck with the dirty work; and if the committee just muddles
through instead of developing ethically sound criteria and procedures, you
can't be blamed.                                                               ↓

However, our discussion of the contractual model and paternalism should    **355**
make it clear why we cannot avoid the "who" question. The unconscious
paternalism that infects nearly all members of the medical profession leads
one easily to forget that there are many decisions that are not the doctor's
to make; and that there are many others for which the doctor must play the
role of information source rather than true participant. While avoiding getting too hung up on the problem, the ethical physician must continually be
asking himself "who?" lest he deprive a patient of his ethical rights.        ↓
REVIEW CONTRACT ↑ 131

**356** Here, however, we might reemphasize some important characteristics of the "what," or the decision that is to be made. First, recall that the decision is made in a state of relative ignorance, which can be reduced but never eliminated. Even if, in principle, we could gather all the data that is relevant to the decision — which we cannot — the time for the decision would be ↓ long past after we had done so.

REVIEW UNCERTAINTY ↑ 38

**357** Second, recall that any ethical judgment is based in part on predictions concerning the future — the consequences of the alternative actions. While these future predictions are only one ingredient in the decision-making process, they are essential; if they are faulty, the decisions will be flawed as ↓ a result.

**358** Because of these two aspects of decision making, we can conclude a third: Some of our decisions will be based on the best information we can collect at the time and will still turn out to be wrong. Looking at the matter in retrospect, we cannot conclude that the decision-making procedure was faulty just because a wrong answer was obtained; and we cannot conclude that the right procedure was chosen just because an ethically valid action was the result. The best we can do is test out the various alternative procedures, pick the one that has the most potential for choosing valid actions, and then work on applying it to the best of our ability, learning from our ↓ mistakes as we go.

**359** The other ingredient needed for ethical decisions, of course, is the set of values against which the consequences are to be weighed. If we could assume that the physician had roughly the same value set as the patient, we might conclude that because the physician will also have the best grasp of the likely consequences, he will be the best person to make decisions on ↓ behalf of the patient when the patient himself cannot choose.

**360** But there are two major arguments against this conclusion. First, it is rarely the case today that the physician can be assumed to share the value outlook of the patient, since most physicians inhabit a different social class and cultural milieu from their patients. (This may be less true for nurses and other health professionals, but is still a factor with them as well.) Second, while the physician may have a superior grasp of the purely medical consequences, he seldom knows the patient's life style well enough to be able to say what those consequences actually mean in terms of the patient's daily life. How many doctors, for example, know in any detail how their patients spend their days, and what their jobs entail? The physician may know that a certain operation carries a 30 percent chance of causing left arm weakness; but does he know what that would mean for the patient's employability ↓ and life style?

Perhaps decades ago, when most doctors lived in the same neighborhoods    **361**
as their patients and commonly made house calls, physicians did share their
patients' values and did understand the consequences of illness from the
patients' viewpoint. In that world, physician paternalism may have been a
rational policy. But in today's world, for better or worse, it makes less sense. ↓

We can now start dealing with the "who" question, since we have just be-    **362**
gun by casting suspicion on the notion that the physician, as a rule, ought
to be the primary decision maker. The next party we might want to consider is society. It is generally agreed that society has a stake in many if not
in all of the kinds of decisions we have been discussing. However, society
(whatever that is) certainly cannot participate directly in any decision making (although, of course, it participates indirectly by shaping our values).
We are then left with sticky questions about which individual or social institution can speak in place of society for any given case.    ↓

Regardless of who speaks for it, it seems clear that society does have a    **363**
stake. All individuals are part of society, and stand to suffer if society as a
whole suffers. Thus we can say in principle that if a person does something
that is not in the best interests of society, he himself, along with everyone
else, will eventually suffer the consequences. However, even if we recognize this to be the case in the long run and in the broader view, we cannot
exclude the possibility, and indeed the probability, that there will be
conflicts of interest in specific instances, where, according to our analysis,
the best interests of the person, both short- and long-range, can best be
served by doing something that seems to be at variance with socially legitimate dictates.    ↓

When faced with such a conflict, our general tendency is to go along with    **364**
the individual, on the grounds that society can stand a small insult better
than the individual can stand a large one. (This assumes a particular sort of
relationship between the individual and society, which we will describe in
more detail in Chapters 17 and 18.) However, we cannot accept this as a
rule. As we saw in the section on professional confidentiality in Chapter 4,
there were several instances which seemed to call for maintaining a
confidence even where society could benefit from disclosure, and other instances where a disclosure seemed ethically valid despite the patient's own
interests. We cannot treat individual–society conflicts as simple cases,
therefore, and must proceed by carefully investigating the consequences of
each particular case. The identification of such an apparent conflict should
serve as a red flag to warn us that we are going to get into trouble if we try
to solve the matter simply by habit or by inclination.    ↓

**365**    How about other individuals in the decision-making process? We have already established the rights of the patient under the doctor–patient contract so long as the patient is competent. In Chapter 4, we recognized several categories of incompetent patients, whom we could exclude from decision making without violation of the contract. These were:

1. *The unconscious patient.*
2. *The conscious but irrational patient.*
3. *The child patient, below the age of understanding.*

For those instances in which we want to consider abortion as possibly being in the best interests of the person-to-be, rather than abortion strictly on behalf of the mother or of society, we can add:

↓ 4. *The unborn patient.*

**366**    For social and legal purposes, we recognize by convention persons who can speak for patients in all these categories — the spouse or next of kin in the first two, the parents in the second two. (These conventions are not absolute. For example, in human experimentation, the question has arisen of whether parents can consent for their children to take part in an experiment from which the children get no therapeutic benefit. There is a growing sentiment that parents "have no right to make martyrs of their children," and that only the court can give consent for the child in such a case. Courts have also ruled that Jehovah's Witness parents cannot refuse blood transfusions for their children.)

Are these customary representatives adequate also from a medical-ethical viewpoint, or must we seek another way of obtaining a proxy deci-
↓ sion?

**367**    We assume that when a patient makes his own decision, he is acting for his own best interests, and in accordance with his own set of values (assuming the decision to be well thought out and rational). When we see an individual make a rational decision to do what we feel to be contrary to his best interests, what we are saying is that if we were in that situation, that decision would be contrary to our own values; so this other person must have some different values from our own in order to make that decision. Our disagreement cannot be taken as evidence that the action was not in his best interests. The only one who can say that is the person himself, if in the future he looks back upon the decision and sees that it was faulty in the
↓ light of new information.

So what we seem to need is an individual who has the same personality and   **368**
set of values as our incompetent patient, but who is conscious, rational,
above the age of comprehension, and born. Clearly this individual is a hypothetical fantasy. How closely can he be approached by the parties alluded to by social convention?                                           ↓

First take the case of parents. While many of the laws and conventions of   **369**
society reinforce the notion that parents know better what is in their child's
best interests than anyone else, psychological investigation of the family
relationship fails to bear this out in any general way. Why do parents have
children? The strictly altruistic, and ethically ideal, motive of wishing to
give life to and assist in the nurture of a unique individual with his own
needs and values, is most often combined with or totally replaced by self-
centered motives. While we may not be so crass as to want children in order to have more hands to work and make money for the family, we might
very well subconsciously want children because of the emotional grat-
ification — reinforcement of a virile or feminine self-image. We might also
subconsciously seek to direct the child's life in order to compensate for
deeply felt unmet needs or ambitions of our own, instead of allowing the
child to choose a course consistent with his or her own individuality.   ↓

Now consider the next of kin, say in a passive euthanasia case such as those   **370**
described in the last chapter. When a person is near death, a very common
emotional reaction of the immediate family is to feel guilty about the real
or imagined things that they should have done for that person and now
cannot do. As a means of assuaging their guilt, they might well become
suddenly oversolicitous and overprotective. Possibly having secretly
wished for the death of their parent or spouse over the past few years, they
are now led by their guilt and emotional confusion to demand that all possible means be used to keep the person alive. None of these motives bear
any relation to the question of whether the person himself would be better
off alive or dead.                                                        ↓

This train of argument may well be bothering you. If these socially desig-   **371**
nated proxies can't make the decision in the patient's best interests, who
can? The doctor? Or do you have to get a court order in every such case?

Clearly the court solution is impractical, and one might well object that
having the doctor decide is paternalistic. After all, medicine is practiced in a
social context, and it would be arrogant of doctors to imagine that they are
independent of the usual social constraints. So if these designated proxies
are good enough for the rest of society, they ought to be good enough for
us, without the need for us to ask them prying questions to determine their
competence. Absolute acceptance of the proxy eliminates the problem —
except in the all-too-frequent cases where the next of kin ducks the responsibility completely and leaves it back on the doctor's shoulders.         ↓

**372** No matter how much we might want to avoid paternalism, though, there is a second danger that we cannot ignore. That is the danger (alluded to previously in Case 12) of forgetting who is the patient.

The doctor can communicate with the parent or spouse, while with the incompetent patient, he either cannot communicate at all or can do so only at an unsatisfactory level. When the doctor does what is satisfying to the parent or spouse, they can verbally express their appreciation, while the patient cannot demonstrate any gratitude. There is, therefore, the obvious danger that the doctor will come (unconsciously, of course) to prize the satisfaction of the parent or spouse above the presumed best interests of the patient. There is no problem where the interests of the two parties do not conflict. But as we just saw, there is no guarantee that that will be the case.

↓ REVIEW CASE 12 ↑ 219

**373** The concern that lies at the base of all this is the duty of the physician to consider the interests of the patient as an individual as his primary concern. As we noted in Chapter 4, there are times when social responsibilities may outweigh this duty. Future physicians will be called upon increasingly to temper their actions with a greater awareness of society's needs and priorities. But if medicine as a profession ever began to put the consideration for the individual in a secondary position, it would cease to be the institution it ↓ is supposed to be now, and would become something completely different.

**374** If the doctor wishes to follow this duty to the individual patient, it would seem that the duty does not cease just because the patient is unable to communicate his own perception of his best interests. The next of kin may in fact be well suited to speak for the patient. Even if this is not the case, the next of kin is a valuable source of data about the patient's values and desires — or, in the case of the unborn patient, about the quality of life that the person-to-be might expect to experience. Therefore the doctor should never hesitate to consult with the next of kin; and, if satisfied with the results, willingly yield to his decision. But the doctor, to protect his patient, must listen critically and be alert for any signs that might indicate a conflict ↓ of interests.

All this discussion has led to the following general conclusions about rights    **375**
of participation:

1. *The primary decision-making responsibility rests with the patient, so long as he is competent.*
2. *When the patient is incompetent, the socially designated next of kin and other close relatives should be allowed to speak for the patient.*
3. *If the physician has reason to doubt whether the above individuals are representing the patient's best interests, he may choose other individuals to involve in the decision process, or as a last resort may make the decision himself; however, he assumes the responsibility for demonstrating that his doubts were based on reasonable evidence.*
4. *Any of the above individuals, except the doctor, may opt out of the decision process by being unable to decide or by refusing to take responsibility. In such a case the doctor must seek the opinion of an alternative patient representative (such as a court order or a more distant relative) if there is time, or make the decision himself if there is not. The doctor cannot opt out of the process.*
5. *As a general rule, all the above individuals must act within the usual constraints imposed by society. Where these constraints have become so rigid as to constitute a conflict between society's best interests and the patient's best interests, the case must be decided individually by careful consideration of the consequences.*    ↓

The criteria just listed, if followed, will help ensure that the doctor has in-    **376**
cluded the appropriate participants in the decision process from the ethical standpoint. He has another task as far as his legal responsibility goes; the list above does not address this other responsibility. In some cases his legal duties can be fulfilled by doing less than what the ethical rules would suggest; an example was Case 12 where the doctor is legally covered by the mother's informed consent, but is ethically required to obtain informed consent (or at least to inform) the minor child as well. In other cases, where the physician is wary of a lawsuit, he may want to do more than the ethical guidelines would require in order to protect himself. An example is a case where the patient is senile and his mental status might be open to question, but appears to the doctor to be competent. If the doctor fears that some relatives might later disagree with the therapy given, he might want to get some other relatives to give consent in addition to obtaining it from the patient. ↓
REVIEW LAW VS ETHICS ↑ 69–71

We can now start to apply these guidelines to cases, and we can start with a    **377**
simple and a common one.    ↓

## CASE 27

**378**    Mrs. L.K., a 74-year-old widow, has been your patient for 15 years. Recently she has been getting confused and forgetful, but she is aware of her surroundings and you would hesitate to label her mentally incompetent.

Some of Mrs. L.K.'s recent symptoms have worried you enough to put her in the hospital and run some tests. You are now quite certain that she has a metastasizing carcinoma and that she probably has 6 months to 1 year to live. You really cannot offer her any realistic hope of palliation by chemotherapy or radiation.

Before discussing your findings with Mrs. L.K., you reveal the bad news to her two children. They are immediate and unanimous in their response: "Don't tell Momma she is going to die. Tell her these are just nonspecific symptoms of old age. Let her live out the rest of her days in peace."

↓   What do you do with the information you have?

---

**379**    While you are always free to disagree, you should have no trouble guessing what we are going to say about this case. Mrs. L.K. is not incompetent. She came to you as a patient and your doctor–patient contract is with her. Her impending death is morally relevant information to her; maybe there is something she very much wants to do before she dies. At any rate, even if you "don't tell Momma" (and if Momma doesn't know already), her children, in their concern about keeping up the concealment, will soon communicate to her nonverbally that something is being kept from her. The likely result will be resentment and concern rather than "peace."

At any rate, all the above suggests that the children have no right of participation in this instance. Since you had no intention of following their advice if they suggested concealment, you might have avoided ill feelings by saying something like, "Your mother has to be told this in the near future. I want your opinions on what would be the best way and the best time
↓   to do this."

**380**    Going back to our discussion of what constitutes a good decision maker, we have, in effect, faulted the children in Case 27 on both counts. By rushing to speak for a person who is still able to think and to communicate, they have raised doubts about the extent to which they actually share the values of that person. And they have shown themselves as having a faulty view of the future by assuming that peace will automatically result from an attempt to conceal important information. It is clear that their own emotional responses have interfered with their ability to be good ethical deci-
↓   sion makers.

In the next case we will look more closely at the problem of consent on     **381**
behalf of a child. While we have thus far loosely referred to this kind of
consent as "proxy" consent, this terminology may create misunderstanding.
A true example of proxy consent is a person who wants to attend a stock-
holders' meeting to vote on an important motion, but cannot be present; so
he appoints a proxy to vote for him as he directs. In this situation, the person has both chosen the proxy himself, and indicated the interests that the
proxy is to uphold. But no child has freely chosen his own parents; and in
what sense does the child have interests that the parents may or may not
protect?                                                                    ↓

---

## CASE 28

Michael W., 4 years old, is currently hospitalized with severe edema caused    **382**
by recurrent idiopathic nephrotic syndrome. This kidney ailment has come
back in the past despite high doses of steroid drugs, and the pediatricians
caring for Michael recommend a trial of another drug — cyclophosphamide
— commonly used in cancer chemotherapy. The major side effects of cyclophosphamide are bone marrow suppression in the short term and probable sterility in the long term, as well as a questionable but hypothesized
increased risk of developing cancer in later life.

On the other hand, if cyclophosphamide is withheld, the only alternative
is continued high doses of steroids, and this treatment is likely to lead to
growth retardation. The pediatricians foresee the risk of severe psychologic
trauma to Michael should either the sterility or the short stature be chosen
for him; but they are leaving the final choice up to Michael's parents.

What treatment should Michael receive?                                       ↓

---

Before looking at the medical decisions, consider the problem from the       **383**
standpoint of the parents. What rules might govern their attempt to choose
the best treatment for Michael?

Blustein (1978) has recommended that two basic ethical guidelines
should govern parental consent. First, parents should try to secure for their
children a maximum of basic "goods" such as food, shelter, financial security, education, and health — that is, things the children will want to have,
no matter what else they may want to have. Athletic prowess may be a
"good" for somebody whose major goal is to star in the Olympics, but not
for someone whose goal is to write poetry. On the other hand, a similar
level of health would be good for both of them. Securing these basic goods
for your children leaves them free to choose their own goals in life, and
does not determine for them the specific goals they should have.           ↓

**384** Second, parents should treat their children as beings in the process of becoming autonomous and should try to develop in their children the capacities for autonomous choice. This guideline is important for older children, but 4-year-old Michael has a very limited capacity for autonomy, and so his parents may properly choose to decide on his behalf on the basis of the first guideline. The question is a difficult one for them, because recovery from his present illness, attaining a normal height, and being able to father children are all very basic goods.

**385** In choosing which goods to seek and which to do without, the parents ought to be guided by Michael's interests. But the interests of a child are not fixed. In particular, a child's interests are in part shaped by his or her environment and training, and parents have a good deal of control over those factors.

Supposing the parents choose steroid therapy, knowing that short stature will result. They may then work to develop whatever talents Michael has that do not depend on physical size, and to give him a sense of self-respect and security so that the taunts and thoughtless behavior of others cause him minimal distress. In this way they would be shaping Michael's interests to conform to his condition — making their choice of drugs, in retrospect, an appropriate one for him. By contrast, were they to continually belittle him for his size and compare him unfavorably to his playmates who are basketball stars, they would be undermining their own choice.

**386** It is part of the nature of being a child to have one's interests in a state of flux, and to have parents who are, in effect, appointed by society to shape those interests to a large degree. This, combined with the child's inability to exercise true autonomy, makes it impossible for proxy consent on a child's behalf to exist in any real sense. The parents are consenting <u>to</u> a procedure to be done on the child, and we hope in doing so they are keeping in mind Blustein's two ethical guidelines. But they are not really consenting <u>for</u> the child.

**387** The fact that parents shape their child's interests does not justify any parental decision. If the W. family in Case 28 decided to use neither drug, because they didn't want to pay the costs, then (assuming the nephrotic syndrome to be a life-threatening condition) the parents could be found guilty of child neglect. It is assumed that all children, whatever their other interests may be, have interests in such basic necessities as life, food, shelter, and freedom from physical harm; and child abuse and neglect statutes recognize these interests as legal rights. But when less basic interests are at stake, the traditional presumption on the side of family privacy prevents the legal system from intervening in most cases.

The second question in this chapter refers to the case of a patient in which     **388**
other individuals have a significant stake in the outcome and, hence, a right
to participation in the decision. The key word here is <u>significant</u>. In some
sense, all of society has some stake in the outcome of any medical decision.
However, since we tend to regard medicine as having primary obligation
toward the patient as an individual, we usually demand proof of a very substantial interest before we will allow another party to overrule the patient's
wishes.                                                                                    ↓

Refer back to Case 23 in Chapter 6, where the court ordered a transfusion     **389**
for a Jehovah's Witness woman on the grounds that failure to transfuse
would be tantamount to the woman's committing suicide. Another court,
in a similar case involving a Jehovah's Witness mother who had a 7-month-
old child, raises the question of whether an individual has the moral right to
desert his family through suicide. We must then ask, if the person has already determined to refuse treatment, whether the physician is morally
justified in either aiding or opposing him.

   To the court, however, the case was clear. The 7-month-old daughter had
such a significant stake in the outcome that she had not only a right of
participation, but also the right to summarily overrule the mother.          ↓

In medical ethics, the one case where the right of another's participation is     **390**
most clearly upheld is sterilization of a married individual. It is almost universally agreed that the consent of the spouse as well as the patient is ethically required.

   Note that an analogous right does not extend to abortion. If the motive
for abortion is the presumed best interest of the fetus, then the father does
not necessarily have a final say. If the motive is the "right of the mother to
have control over her own body," then the father has no right to make a
woman carry and bear his child against her will.                             ↓

Many cases, however, are not so clear-cut. The physician may find a large     **391**
cast of characters surrounding the patient's bed, producing mutually contradictory statements, and each demanding to have his say. The physician
then has to sort out those who have a legitimate stake in the matter from
those who merely have useful data to offer and from those who have no
business being around at all.                                                ↓

## CASE 29

392 A four-day-old infant is being maintained on a respirator because of severe respiratory deficiency. While there has not been time for chromosomal analysis by karyotype, all evidence points to a diagnosis of Trisomy 18, a genetic disorder leading to severe mental retardation, growth failure, and numerous anatomical abnormalities. While there have been scattered reports of patients with this anomaly living to adulthood, 87 percent die within the first year of life.

A conference is being held to decide what to do with the infant.

The chief of pediatrics reports several conversations with the father, who said, "If you cannot guarantee that my child will be normal, I don't want you to do anything for him." The chief says that he sympathizes with the father and has told him, "I promise to do everything in my power to see that your wishes are carried out."

A psychiatrist has also had several conversations with the father, and feels that the father is presently in a state of acute denial; however, if the respirator were turned off at the father's initiative, later guilt feelings could create psychiatric problems for him. He also noted that parents who bring a retarded child home only to have it die later might well suffer guilt over that as well.

The psychiatric social worker contradicts the psychiatrist and states that she feels that the family would be put under extreme stress if the infant were brought home.

At this point, the nurse, who has been most directly responsible for the care of the infant, interrupts with an obvious sense of outrage. She insists that the infant has every right to live and should not be allowed to die by the hand of man. In fact, if necessary, she says she is willing to try to adopt the infant and care for him herself.

A pediatric resident calls attention to a patient of his own, who has a slight respiratory difficulty but cannot be put on a respirator because the Trisomy 18 infant is using the last available machine. Without the respirator, the other infant, who is otherwise healthy, may run a 50 percent risk of some brain damage.

Who should decide? What should the decision be?

(Adapted from R. M. Veatch, "Case 6." In *Case Studies in Medical Ethics.* Cambridge, Mass.: Harvard University Press, 1977.)

---

393 Note on Case 29: Did you notice that no mention was made of the infant's mother anywhere in the case history? When this case was presented to 200 nurses in a New York hospital, fewer than a dozen noticed this point.

For the remainder of the discussion, assume that there was some pressing reason why the mother could not be available to register an opinion. Also, assume that the father's view represents the view of both parents.

The question of who should decide was asked when this case was printed **394**
in *Medical World News* (Sept. 12, 1972). The following is a compilation of
the responses by readers:

46    the child's physician
41    "the parents" or "the father"
 4    the physician plus the parent(s)
 2    the physician plus the psychiatrist
 1    a committee of professionals and laymen
 1    the hospital administrator
 1    a clergyman
 1    a medical panel
 1    the parents plus the health workers
 1    none of the above                                           ↓

These tabulations indicate two things — first, why the idea of making ethi- **395**
cal decisions by majority vote is so poorly received in general; and second,
the fact that very few nurses and psychiatric social workers read *Medical
World News*.

  In determining who should decide in one particular case, how much is
one's opinion swayed by the course of action preferred by the various parties? That is, how likely is one to choose as decision maker one of those
who agrees with one's own choice of solution? If the professional titles of
the various characters had been listed without reference to their views on
the case, how might the tabulated results have been different?           ↓

Another interesting feature of the *Medical World News* poll was the wide **396**
range of weights given to both the chief's promise and the father's wishes.
Responses ranged from the position that a great weight should be put on
them to the position that they should be ignored. On the chief's promise,
comments included: "It's not binding; it's thoughtfully vague." "A promise
is a promise." "It's meaningless reassurance." "It was a mistake." "A rash
promise, and he should admit it."                                        ↓

Anyway, let's forget medical sociology and move on to medical ethics. The **397**
decision to be made here falls under the categories listed in Chapter 6. Do
you think that a child with Trisomy 18 is so severely retarded that he will
never possess the minimal capacities needed to become a person, and so
morally may be considered to be in the same category as Karen Quinlan?
Or do you think that this child is a person, albeit one with a very restricted
quality of life, so that the decision must be made on quality-of-life
grounds?

  If the first answer is correct, the decision can be made strictly on the basis
of what is best for the family unit; the child cannot have interests that matter in a strict sense. If the second answer is correct, the child does have
interests that must be taken into account. What are those interests, in that
case, and who best speaks for them?                                     ↓

REVIEW PERSONHOOD ↑ 280–290

**398**    Notice that in this case there might not be a conflict between the best inter-ests of the child and the emotional needs of the family. If the latter would best be served by allowing the child to die, it might also be that the quality of life to be anticipated by this child is low enough to justify passive eu-thanasia on the basis of the child's own interests.

**399**    There is, however, a clear conflict between the ethical duties assumed by two members of the health-care team — the chief's promise to the father vs. the nurse's perceived obligation to uphold her own sanctity-of-life impera-tive. Recall that at the end of Chapter 4 we pointed out the artificiality of viewing the doctor–patient relationship as simply a one-to-one situation. We noted that in the future, the decisions to be made would increasingly be assumed by a health-care team instead of the solo physician. Here is a working example of the problems that can arise.

**400**    Did the nurse's outburst sound to you to be ridiculous, naive, or irrelevant? If so, note the following passages from the Code of Ethics for nurses:

> The nurse's primary commitment is to the patient's care and safety. She must be alert to take appropriate action regarding any instances of incompetent, unethical, or illegal practice by any member of the health care team, or any action on the part of others that is prejudicial to the patient's best interests.

And:

> The nurse's respect for the worth and dignity of the individual human being extends throughout the entire life cycle, from birth to death . . .

**401**    Even if we must respect the basis for the nurse's ethical concern, however, we are forced to regard her proposed solution as ethically naive. Is she go-ing to adopt and care for every mentally retarded child that is not wanted by the parents?

**402**    The conflict is such that no matter what is done with the infant, either the doctor or the nurse will be placed in a position of having to violate what he or she feels is the proper ethical duty. (Even if a compromise between their two positions were possible, it might not coincide with the best interests of either the infant or the family.) Does this mean that one or the other is being forced to abandon his own moral integrity? If we say that the moral integrity of individual members of the health-care team is of secondary concern as opposed to the needs of the patient, are we in danger of slip-ping into the engineering model of the health-care team–patient relation-ship? And if the moral integrity of the individual health professionals must be protected, how can this be done if the team is still obligated to act in unison?

**403**    We can dodge these difficult questions here simply by having all team members agree that the parents are best qualified to speak on behalf of the

infant, and that the team will abide by the parents' decision. The questions    **403**
do not disappear, however; we can easily imagine a similar case in which    cont.
the parents are either unable or unwilling to make any decision on their
own.

↓

We must also consider, however, that there will be cases in which the par-    **404**
ents' decision seems so far out of line with the realities of the case that we
would be willing to try to overturn it — even to the extent of going to court
to get a guardian appointed for the child.

↓

As Shaw (1973) and others have pointed out, there is a spectrum of cases    **405**
involving life-prolonging treatment in children, according to how ill or impaired the child is and will be if life is preserved. At one extreme of this
spectrum are children with severe birth defects such as anencephaly (absence of any higher brain function) and Trisomy 18. By our definition of
severe birth defects in Chapter 6, the more severely afflicted children at this
extreme will never be persons. In such cases we would be willing to try to
persuade the parents not to request any life-prolonging treatment. In the
future, if scarcity of medical resources becomes a priority consideration, we
might follow Robertson's recommendation (1975) and refuse treatment for
these classes of infants on that basis.

↓

At the other extreme are children who have the capacity for full mental    **406**
development and a good chance for recovery, but whose parents refuse
treatment on religious grounds, or for other reasons regarded as idiosyncratic in our society. In one widely publicized case in Massachusetts in
1978, the court ordered continuation of standard chemotherapy for a
4-year-old boy with childhood leukemia in remission. The physicians felt
he had a chance for complete cure if he remained on chemotherapy; the
parents wanted to reject standard medical treatment in favor of the unap-
proved drug, Laetrile, and nutritional therapy alone.

↓

Another case receiving wide publicity involved a baby born with Down's    **407**
syndrome (mongolism) and duodenal atresia. The parents refused surgery
for the bowel condition and the infant, as a result, starved to death. As we
noted in Case 25, Down's syndrome is associated with a wide range of mental capacity, and we cannot predict in advance how severely retarded a particular child will be. Thus, as Gustafson (1973) argued, the physicians would
have been justified in seeking a court order to overrule the parents in this
case.

COURTS VS. PARENTS * 408    ↓ **409**

---

* An emotional issue is often raised when courts order treatment for a se-    **408**
verely deformed infant: "If the court orders the treatment, why doesn't the
judge have the responsibility to raise the child afterward?" It may seem unfair for the court to impose such a burden on a family; but, if children have

**408**
**cont.** rights, and we are to take rights seriously, we must be willing to accept this outcome. The family may give up the child for adoption, or the child may have to be placed in a public institution; but for a child who is not totally a ↓ "vegetable," such a life may still be better than no life at all.

**409** In between these two extreme sides of the spectrum, however, exists a gray zone of difficult cases — possibly involving the greatest number of cases. Such children will be markedly retarded or physically handicapped, but have some capacity for a decent quality of life. Their chance to develop such a capacity, however, may in large part depend on the ability of their families to give them the special care and emotional support they require; and families differ dramatically in their ability to provide such care. A retarded child who would be a great joy for one family unit might completely destroy another.

In this gray zone, where the interests of the child-patient are so closely bound with those of the family, it is least likely that a health professional who is not actually a part of the family will be able to decide unilaterally what is best. For gray-zone cases, Duff's (1979) policy of allowing maximal parental autonomy in reaching the decision seems the wisest choice. The health professionals must then undertake the commitment to support the ↓ parents, no matter what choice is made.

**410** The following cases are included for discussion of this spectrum of cases involving infants and children; you will want to decide where along the spectrum these cases fall. Case 30 raises the question of parental refusal to be involved in decision making and to care for the child; Case 31 illustrates a problem in which the infant's life or death is not at issue, but in which the ↓ later health of the infant is at stake.

## CASE 30

**411** Infant Jones is doing poorly in the neonatal intensive-care unit. Though she was born very prematurely and weighed under 2 pounds, she was without physical defects; but she has developed respiratory distress syndrome over the past 2 days and now will require a respirator to survive. This problem will require prolonged treatment in the intensive-care unit, and other, secondary problems are likely to develop; but if Infant Jones survives all this, she is likely to be a normal or near normal child. (It is also possible she might develop permanent lung scarring and never be able to survive without the respirator.)

The mother, unmarried and 14 years old, did not seek medical attention **411** during her pregnancy and has not been in to visit the baby since birth. The cont. hospital bill will be paid by Medicaid and is expected to be a minimum of $20,000. One house officer is opposed to a respirator for this "preemie," saying, "If she survives she'll be handicapped anyway, socially if not physically." Another physician argues, "If we don't treat aggressively and she does survive anyway, her handicap will be all the more severe."

Consider the following questions:

1. What rights does the mother have in determining care for this infant? Should she have a role in the decision making?
2. To what extent ought the baby's "social handicap" — having a neglectful, unwed, teenage mother — be used as a criterion as to whether she should live or not?
3. Would your decision be different if the mother were married and actively concerned about the child? Or if the mother had declared her intention to place the baby for adoption?
4. If the factors in the above question influence your decision, can you defend your consideration of these factors in terms of the <u>child's own</u> interests? If not, what morally compelling reasons are there to include these considerations?

(Case report [unpublished] courtesy of Sharon L. Hostler, M.D.)   ↓

---

## CASE 31

Suzie is the first child born to college student parents. She was born with a **412** significant clubfoot deformity of her right leg. You are the orthopedic specialist who is seeing her at 3 months of age; the distraught parents, originally frantic that "everything should be done to make her whole again," are now clearly joyful over her otherwise good growth and health.

You explain two possible courses of action. Suzie could undergo surgery repeatedly over 10 to 21 years, requiring hospitalization and prolonged casting each time; and the <u>best</u> possible result would still leave her with some impaired function and physical deformity. Alternatively, you could do below-the-knee amputation at 1 year of age, fitting Suzie with an artificial leg in time for her to have normal development of toddling and walking. No further surgery would be involved, and her ability to function with the leg would be excellent, but she would have the prosthetic limb.

You are somewhat chagrined when the parents express dismay over the very idea of amputation for their beautiful little girl and again ask plaintively what can be done "to make her whole again."

**412**
cont.

Consider the following questions:

1. Does a decision have to be made now? Do you think the parents will respond more appropriately if you delay the decision for a few weeks?
2. What value judgments underlie the parents' and the physician's position?
3. Are the parents currently protecting Suzie's best interests? If not, what basis do you have for questioning their judgment? (Recall the fact that you would choose differently for your own child is not, in itself, grounds to dismiss the choice of these parents, unless we are to do away altogether with parental autonomy.)
4. If the impasse persists between the orthopedist and Suzie's parents, what should be done next?

↓ (Case report [unpublished] courtesy of Sharon L. Hostler, M.D.)

---

**413** We have considered the case in which the competent patient is called upon to share some of the decision-making responsibility because another individual has a significant interest in the outcome. There is another side to the coin. Are there some cases in which a competent patient may be deprived of part or all of his usual decision-making responsibility, because of some peculiar features of the case itself? One type of case that has been proposed as an example is the sticky situation presented by a possible self-fulfilling prophecy. Case 32 illustrates a way in which this problem might
↓ arise.

---

## CASE 32

**414** Mrs. A.B., a 41-year-old mother of two, has become pregnant again. Because at her age there is a higher risk of her having a child with Down's syndrome, you, as her physician, have suggested amniocentesis — withdrawal of an amniotic fluid sample from around the fetus to obtain a few fetal cells, which can then be analyzed to see if they contain the normal 46 chromosomes, or the 47 that would be indicative of Down's syndrome or another genetic anomaly.

Mrs. A.B., a high school teacher, wants to have this child, but she has indicated to you that she wants to consider an abortion if the child has Down's syndrome. There is not much time to decide since the pregnancy is in the eighteenth week before the results come back.

The report of the karyotyping shows that the fetus has no extra chromosome of the G group and thus is free of Down's syndrome. But the fetus is not normal. Instead of the usual XX chromosomes of the female or XY of the male, the fetus' sex chromosomes are of the XYY composition.

You are familiar with the research on the XYY genotype and know that it is inconclusive. Studies of the inmates of institutions for those who have

committed violent and antisocial acts indicate that persons with the XYY    **414**
genotype are found among these groups more frequently than would be    cont.
expected by chance — giving rise to theories that XYY individuals are more
prone to violent or antisocial behavior. At the same time it has been shown
that there are many XYY individuals who lead perfectly normal lives with no
indications of sociopathology. There are no physical or mental abnormalities of significance that have been directly tied to the XYY genotype.

What do you tell Mrs. A.B. about the results of the karyotype? Is she entitled to participate in the decision of whether to abort or not?

(Adapted from R. M. Veatch, "Case 41." In *Case Studies in Medical Ethics.* Cambridge, Mass.: Harvard University Press, 1977.)                              ↓

---

This case is what Robert Veatch calls a "condition of doubt" situation — the    **415**
doctor "has to decide not only which facts to communicate, but what the
facts actually are. . . . Some day there may be more evidence, but the decision is demanded today." This condition of doubt has a direct bearing on
the ethical decision.                                                       ↓

A person could argue against telling Mrs. A.B. about the extra Y chromo-    **416**
some as follows: From a technical view, your doctor–patient contract with
Mrs. A.B. was to tell her whether or not the child will have Down's syndrome, so you are not obligated to pass on any further information you
learn coincidentally. Furthermore, if you consider Mrs. A.B. as your patient,
you would be doing harm by generating a considerable amount of anxiety
about the future for her child — an anxiety for which you do not have any
hard data to ease her mind.                                                 ↓

If you broaden your view of the patient to include the entire family struc-    **417**
ture, the case is even more compelling. Suppose you tell Mrs. A.B. and she
elects to have the baby. From then on, she will be unable to avoid thinking
of the child's possible fate, and will always be searching every aspect of the
child's behavior, looking for the slightest clue toward any personality disorder. She might be led to go overboard either as a strict disciplinarian or in
showering affection on the child, in hopes of preventing later problems. Is
there any situation more likely to produce a child with a behavior disorder,
even if no tendency toward such disorder existed at the start? This is the
problem of the self-fulfilling prophecy, where the attempts to avoid something end up producing it.

Or suppose you tell Mrs. A.B. and she then decides to abort. The chances
are good, based on present statistics, that you will be aborting a "normal"
fetus with no sociopathic tendencies.

(To be fair, we have to add that if you do not tell Mrs. A.B., she might still
learn of the XYY later. Then her anxiety at that time will be further com-
pounded by her knowledge of your concealment.)                             ↓

**418**  Before considering the arguments on the other side, note what the self-fulfilling prophecy argument boils down to: that Mrs. A.B. has no right of participation because this right would demand information in order to be exercised; and the possession of this information would mean that Mrs. A.B., in spite of herself, would be very likely to produce the undesirable outcome through her own actions. This might sound like a rather extreme position. However, it serves to remind us that the participants in these sorts of ethical decisions are not spectators on the sidelines. They are active parties in what will follow the decision, and they are changed as persons by the act of participating in the decision. (Call this the Heisenberg uncertainty principle of medical ethics if you will.) The change brought about by the decision process itself ought to be taken into consideration when figuring the consequences of an ethical action.

**419**  Now the arguments in favor of telling. If we go back to our basic premise we have to ask one question: Is the decision to abort or not to abort an ethically relevant one for Mrs. A.B., and is the information about the XYY genotype a piece of information that could figure significantly in the decision? We pretty much have to answer "yes" on both counts. It then follows that we are obligated to tell Mrs. A.B. and, within the confines of our own ignorance, give her what assistance we can in helping her to understand the implications and in helping her to deal with her natural anxiety.

Note that, since the information is by its very nature confusing, Mrs. A.B.'s decision to abort or not may very easily be swayed by the way we present the information or even by our tone of voice. This is one situation in which whether we say "the glass is half empty" or "the glass is half full" may make a very significant difference. How would you handle this problem?

**420**  It is also possible to approach Mrs. A.B.'s case from a different angle: consideration of social values over consideration for the individual. Given especially that Mrs. A.B. already has two children and would have been willing to abort this fetus anyway had it had Down's syndrome, we might argue that society already has enough problems without taking the chance, however small, of another murderer or rapist being born. This argument might lead us to say to Mrs. A.B., "The tests show that the chromosomes of the child are abnormal" (or even, "The tests show that the child has an extra chromosome"), knowing full well that she will then elect to abort. In this way you fulfill your social obligation without "really" lying to your patient. How do you feel about this line of reasoning?

This is beginning to get a bit confusing, so perhaps it would be well to go **421** back to the ethical decision-making method and state more clearly what moves we have been making. (This is analogous to the old rule on how to run laboratory equipment: "When all else fails, read the directions.") Back in Chapters 4 and 5, we evolved an ethical rule that could be stated as: "The doctor ought to inform the patient and allow the patient to make the decision in any matter that is of ethical significance to the patient, unless the patient himself has given indication that he does not wish to be told." (For shorthand, we'll state this rule as, "Inform . . ."     ↓

MAY SKIP TO CH. 8 ↓ 436

--------------------------------------------------

A consequence of this ethical rule is that Mrs. A.B. ought to be told about **422** the XYY karyotype. But it's telling Mrs. A.B. that seems to bother us. If in fact this consequence is contrary to some important value that we hold, this would be an indication that the rule is invalid as stated and is in need of revision. But so far we just know we are bothered; we have not determined what value has been challenged and in what way.     ↓

Two proposals have been put forward. One is the condition-of-doubt label. **423** This assumes that we place a low value on confusion and anxiety, and hence are unwilling to produce such feelings in a patient. We have refined this view to hold that anxiety is unavoidable when the facts are unpleasant, and that the patient's right as decision maker overrules the value judgment in a normal case. However, in a case in which the facts are confused (thereby rendering the patient less capable of exercising his right effectively), the negative value placed on anxiety assumes primary importance. Therefore, we ought to change the rule to, "Inform . . . unless there is a significant amount of inherent doubt in the data, and the patient is likely to suffer considerable anxiety as a result."     ↓

The other proposal is that of the self-fulfilling prophecy, which holds that **424** by telling the mother, we will have two bad consequences: (1) the raising of an emotionally disturbed child, and (2) the misery of the mother who is producing the emotionally disturbed child but cannot help herself (in both cases assuming that she did not elect abortion; if she did, that would be a different bad consequence). The values in play here are obvious; few of us positively value misery and messed-up kids. This proposal, then, would have us modify the rule to: "Inform . . . unless doing so would set into motion a situation, outside the conscious control of the patient, which would produce misery for the patient or for another participant."     ↓

Before we decide to make one (or both) of these modifications of our rule, **425** we have to decide whether it really is a bad thing to tell Mrs. A.B. the whole truth. If it is, then we still have to determine the consequences of adopting either of the alternative rules. If, however, it is not, then we can maintain our original rule.     ↓

**426**    We have already listed many of the good and bad consequences of telling Mrs. A.B. everything. The problem is complicated by two uncertainties: whether Mrs. A.B. will get an abortion, and whether XYY individuals do really have a genetic tendency toward violent behavior.

We can construct a table to consider all these possibilities and classify the consequences accordingly. For this we will assume (1) that in telling you do as much as possible to avoid swaying Mrs. A.B. toward either choice; and (2) that if you do not tell Mrs. A.B. there is a 100 percent chance that she will go ahead and have the child. We will also assume for the moment that not telling Mrs. A.B., and instead making up something to tell her that will persuade her to have an abortion, is farther than we are prepared
↓ to go. These assumptions result in Table 2.

**427**    We have set up a matrix like the example of Bayesian decision-theory in Chapter 2; in theory, we can now plug in numerical values for the probabilities and desirabilities of each of the squares, and obtain a preference ranking. However, we have so little data on which to base the numerical values that the result of this procedure would probably be what the computer programmers call "garbage in, garbage out"; we would be using numbers to cover up our ignorance. Therefore, let's keep the matrix but instead try a
↓ qualitative approach.
        REVIEW BAYESIAN THEORY ↑ 102–113

**428**    We can start by making some assumptions. First, presumably you are prepared to tell a lie if it can be shown that this will benefit Mrs. A.B. (If you accept the rule, "Never tell a lie," and admit no exceptions, you are not following our ethical method.) So whether you tell a lie or the truth must be of lesser consequence to you than the outcome for Mrs. A.B.; we can
↓ assign a zero value to your truth-telling, as being ethically neutral.

**429**    Next, note that we cannot predict in advance whether Mrs. A.B. will place a high value or a low value on her right of participation, until she is actually put on the spot. We also cannot know whether she is the sort who handles anxiety in stride or who tends to fly off the handle. However, it would be very inconsistent with everything we have said up to this point about the doctor–patient contract if we did not place a higher positive value on participation than the negative value on anxiety. After all, the anxiety can be lessened by judicious handling and emotional support by the physician; deprivation of rights cannot be so easily made up. So we can assign a moral value of "+ +" to granting the right, and "− −" to withholding it without consent, while we assign a value of "−" to creating anxiety by telling Mrs.
↓ A.B. and "+" to preventing anxiety by not telling.

**Table 2**

|  | Causal Connection Between XYY and Sociopathic Behavior | No Causal Connection Between XYY and Sociopathic Behavior |
|---|---|---|
| Tell Mrs. A.B. and she decides to have abortion | 1. You told the truth. Mrs. A.B. got her right to participate. Mrs. A.B. is made anxious. Society is spared possibility of birth of sociopath. Mrs. A.B. has no baby. | 4. You told the truth. Mrs. A.B. was given right to participate. She is made anxious. She has no baby. Society has one less mouth to feed, but also loses one "normal" productive member. |
| Tell Mrs. A.B. and she decides not to abort | 2. You told the truth. Mrs. A.B. was given right to participate. She is made anxious. She has a baby which may be normal or sociopathic, with social consequences as above. | 5. You told the truth. Mrs. A.B. was given right to participate. She is made anxious. She has "normal" baby which she then may make abnormal by self-fulfilling prophecy mechanism. |
| Don't tell Mrs. A.B. | 3. You told a lie. Mrs. A.B. was denied her right to participate. She is not made anxious. She has her child, with same risks and consequences as above. | 6. You told a lie. Mrs. A.B. was denied her right of participation. She is not made anxious. She has "normal" baby and presumably will raise it normally. |

Note: In Squares 1, 2, and 3 the risk of the individual being a sociopath is related to how many XYY individuals develop that way (we know not all of them do) and how amenable the trait is to environmental correction. In Squares 4, 5, and 6 it must be remembered that the "normal" baby might still develop into a sociopath, by mechanisms other than the XYY genotype. The risk of this would be equal to the percentage of sociopaths in a randomly selected population.

We can now assign arbitrary values to the other consequences. From the mother's view, call the consequence of aborting the child a $--$, while having the baby is $++$. If society is spared the risk of the birth of a sociopath, we cannot call this more than $+$ because one individual more or less cannot matter that much. The nonbirth of a normal individual might otherwise be seen as $-$, but since we are having a population problem, we might want to call that 0 instead. If the baby is born and there is a risk of it becoming a sociopath, we know that the risk is less than 100 percent, and it is most probably significantly less than 50 percent. Under those circumstances the bad effects on society cannot be more than $-$, while for the mother, this would be a severe personal tragedy, so for her it would be $--$. Because we have argued that the self-fulfilling prophecy is preventable, given that the mother is warned and that you or another doctor give good follow-up care, we can label this consequence a $-$, instead of making it worse. If we know the mother will raise the child normally, call this $+$.  ↓

**430**

**Table 3**

| | Causal Connection Between XYY and Sociopathic Behavior | | No Causal Connection Between XYY and Sociopathic Behavior | | Sum |
|---|---|---|---|---|---|
| Tell Mrs. A.B. and she decides to have abortion | 0<br>+ +<br>−<br>+<br>− − | [0] | 0<br>+ +<br>−<br>− −<br>0 | [−] | − |
| Tell Mrs. A.B. and she decides not to have abortion | 0<br>+ +<br>−<br>+ +<br>−<br>− − | [0] | 0<br>+ +<br>−<br>+ +<br>− | [+ +] | + + |
| Don't tell Mrs. A.B. | 0<br>− −<br>+<br>+ +<br>−<br>− − | [− −] | 0<br>− −<br>+<br>+ +<br>+ | [+ +] | 0 |

**431**    Table 3 shows all these weighted-desirability values inserted into the appropriate squares in the table. Also in each square is the sum of the consequences in that square; the sum for each row of squares is shown in the last
↓   column.

**432**    Table 3 gives us the following preference ranking:

    Tell followed by no abortion
    Don't tell
    Tell followed by abortion

However, assuming that we try to tell Mrs. A.B. in a way least likely to sway her opinion one way or the other, we cannot know in advance which course of action she will choose. Therefore, we have to add the desirabilities for the two "tell" rows together. This gives us the new preference ranking:

    Tell
↓   Don't tell

We conclude, based on the values that we have placed on the various   **433**
items, that we are better off telling Mrs. A.B. Therefore, our original rule can
stand up; we need take into account neither the condition-of-doubt objection nor the self-fulfilling-prophecy objection in the rule itself (although
we want to use both as warnings to ourselves to remind us of our responsibility).

If you disagree with our conclusion, you can go back and change some of
the value assignments to make the sums come out in your favor. One way
to do this is to put less weight on the right of participation; but, as we
noted, this can be seen as the equivalent of putting a low-priority judgment
on the entire doctor–patient contract as we described it in Chapter 4.
Therefore, you should be willing to accept the various consequences, including paternalism, possible increase in patient mistrust, and all the others
mentioned in that chapter.                                                ↓

We have devoted this much space to Case 32 not because it had a great deal   **434**
to do with the topic of this chapter, but more because it gave us a good
chance to illustrate some of the ethical decision-making methods we described in Chapter 2. However, consideration of this case has shown us that
we want to be very careful before we decide that a competent patient is to
be deprived of participation in a medical decision that has important ethical implications for him or her. Some significant reasons, such as condition
of doubt and the self-fulfilling prophecy, can be given for denying participation, but in the final analysis these can generally be shown to be of insufficient weight to overturn the doctor–patient contract.                ↓

With this, then, we can conclude our discussion of ethical participation.   **435**
However, this problem will arise frequently in other cases as we go on to
discuss specific issues in medical ethics. As we go on to these, you might
want to refer back to the guidelines we listed earlier in this chapter, to see
how they apply to the new cases.

CH. 8 ↓ 436

# Specific Issues 8 in Medical Ethics

We have now completed discussions of the four fundamentals of medical ethics that we proposed back in Chapter 3. Armed with this much practice and with the ethical decision method from Chapter 2, you should be able to deal with any medical-ethical decision. As we have seen, that does not mean coming up with an infallibly "right" answer; it means coming up with a persuasive and rationally justifiable answer given the limited data available.

436

↓

Still, we have good reasons not to stop here, but, instead, to go on to deal with specific, troublesome issues. There are three clear reasons to do so.

First, ethical decision making, like other skills, improves with practice. The more cases you have worked through, and the greater the variety of cases, the better equipped you will be to deal with a new dilemma.

437

↓

Second, even though values cannot come directly from facts by simple deduction, certain kinds of facts illuminate value judgments. (We saw, for instance, how knowing the statistics on what both doctors and patients think of telling the true diagnosis to a cancer victim helped to highlight the ethical argument.) These facts are best learned in the context of the particular issue. If you don't know what different techniques are used for behavior control, you will have trouble reaching valid ethical conclusions.

438

↓

Third, no ethical decision-making scheme or set of ethical principles is perfect. As we try out our method on these new issues, we may find cases where it fails to work as well as it should — even more important, these failures may suggest new modifications we can make in the method. We have noted that developing a coherent ethical framework requires always going back and forth between general theories and specific cases.

439

↓

Each of the eight specific issue areas we will take up in subsequent chapters can be broken down in terms of some of the fundamentals of medical ethics, as we have been reviewing them in the last four chapters. We may add an additional feature by expanding our notion of quality of life to fit other situations besides terminal care. Where life or death is at stake, we of course want to be very conservative about what we call an unacceptably low quality of life. But for other purposes, we can use the concept of quality of life in a looser, relative sense. For instance, if a patient's quality of life under treatment A is better than under B, we ought to choose A. (We still need to specify what our criteria are for making the quality-of-life judgment, and to show that the criteria reflect that person's own views, not the views of someone else.)

440

↓

**441** *Behavior Control.* The problem of behavior control cuts across all four areas that we have discussed. Perhaps most basic is the question: To what extent is our concept of our quality of life dependent upon freedom from obvious restrictions on our ability to make voluntary and self-aware decisions; and in what way would our self-perceived quality of life be altered if we no longer had control over our own actions or thoughts? Also, our whole understanding of the doctor–patient contract and of the meaning of informed consent must be modified when we take into account the fact that behavior-control techniques are already being used in medicine.
↓ BEGINS ON ↓ 451

**442** *Control of Reproduction.* This has always been an emotionally charged issue, since we are making very significant quality-of-life decisions — both with regard to a person-to-be when we decide whether or not he is to be conceived, and with regard to the parent when we decide whether or not she shall bear a child. Also, this is another area where rights of participation have tended to be unclear: Does society, either in its own right or as spokesman for the interests of the unborn, have anything to say, and if so, how is it to be heard?
↓ BEGINS ON ↓ 536

**443** *Research on Human Subjects.* This has also been an emotional issue for medical researchers, looking back as they do upon the vast progress made by medical science in this century. This has not prevented thoughtful investigators from raising tough questions — how is the doctor–patient relationship altered if the doctor is also an experimenter? And how can informed consent be meaningfully applied where there is so much uncertainty involved, as when the investigator himself does not know whether patient X is getting the experimental drug or a placebo? And can there ever be voluntary informed consent in the case of minors or prisoners, both of which groups now make up significant pools of experimental subjects?
↓ BEGINS ON ↓ 622

**444** *Allocation of Scarce Resources.* We have already shown that allocation of scarce resources is, to some degree, an element of any ethical decision. The most significant resource-allocation problems, however, have to do with scarce social resources such as money, technically sophisticated equipment, and trained personnel. Since society has a stake, what is its right of participation in these medical decisions — and what is the mode by which it is to be represented, since "society" is only an abstraction? How does the doctor–patient relationship change as the doctor is brought increasingly under resource-allocation constraints?
↓ BEGINS ON ↓ 713

*Active and Passive Euthanasia.* These issues pick up on issues raised in    **445**
Chapter 6. If we can decide, based on personhood or on quality-of-life
grounds, that some patients are better off dead, how far are we willing to go
in implementing this decision? What would informed consent require in
such a case? And is there any moral difference between allowing a patient
to die (passive euthanasia) and actively killing a patient (active euthanasia)?    ↓

BEGINS ON ↓ 783

*Mass Screening Programs.* Another area in which social interests have    **446**
threatened to come into conflict with individual freedoms is the area of
mass screening programs, such as genetic screening to locate carriers of
sickle-cell genes in the black community. What sort of voluntary consent is
to be required for such programs? Has this sort of program turned society or
some agent of society into the "doctor" in the doctor–patient relationship
– and if so, how has the contract been rewritten as a result? How much
governmental knowledge of our medical status as individuals is consistent
with our ideas of quality of life?    ↓

BEGINS ON ↓ 854

*Genetic Engineering.* Medical people have always made value judgments    **447**
about which hereditary traits are good and which are bad, but until the
development of recent technology, there was no way to attempt to implement any of these judgments. The issue of genetic engineering is analogous
to euthanasia, in that the question arises of how far we will allow medical
scientists to put their quality-of-life judgments into actual practice. Only
here, the judgment affects not just one individual, but entire generations of
unborn individuals – possibly the entire species. We saw how difficult it
was to decide what constituted informed consent on behalf of a fetus in
utero. Who can give informed consent on behalf of posterity?    ↓

BEGINS ON ↓ 908

*The Social Responsibility of the Health Professions.* Among the social con-    **448**
straints that have the capacity to put significant strain upon the contractual
model of the doctor–patient relationship are certain aspects of the social
responsibility of the health professions. While the physician may (wrongly)
feel that he is not responsible for what society as a whole or what the government tells him he has to do, he is less able to cop out when the offending party is his own profession. If certain aspects of the medical profession
itself, present or future, constitute part of the problem, at what point is the
doctor ethically justified in refusing to participate? We stated that the doctor is released from his contract with the patient if following the patient's
requests would entail an act that the doctor finds morally abhorrent. What
is the nature of the individual practitioner's contract with his profession?    ↓

BEGINS ON ↓ 973

**449**    After dealing with these eight issues, we will conclude with two chapters on important basic considerations. The first involves the definitions of health and disease, and the role value judgments play in these basic medical concepts. If we can show that our definitions of health and disease are based as much on values as on empirical knowledge, we will gain increased respect for the notion that medicine is an inherently value-laden enterprise — and we will have a strong rebuttal for those who argue that value matters
↓  are merely peripheral to medicine.

**450**    Second, we have to face the fact that we have been referring all along to one's values, without showing how values are grounded and evaluated — why it is that the values of Mahatma Gandhi are better than those of Attila the Hun. We have rejected the views that empirical statements are the same as ethical statements, and that we can derive values from facts by a simple deductive process. But in rejecting those positions (which philosophers call the "naturalistic fallacy") we may still hold that there are less precise connections between facts and values, and that certain facts about the world lend increased plausibility to some values — that is, that the empirical world in some way can act as a check on our value judgments, even if facts can't be substituted for values directly. We will take up this complex but important topic in the last chapter.

**451** ↓ CH. 9

# Behavior Control 9

Presumably all of us, to some degree or other, control our own behavior.   **451**
Behavior control becomes a matter of medical ethics either when the
means utilized to control one's own behavior fall into the category we term
"artificial," or when one person undertakes to control the behavior of another. These may be accomplished by a number of techniques.   ↓

Possibly the oldest form of behavior modification by artificial means is the   **452**
use of psychoactive drugs. (Alcohol may have been the oldest such sub-
stance in general use — of course the number of compounds available for
such purposes has increased considerably in recent years.) This category
must include commonly abused street drugs, drugs used in psychiatry such
as tranquilizers and antidepressants, and substances such as alcohol, coffee,
and tea, which in the public mind are usually not classified as drugs at all.   ↓

A second group of behavior control techniques could be classed as "per-   **453**
suasion," in which there is no physical-chemical contact between the con-
troller and controlled. Psychotherapy fits into this category, as do the newer
methods of behavior modification and operant conditioning; we also have
to include mass-control techniques such as propaganda and advertising.
Sometimes these are used in combination with other techniques. For example, the drug succinylcholine in certain doses gives the subject a very unpleasant sensation of drowning. This drug has been used in behavior
modification, to negatively condition persons such as alcoholics by at-
tempting to associate the unpleasant sensation with the unwanted behavior.   ↓

A third and particularly controversial technique is psychosurgery, which is   **454**
distinguished from neurosurgery in that the brain to be operated on in the
former has no identifiable pathological lesion. The first such technique was
lobotomy, pioneered in the 1930s, which fell into disuse when it became
obvious that the result was usually an almost complete blunting of the
victim's emotions and higher functions. Psychosurgery is now on the rise
with new techniques that are claimed to be more specific than the old lobotomy. A new development is the implantation into specific brain areas of
micro-electrodes, which can then be electrically stimulated at will.   ↓

**455** All the techniques mentioned have been shown to be effective in producing changes in behavior — how precisely, we shall come to later. The next question is what motives a person might have for wishing to control the behavior of another person by these means. We might distinguish three general types of motives.

1. Therapeutic. The assumption is made here that the control is being offered to correct some defect, which the person to be controlled recognizes as such, or would recognize if he were rational. The therapist is acting as an agent of the patient; this is merely an extention of behavioral self-control.
2. Social. It is assumed that certain types of behaviors are detrimental to society and thus to the good of all the individuals that make up society. Behavior control may be used to prevent or correct these behaviors.
3. Manipulative. Person A controls the behavior of person B without regard for person B's best interests, because the result is beneficial in some way to A.

↓

**456** Before examining the ethics of each of these motives, we might note that often elements of all three are operating in any given case. Since the line of argument used to justify the act will be partly determined by the motive, as in the case of abortion, it is easy to see how this mixture of motives leads to lack of clarity in ethical debates on this subject. For example, one of the most slippery concepts in use today is the idea of "rehabilitation" of criminals, in which the motives of therapeutics and of benefit to society are combined in a tangled and sometimes self-contradictory manner. Also, in any instance where one person (such as the doctor) is in control of either the therapy or the social benefit, the problem of manipulation is almost ↓ bound to arise, even if only to a slight degree.

**457** We might now wish to attach ethical values to the three motives — saying for example, that the manipulative is to be condemned; that the social is to be condoned in certain special instances, but that we ought to have stringent safeguards to prevent its misuse; and that in most instances, with minor safeguards, the therapeutic is acceptable.

However, this argument is premature, unless we show that there is some viable alternative to the use of the behavior control techniques that we wish to prohibit. As we saw in Chapter 2, there can be no ethical decision if there is no real choice among alternatives. One line of argument, put forth most ably by the psychologist B.F. Skinner, calls for increased use of behavior-control techniques precisely because this choice is not a real one ↓ in this instance.

Anyone arguing why behavior control is wrong is most likely to fall back on **458** arguments appealing to the freedom of the individual to make choices, or to the dignity of the individual human being. Skinner (1972) retorts that in fact, concepts such as freedom and dignity are empty and outmoded. Just like primitive man might invent a rain god to explain a natural phenomenon of which he has no real understanding, we have invented freedom and dignity as pseudo-explanations of human conduct whose motives are hidden from us. Freedom and dignity are concepts not of reality but of ignorance. ↓

By following the freedom-and-dignity ethics (Skinner says), we withhold **459** praise from a person who does something for some obvious motive, such as money, while praising someone else who does the same thing for "the good of humanity" or some other altruistic motive. If we really looked into the matter, Skinner contends, we would find that the second person was also acting out of a motive, such as some psychologic force in his character, and was just as powerless to disobey that motive as was the first person. Therefore neither person has done anything intrinsically worthy of praise or blame, and the concepts of freedom and dignity do not apply in either case. ↓

In Skinner's behaviorist view, all behavior is conditioned — we do what we **460** have been positively reinforced to do and avoid what has been negatively reinforced. If the language of freedom and dignity has any meaning, it is because many of us have been conditioned to those words, so that they reinforce our acting in socially useful ways. But they lose this usefulness if they lead us to praise or blame people, or to question motives, instead of seeing that behavior modification through conditioning is the only effective way to go.

↓

Once we see the emptiness of the freedom-and-dignity way of looking at **461** things, Skinner argues, we come to realize that our behavior is always being controlled or shaped by forces outside of our power. Society condones this, as with advertising and Madison Avenue techniques. In some places society even places a very high value on it, such as the behavior modification and control that we call "going to school."

↓

Even though we control others' behavior and others control ours, the whole **462** system is very inefficient, precisely because we try to deny what we are really doing by hiding behind the freedom-and-dignity concepts. The real challenge, Skinner says, is to replace these ineffectual techniques with scientifically proven methods. In particular, we must look into the matter of behavior counter-control. If these things are done, the "good guys" will be able to control behavior to achieve the greatest social good and individual happiness; and they will also be able to prevent the "bad guys" (who are now threatening to run the show) from taking over the behavior-control system for their own manipulative ends.

↓

**463** Skinner's views can be (and have been) attacked on a number of philosophical grounds. However, at present they represent one of the most formidable obstacles that an argument opposed to the more widespread use of behavior control must overcome. They also illustrate a point that we have alluded to earlier — that the kinds of ethical decisions one makes are closely tied with one's personal view of the future. Clearly Skinner is envisioning a utopia that has many features that we might not want to include in our view of the future world, and this is the basis for much of the debate.

**464** What has been said against Skinner's arguments? The best critics of Skinner generally agree that the environment plays a large part in shaping our behavior and our values, but object that Skinner's views place too much emphasis on externally observable behavior while neglecting the internal workings of the mind.

What proof can be offered that these internal workings exist? One line of thought, on philosophical lines, is related to the views of existentialism. Simply put, this concept denies that free will is something that either exists within us or does not. Rather, freedom is something we achieve through our own actions — we become free through the process of making choices.

**465** Rhinelander (1974) launches a more direct philosophical attack by showing where we might catch the Skinnerian attributing his behaviorist model to others but not to himself. For instance, by Skinner's theory, it would be incorrect to say that one is a behaviorist because one believes that it is true; that is a motive and assumes one has the freedom to choose what to believe. One must simply say that the behaviorist has been positively reinforced by behaviorist theory. But we might well expect to find the behaviorist wanting to insist on more than that, which he cannot do without denying his theory.

**466** Another somewhat less abstract view is offered by Platt (1972), who seeks a compromise position between the two extremes of the freedom and dignity ideas and Skinner's total rejection of them. Platt does this basically by preferring the phrase "self-control" to the idea of free will. *This recognizes the existence of an individual, internally experienced "self," which is what the humanistic critics of Skinner are anxious to maintain; on the other hand, by omitting the word "free," it reminds us of Skinner's point that the behavior of the self is determined in large share by environmental factors.*

**467** Platt also adds a note to remind us that "largely determined by environmental factors" does not mean "completely determined" in the sense of allowing accurate predictions of all behaviors from outside observations. Because of the complexity of the brain structure and the random nature of mental processes, there will always be a level of uncertainty in our knowledge of the workings of the mind. Thus, at least some of the privacy that the humanists want to protect seems to be safe.

This is, after all, a book on ethics; and so we should give emphasis to the **468** fact that any real system of ethics is impossible given Skinner's radical behaviorist philosophy. Ethics entails being responsible for one's actions, and — just as much — regarding others as responsible for their actions. There is something reciprocal about an ethical community — we praise or blame others as they act ethically or not, and we likewise expect their praise or blame for our own actions. But if all behavior is independent of will, and is caused by reinforcements of one kind or another, then the very words "praise" and "blame" make no sense, any more than we would praise or blame a wire for glowing when an electric current passes through it. ↓

The reciprocity of an ethical community suggests an even more basic flaw **469** in Skinner's philosophy. Suppose we were convinced by him, and decided henceforth to act toward other people as if their behavior was never the result of free will and was always caused by reinforcements. Would we even know how to begin to do this? Our entire way of life, as well as our language, is based on regarding both ourselves and others as persons acting from free will.

Certainly, we make exceptions. When we discover that a criminal acted out of impulses due to a mental illness, we tend to regard that individual less as a subject of blame and more along the lines of a robot that was programmed to act the way it did. But this case makes sense to us precisely because it is an exception to the rule. Could we imagine regarding everyone, ourselves included, as robots in this sense? Skinner's views require us to turn the exception into the rule; but without that rule we cannot make sense of the exception. ↓

We should also note, however, that Skinner has given a practical warning in **470** his emphasis on counter-control. Behavior control can work; and if we assume that various evil people may at some time want to use it against us, our only defense is to know enough about the techniques of behavior control to be able to detect this — or, even better, to be able to use morally acceptable means of control to reform those evil people. Therefore, in this as in many other areas of experimental biology, we might want to encourage basic research in behavior control, even while we are opposing behavior control as applied technology. ↓

We have now examined the motives for employing behavior control. Ac- **471** cording to our ethical method, this discussion has only set the stage for the major task, which is to determine the consequences of behavior control — in particular, the side effects that are not part of the intended consequences and which may not be immediately evident. In keeping with our views of the future, we also want to inquire particularly into the long-range effects for society. ↓

**472** The specific side effects of each individual drug or psychosurgical procedure would have to be listed separately; however, some general observations are possible. While psychology and neurophysiology have hardly scratched the surface when it comes to understanding the mind and the sources of behavior, it does seem to be a legitimate conclusion that mental functions are complexly integrated and involve feedback circuits among a large number of subcomponents of the system. *Just as killing off a species of insect or drying up a pond can eventually disrupt an entire ecosystem, the alteration of one of the mental subcomponents by chemical or physical means must eventually have an impact upon many other, seemingly unrelated mental functions.*

It is of interest that the scientific justification offered, implicitly or explicitly, for modern psychosurgery is the idea that specific emotions or behaviors, such as rage or pleasure, are located in specific areas of the brain. It is ironic that at the same time that neurophysiologic theories of brain function are becoming increasingly complex, the psychosurgery researchers are
↓ going back to this less sophisticated view.

**473** This account of the complexity of the mind leads to the conclusion that, while we might have to do research to determine the unwanted side effects of any particular technique, these unwanted side effects will almost certainly exist. It might also suggest that the ethical problems will be greater where the number and magnitude of these side effects are greater. (One could also argue the other way: We were able to mobilize medical opinion against lobotomy in the 1940s precisely because the effects were so grossly observable. The newer methods are more dangerous and more open to misuse precisely because they are more subtle.)

The side effects we are particularly concerned with might be described as "lessening of consciousness" or "lessening of choice." These occur with lobotomies or the use of tranquilizing drugs, which seek to eliminate the particular unwanted behavior either by lessening the subject's power to perform a whole series of behaviors, or by making him less aware of a variety of external stimuli, some of which had acted to trigger the unwanted
↓ behavior.

**474** It is important here to recall the values we placed on self-respect and individual autonomy. One thing that enhances our self-respect and sense of autonomy is to make plans and then to put them into practice. If drugs or other control techniques interfere with our acting on our plans, or cause us to behave in ways we have not intended, we lose a sense of our behavior as
↓ ours and hence we lose self-respect.
REVIEW AUTONOMY ↑ 79–84

It should be noted, however, that some experts, who agree that the lobot-   **475**
omy procedure of the 1940s and 1950s had too many adverse side effects to
be used justifiably, nevertheless feel that the emotional and political reaction to these old techniques has gotten in the way of recognition of genuine advances in the form of the new techniques, which produce much
smaller and more specific lesions. In reviewing the current literature, Sweet
(1973) cites in particular one study in Australia that performed a limited
psychosurgery technique called cingulotomy on 48 patients with severe depression, all of whom had been treated unsuccessfully with medical therapy for at least 5 years. Sweet quotes the investigators as reporting that 88
percent had "remission of all symptoms and ability to work at the pre-illness
level or better," with "no instances of impairment of social awareness or
deterioration in ethico-moral behavior after operation." *                    ↓

Sweet also questions the universal assumption that any psychosurgery is an   **476**
irreversible procedure: "Although it is true that new neurons do not replace
the ones destroyed, those that remain possess extraordinary capacity to
reestablish new connections or take over functions that they did not have
before."

Sweet concludes his survey by noting that the results of limited psychosurgery in a number of English and Australian studies, on patients who have
not responded to other therapy, are good enough so that new controlled,
randomized studies ought to be carried out in the United States. Thus, he
feels that psychosurgery might well be employed ethically in at least one
class of patients — those unresponsive to all other therapy. However, the
physiologic rationale that he offers for why limited psychosurgery works is
essentially no more sophisticated than the one given above — the equation
of specific brain areas with specific mental functions.                      ↓

If we are concerned that this approach to behavior control will lead to un-   **477**
desirable side effects, we ought to note that having a diminished range of
alternative behaviors and being less able to respond to environmental stimuli, will generally lead to a diminished quality of life (as Margolis [1976]
argues, to being less of a person, since the capacity for purposeful behavior
is a key feature in our concept of personhood). These behavioral side
effects, it is claimed, commonly follow psychosurgery, and certainly result
from the use of major tranquilizers.

Sweet (1973), however, contends that many of the candidates for psychosurgery are repetitively and compulsively overresponding to internal instead of external stimuli. While our quality of life might be lessened by the
side effects of psychosurgery, it can be claimed that for this special class,
quality of life would actually be enhanced compared to existence in a
chronic-care institution.                                                     ↓

REVIEW PERSONS ↑ 280–290

* Reprinted, by permission. From W.H. Sweet, Treatment of medically intractable mental disease by limited frontal leucotomy: Justifiable? *New England Journal of Medicine* 289:1117,
1973.

**478** If we focus on some of the possible long-range consequences, we may use a biological analogy and anticipate some of the points we will discuss under bioethics in Chapter 18. If we look just at the survival value of different behaviors in the natural world, we are drawn to the conclusion that variability and adaptability are two qualities that give a species an increased chance for survival. If it turns out that behavior-control techniques tend to limit the individual's adaptability, and tend to produce uniformity of behavior by blunting individual differences, we might be fearful that such techniques would decrease the survival capacity of man as a species. (However, how widespread must the use of such techniques become before this would occur?) We might argue as an alternative that we ought to try to solve our problems by creating new, more sophisticated behaviors, rather than seeking to eliminate or mask existing behaviors in hopes that the prob-
↓ lem will go away.

**479** Note that behavior control usually is not aimed at behavior alone; behavior is not bad unless it occurs in a particular context or setting. The problem is not bad behavior, but rather behavior that is inappropriate for the environment in which it occurs.

*Therefore, as it relates to quality of life, one of the central questions on behavior control is: Do we want to live in a future where these conflicts are resolved by changing persons' inner selves, or one where they are resolved by changing the outer environment? If our answer (as we would expect) is some of each, the question then becomes how much of each and in what situations.* We can see arguments of this sort today. Those who would rather manipulate environments than people urge eliminating poverty as a solution to the problem of crime, while those who prefer a different future
↓ want to throw the criminals in prison.

**480** Take another, more extreme argument against behavior control. This argument would say that the possible tyrannical uses of these techniques outweigh any good that we might derive from them; and that if we allow even the so-called harmless uses now, we are just opening the door to future abuses.

This argument ought to look familiar. We called it the domino theory when we examined it in the context of sanctity of life. We saw there that it made the error of assuming that the entire decision, for now and ever after, was being made in one sweep; and of denying that there would be many times in the future when we could step in and say, "Okay, we have now gone far enough." (One author, tongue presumably in cheek, stated this in
↓ the form of a rule: "Never do anything for the first time.")
REVIEW DOMINO THEORY ↑ 258–261

However, there may be reasons to give the domino argument more weight **481** in the matter of behavior control than in other contexts. That is because some sorts of behavior control, by their nature, make one less able to make free choices in the future. We can reject the argument that we should never legalize abortion because it would lead to infanticide — if we legalize abortion now, and later somebody proposes infanticide, there is nothing to prevent us from rejecting the proposal. On the other hand, if we submit now to certain sorts of behavior control, our capacity to detect and object to abuses in the future might be diminished.

Therefore, the domino argument, in the behavior-control context, warns us to be particularly sensitive to long-range consequences, both for individuals and for society as a whole.                                                                      ↓

---

## CASE 33

R.J. is a 33-year-old man who has been diagnosed as having temporal lobe **482** epilepsy, which occasionally causes him to exhibit involuntarily violent behavior when he has an epileptic seizure. On two occasions he has physically assaulted members of his family, and he is very concerned about what he might do in the future. You are aware that this sort of problem has been traced to specific organic lesions in the brain. So far your attempts to treat him with drugs have had limited success. You are considering referring R.J. to a neurosurgeon who has had some success in treating such cases. You have explained to R.J. what would be involved in such surgery, and he has indicated his desire to go ahead.

However, when you chanced to mention this case to your minister, he raised objections to such neurosurgery on moral grounds. He contended that the essence of man was free choice, and that it was immoral to surgically tamper with a man's brain so that he would act in the way we wanted.

What do you do in R.J.'s case?                                                                              ↓

---

First, is this a psychosurgery case? Recall that we defined psychosurgery as **483** surgical intervention in the brain in the absence of demonstrable organic pathology. While we have not made sections of R.J.'s brain for histologic examination, we have presumptive evidence to believe that if the diagnosis of epilepsy is correct, such pathology is likely to be present. Therefore, the label neurosurgery is justified.

Second, which of the three motives is operative here? The case was written so that the cards were heavily stacked toward the therapeutic motive. We have the patient's voluntary and presumably informed consent. As primary physician, you are not even going to get any fee for the surgery, while you would get a fee if you continued to treat R.J. medically.

The answers to these questions show why R.J.'s case presents fewer ethical problems than many other cases we could envision.                                                                    ↓

**484**  How do you evaluate the minister's argument? It is not too hard to overcome because it represents a mockery of the facts of the case. R.J.'s problem is precisely the lack of free choice. When he has a seizure, he commits violence whether he wants to or not. With the surgery, if performed correctly, there is at least hope that he will no longer have these seizures, though he will still be capable of violent acts if provoked for other reasons.

This argument ought to reinforce the notion that control of behavior and free ethical choices are by no means contradictory notions. If we could not control our own behavior, how could we act ethically? We would never know if our bodies would implement the ethical judgment we had made, or whether our bodies would, of their own accord, do exactly the opposite.

**485**  All of our discussion of Case 33 assumes that there is such a thing as temporal lobe epilepsy and that it has been correctly diagnosed in this case. Opponents of psychosurgery have charged that this diagnosis is abused in such cases — that such a diagnosis is made where no organic lesion has in fact been identified, in order to justify the surgery. This debate has become so polarized that two authors, Breggin (1972) and Mark (1973), have described the case of the same patient in radically different terms. Mark describes a patient with symptoms similar to those in Case 33 and states that after surgery he returned to essentially normal function. Breggin states that he is familiar with that case and that the man actually ended up back in a mental hospital in much worsened condition. You will have to read the arguments of Mark and Breggin and take your pick.

**486**  Disputes such as this have led to calls for regulation of psychosurgery and related research. The issue was debated by the National Commission for the Protection of Human Subjects of Biomedical and Behavioral Research. Their report, released in 1976, suggested that they were swayed both by unquestionable successes in psychosurgery and the absence of rigorous research methods in most studies on the subject. The Commission refused to ban psychosurgery, but did restrict its use and proposed stringent guidelines for consent and ethical review.

**487**  While we have emphasized how defenses of psychosurgery may be overly simplistic, we should also be alert to errors on the other side. One suspects that some opponents of psychosurgery may be guilty of an uncritical "sanctity-of-the-brain" stance analogous to the sanctity-of-life stance we found fault with in Chapter 6. If future studies show good results when psychosurgery is used on carefully selected patients and also show the absence of the feared side effects, we should not continue to oppose psychosurgery just because it involves tampering with the brain.

## CASE 34

As a public health physician employed by the metropolitan school system, **488**
you are aware that there is a disorder in children known as hyperkinesis,
which produces hyperactivity beyond the conscious control of the child.
Such children are unable to pay attention for any length of time and thus
do poorly in school, out of proportion to their actual intelligence. Because
there has been no organic lesion identified, although the disease is presumed to have an organic basis, the condition is also referred to as "minimal brain dysfunction."

You also know that amphetamines, which are called "speed" because
they tend to produce increased activity and alertness in people who use
them, have a paradoxical effect on hyperkinetic youngsters — the drugs
slow them down and allow them to sit still and pay attention. One such
drug commonly used is methylphenidate, manufactured under the trade
name of Ritalin.

Your school nurses want you to write a blanket prescription for Ritalin for
any children found to need it by the teachers. They argue that the teacher
sees the child all day and thus is best qualified to judge those children who
would benefit from the drug.

What do you do?                                                             ↓

---

This case represents more than a strictly medical decision — it asks one to   **489**
determine a matter of public policy as regards a technique of behavioral
control. How ought one to approach such a determination? You might wish
to begin by taking a specific proposal and examining it according to questions such as:

1. What are the criteria for the "disease" that you are treating? Who has
   determined these criteria?
2. Who is going to assess the individual subjects based on these criteria to
   see which ones have the disease? Are they competent to do so?
3. Who is going to apply the treatment to the subjects thus selected? Are
   they competent to do so?
4. What is the goal of the treatment? Who is going to assess the subjects to
   see whether this goal has been accomplished?
5. What are the other consequences of the treatment? In particular, what
   are the social consequences for the subjects who have now been labelled as having this disease?                                          ↓

**490**   Taking the proposal as put down in Case 34, we see that no mention is made of the criteria for determining hyperkinesis. In fact, the diagnosis requires careful psychologic evaluation to rule out other possible causes, such as emotional disturbance. We see that the teachers are going to judge which children are hyperactive so that the nurses can give out the Ritalin, ↓ and that no provision has been made for follow-up on individual cases.

**491**   When a plan of this sort was put into effect in Omaha several years ago, it was found in a later survey that 30 percent of the school children were receiving Ritalin. Simply by statistics, it is impossible that that many children were actually suffering from hyperkinesis in the strict medical sense. In retrospect, it was clear that the teachers were simply displaying a low tolerance for the normal activity levels and low attention span of youngsters in the elementary school age group, and they were using their own exasperation with their chaotic classrooms as the criteria to determine use of the drug. The result was that 30 percent of the school children were being made to ingest a psychoactive drug and possibly were receiving significant training for later life — if you have a problem, reach for a bottle of pills to ↓ solve it.

**492**   It is interesting to ask what happened to the medical profession in Omaha during all this business, especially since doctors are traditionally very jealous about their power over the prescribing of drugs. We might also wonder what happened to the parents. It may well have been that the idea that their child was receiving a medicine to help him do better in school was satisfying enough to the parents. This brings back the point about the social context in which behavior occurs. We live in a society that is still dominated by the so-called protestant ethic, which among other things places very high value upon socially useful work. Thus, we might be expected to be much more tolerant of the use of behavior control when it serves the purpose of promoting this kind of "socially useful" behavior. Although caffeine is demonstrably a drug and has a number of known harmful side effects, we hear no social condemnation of the morning cup of coffee that ↓ allows us to wake up enough to trudge to work.

**493**   As far as amphetamines go, it is interesting to review the situations in which these drugs are "medically indicated" and "medically not indicated." The former category involves only two conditions: hyperkinesis, and narcolepsy (in which the victim is subject to falling asleep spontaneously at inopportune moments). Uses of amphetamines not sanctioned by the medical establishment include street users who want to get "high," and the use of so-called diet pills because of their (temporary) effect of curbing the appetite.

   While there are medical justifications for this categorization, it is at least curious that the distinctions correspond almost precisely to the values of

the protestant ethic. Narcoleptics and hyperkinetic kids can't work effec-   **493**
tively, so it is all right to use drugs on them to correct this. Obesity, on the   cont.
other hand, does not preclude useful work, and the fat person ought to
have enough willpower to eat less without using a "crutch." And it is clear
that the person who is high on speed is not being socially useful at all and
ought to be condemned.   ↓

Final note on Case 34: One critic suggested that as long as you were going   **494**
to use some sort of drug to solve the problem, it would have made much
more sense to give tranquilizers to the teachers.   ↓

---

## CASE 35

You are the same school physician. After kicking the nurse who wants to   **495**
dispense Ritalin out of your office, you pick up the latest medical journal
and read that a new drug has just reached the market. Its chemical name is
3',5'-cyclic I.Q., and it is being marketed under the trade name of Precoci-
tabs. Its effect on children is to increase the measurable IQ by 15 to 20
points as well as improving performance on school exams, intellectual
problems, and all sorts of other mental tasks.

    While the drug has not yet been tested on pregnant women, clinical trials
involving 4,000 children over a 2-year period have turned up no significant
side effects from the drug.

Would you want to prescribe this drug for all the children in your school
system? None of them? Some of them?   ↓

---

While so far we have emphasized the use of behavior-control techniques to   **496**
get rid of bad behavior, there is certainly another side to the coin. Such
techniques could conceivably be used to promote good behavior. We
would then be stuck with coming up with some consensus on what good
behavior is. Those who believe that abuses of behavior control can best be
prevented by keeping the number and types of allowed intervention to a
minimum are particularly dismayed by these proposed good uses.

    How does your judgment on this case compare with your judgment in
the Ritalin case (remember the five questions)? If there is a difference, is it
rationally justifiable? Is it possible to make ethical judgments on "psychoactive drugs" across the board?   ↓

REVIEW CASE 34 ↑ 488

## CASE 36

**497**  You are a clinical psychologist specializing in behavior modification through operant conditioning techniques. A middle-age woman, Mrs. B.K., comes to you seeking treatment. She states that she suffers from feelings of anxiety and depression and freely relates these to the fact that her husband is continually involved in affairs with other women. However, Mrs. B.K. is devoted to her family and enjoys the security of marriage, so even though she has decided that her husband will never change, she considers divorce to be out of the question. She wants you to help desensitize her so that she will not have this emotional response to her husband's affairs.

↓  Do you accept Mrs. B.K. for therapy or not, assuming that you have the techniques required to bring about the desired goal?

---

**498**  Let's examine both sides of this case. If you agree to treat Mrs. B.K., you seem to be coming down on the side of those who would prefer to alter the individual's inner self when one could conceivably alter the environment instead. (Or you could argue that the environment is, for all practical purposes, unalterable, since the husband is not willing to seek therapy.) Is this the same as saying that the problem is not in the marital relationship, or in the husband, but rather within Mrs. B.K. herself? And if you are not saying this, then why treat Mrs. B.K. instead of the place where the problem actu-
↓  ally exists?

**499**  On the other hand, suppose you decide not to treat (as did the therapist in the original case), on the grounds that you would only be helping Mrs. B.K. to ignore a very real problem in her environment. You might argue that her desires not to be upset by her husband's tomcatting and her desires for the security of marriage are incompatible, and the sooner she comes to the realization that she can't have her cake and eat it too, the better off she will be.

However, is this a fair assessment of the real situation in which Mrs. B.K. finds herself? Is she all that unaware of what her problem is and what alternatives are open to her? Since she has made this particular choice, isn't it a bit paternalistic of you to decide that you know what is in her best interests better than she does?

If you are not going to treat Mrs. B.K., you would seem at least to have an obligation to steer her to someone else who can help her with her problem, be it internal or environmental. What advice are you going to give her on
↓  this score?

If, instead of coming for behavior modification, Mrs. B.K. went to a psychiatrist with a request for a tranquilizer, you might propose a compromise. You might prescribe the tranquilizer as an immediate step to help gain the confidence of the patient; then, in follow-up visits, you could enter into discussion of the real problem and try to assess how Mrs. B.K. might best be able to solve it.    **500**

The only thing wrong with this course is that once the immediate needs are met by the symptomatic treatment, the patient's motivation to grapple with the underlying problem could be greatly diminished. Thus, your compromise could easily turn into a cop-out, with the patient joining the growing army of chronic tranquilizer users. Of course, you could avoid this by exercising diligence and good clinical judgment.    ↓

---

## CASE 37

A 22-year-old black law student comes to you saying that he thinks he could use the help of a psychotherapist. He states that his problem is constant anxiety, which he attributes to the pressures of competing with his mostly white classmates who have had a better academic preparation than he was able to get at his all-black college. So far he has kept up with his studies, but has lately been worried that the anxiety and the pressure are interfering with his academic performance. He thinks he could do better if he could relax more.    **501**

In the course of your routine questioning, you elicit the information that he is a practicing homosexual and has been for several years. He contends that he is comfortable with his sexuality and that he has had no anxiety or guilt related to any of his homosexual encounters or relationships.

Do you:

1. Try to treat him for his homosexuality, since that is the most likely cause of his anxiety?    ↓ 502
2. Treat the anxiety alone, accepting his reasoning that it arises from academic pressure?    ↓ 503

**502** Are you justified in the assumption that the homosexuality is more likely to be the source of anxiety than the academic pressure? As the case is written, what is the evidence to support this conclusion? Or are you making the assumption that all homosexuals are anxious and guilty as a result of their sexual preferences?

Even if the latter question is answered affirmatively, recall that the student did not ask you to treat his homosexuality; he stated that he was comfortable with his sexual habits. Is it overly paternalistic to attempt to change a behavior that the patient does not want to change? (More pragmatically — ↓ what are your chances of succeeding?)

---

**503** Psychiatrists have recently been sharply divided on the issue of whether homosexuality is abnormal behavior in its own right, or whether at least some homosexuals can be well-adjusted, provided that society gets off their backs. While this is still a controversial issue, the latest Diagnostic and Statistical Manual in psychiatry leaves out homosexuality as a specific psychiatric diagnosis. With homosexual rights being such a hot issue in political circles, it is obvious that this "medical" debate cannot avoid being influenced by broader social values.

At any rate, in this case, you are justified in treating the patient's self-defined problem, without searching for a more obscure source of the anxiety. If treating him to cope better with his academic pressure fails, you can always reassess the situation to see if homosexuality could be a major issue, ↓ after all.

**504** In the actual case, the psychotherapist decided the treatment should be directed immediately at the homosexuality. This led one commentator to note that the unfortunate patient went to the doctor with one problem (anxiety) and came away with two (anxiety plus the "problem" of homosexuality). Furthermore, he was especially bad off in that both his problems have a very poor prognosis — the anxiety because the doctor is refusing to treat it; and the homosexuality because psychotherapy has a very bad track record in treating this "disorder." Presumably, patients do not go to doctors ↓ in order to have their problems multiplied and rendered incurable.

**505** Incidentally, can we make any ethical generalizations about psychotherapy as it is related to behavior modification? Obviously psychotherapy can succeed only if the patient accepts the authority of, and opens himself up to, the therapist. This could be seen as an advantage, since these conditions are unlikely to occur where there is not genuine voluntary consent. Behavior modification enthusiasts, on the other hand, attack psychotherapy on the grounds that it represents an unwarranted invasion of privacy. Through

their own techniques, they claim, the same or better results can be   **505**
achieved in a shorter time without any of this "paternalistic prying."   cont.

This leads to the old question about treating the symptoms rather than
the root causes of mental disorders. The question certainly has important
ethical implications, since the amount of invasion of privacy or loss of self-
esteem to which you might be willing to subject a patient has to be
weighed against the likelihood of a successful outcome with that sort of
therapy. This debate is so complex, however, that it can better be presented
within the context of a psychiatry course.   ↓

The symptom vs. cause argument leads to a more basic question. You may   **506**
have noticed that the list of three motives that began this chapter made no
mention of mental illness, although some such concept has been alluded to
in several places since. Just what do we mean by "mental illness"? The answer to this question is of great importance if we are going to distinguish
the situations where the motivation for treatment is purely therapeutic, social, or manipulative. It is also of prime importance as the answer to the first
model questions we presented for deciding public policy with regard to
behavior-control therapies.   ↓

One view, which has become popular in psychiatry with the advent of re-   **507**
cent biochemical discoveries relating to brain function, holds that mental
illnesses are discreet entities, for each of which a distinct pathological–
biochemical lesion has been or someday will be found. The finding of this
specific lesion for each specific illness will then lead to the discovery of
specific treatment modes, which will probably emphasize chemical means
to correct the biochemical imbalances. If certain aspects of psvchiatry do
not meet these specifications, it is assumed that this is because all the facts
are not yet known.   ↓

The extreme opposite view holds that there is no such thing as mental ill-   **508**
ness. Rather, some people suffer from problems of communication and disorders of human relations; these are considered more or less tolerable by
other people depending on a number of social factors, such as socioeconomic class.

When, because of the social and cultural context, the disorder is viewed
as being particularly intolerable, the responsible person is labelled with the
mythical label of mentally ill. This is not a descriptive term; rather it is a
political move to justify the things that we wish to do to that person. These
may include both good things, such as offering sympathy and removing the
responsibilities of a job so that the person can be treated; and the nasty
things, such as locking the person up in an institution and taking away his
civil rights.   ↓

**509**   It seems clear to everyone but the psychiatrists who support these two extreme views that the answer lies in a bit of both. There may well be a spectrum of mental disorders, ranging from the almost purely organic to the ones for which no pathologic lesion has been or probably will be identified. As a matter of fact, we have to broaden this spectrum to blur over the distinction between physical and mental illness, since many diseases of other parts of the body affect the brain functions, and many mind disorders show themselves as, or lead to, problems in other organs. Given the many intricate interconnections between the mind and body, it would be rather surprising if it were any other way.

**510**   When it comes to formal definitions, one might suspect that the whole problem is related to immediately seeking to define the disease, while the state of health is presumably what we are really interested in. Can we do better by trying to define mental health?

Try out this rather complicated definition, paraphrased from one offered by Robert Neville (from a presentation to the Workshop on Medical Ethics, Berkeley, Cal., July 1973): Mental health consists of maximizing the various mental capacities, in a balanced manner, so that it is possible both to have inner understanding and peace, and to achieve relevant and discerning fulfillment with respect to the outer environment.

**511**   We'll leave it to you, if you wish, to decide what is meant by each specific item in the definition. For now, notice two points. First, this definition repeats our earlier observation that mental health must be assessed with respect to the outer environment in which the behavior is to occur. But in addition, it adds mention of "inner understanding and peace" — in effect adding on an inner environment as well, and demanding that the healthy mind will be in harmony with both environments. It is precisely this "inner world" that is denied by the behaviorist followers of B.F. Skinner and others, who would hold that the externally observable behavior expresses the whole realm of mental function. If one denies the existence of the inner environment, it is not hard to see how Skinner can discard the concepts of freedom and dignity so easily.

**512**   Second, note that this definition has stacked the deck against those types of behavior control that act by a general blunting of emotion or intellect. According to the definition, a person is rendered less mentally healthy by any such means. We noted before, in the discussion on primum non nocere, that medicine has accepted the principle of making a person sicker in order to make him well later, as in surgery. However, in order for this to apply, there must be reasonable assurances that the sickness will be only temporary, and most of the behavior-control therapies fail to offer this assurance.

REVIEW PRIMUM NON NOCERE ↑ 346–347

So far behavior-control techniques have been attacked on the grounds that **513** they are consciousness-limiting, and the impression may have been given that all or most behavior-control techniques fall into this category. Of those drugs used outside of the doctor–patient relationship, alcohol and the opiates do seem to fit this description; but the hallucinogenic drugs seem to be a different case entirely. At least in the view of their advocates, such drugs are used precisely for their mind-expanding capability; in fact, some say, they may even make the user more healthy mentally. (Is this somewhat analogous to the high-IQ pill hypothesized in Case 35?)

Several justifications for the expansion of consciousness by chemical means can be advanced. One is an alternative-religion model, in which utopia is viewed as an aesthetic experience in the present instead of an ascetic afterlife yet to come. Another rejects the possibility of using drugs to achieve a single, cohesive world-view, but rather makes reference to the desirability of variability and pluralism, and sees drug experiences as additions to the variety of one's life. ↓

While several objections can be cited to these views, this seems to be an- **514** other instance of disagreement based on different views of the future. One states that drug use does not lead to real mind-expansion, but only gives an escapist a superficial impression of doing so; and it is really the escapism rather than the supposed mind-expansion that the user seeks. It is hard to see how such a statement can be proved or disproved on empirical grounds; it may boil down to differences in taste and life style. Besides, people are capable of using just about anything as an escapist device, if escape is what they want.

Another objection points to the deleterious side effects of drugs such as marijuana and LSD as reasons not to engage in their use. Again, potential risks must be weighed against potential benefits, and it is clear that the risks must be very great to outweigh the benefits proposed by the alternative-religion or the pluralism-of-experience models, so long as one actually values those outcomes highly. Besides, even the protestant ethic has social consequences that could be termed adverse side effects; the side effects always seem to be minimal if one places a high value on the desired outcome. ↓

In summary, it must be acknowledged that one can build an adequate ethi- **515** cal foundation for the use of psychoactive drugs for the purpose of expanding consciousness.

As noted, this is not a central issue to medical ethics since these drugs are generally obtained and used without the services of a physician. The most important medical-ethical issues concern the position the medical profession is to take on the social policies relating to the use of drugs, and whether there is an obligation to educate the public at large on the possible side effects, or lack of them, arising from drug use. ↓

**516** Related to this public obligation is the work of some groups of investigators who openly admit that they view marijuana as a great evil and want to see that it remains outlawed. They have on occasion announced their research results before news conferences, claiming that they have evidence to show, for example, that marijuana increases the incidence of infection by altering the white blood cells. When the reseach subsequently appears in scientific journals, their original claims are often found to be considerably overstated. Responsible researchers might well ask what the long-range consequences of this sort of policy will be on public trust in statements of the ↓ medical profession.

**517** Before ending the discussion, we might say a bit more about the problem of labeling, which was mentioned in the last of the five public-policy questions. Going back to the views on mental illness, one of the social reasons for diagnosing a person as having a mental illness is so that that person can assume what sociologists call the "sick role" and accept treatment. A little reflection should reveal the numerous social consequences that befall a person once it becomes known to others that a diagnosis of mental illness has been made; the case of the Democratic vice-presidential candidacy in 1972 was a particularly dramatic illustration. *It is not hard to see that in certain cases, the probable future stigmatization might well outweigh the present benefits of undergoing formal treatment. At any rate, the physician* ↓ *will be very careful about what he calls the condition he is treating.*

**518** The labeling problem (like the problem of how to treat a dying patient) is one in which the ethical components are rather elementary; the real problem, initially, was one of awareness that the problem existed. As soon as psychiatrists in general realized that these consequences did occur, and that they had it in their power to do something about it, their ethical obli- ↓ gations were rather speedily agreed upon.

**519** Further warning on the labeling question is provided by a much-publicized study of Rosenhan (1973). His group of psuedo-patients presented themselves at psychiatric facilities in California complaining of symptoms specifically chosen as typical of no known psychiatric entity. They were immediately diagnosed as schizophrenic and admitted, and a few had some trouble getting out. While it would be unjust to psychiatry to overgeneralize these results, clearly it is possible to overestimate the true validity of ↓ diagnoses related to mental disturbances.

## CASE 38

L.B., a 22-year-old woman, is making her sixteenth court appearance in 3    **520**
years on the subject of her commitment to the county mental health facility. As a psychiatric social worker, you have seen the same pattern repeated
— L.B. is brought in by the police after some bizarre behavior on the streets.
She is treated with major tranquilizers and quickly reverts to a semblance of
normal behavior; at this point, it appears to the staff that, if she could only
be kept for an extended period, her condition might be treated effectively
and she could be released to be followed up in an out-patient clinic. Instead, in the 72-hour period prescribed by the new state law protecting the
rights of mental patients, L.B. is brought before the judge and demands to
be released. Since the judge is empowered to order prolonged commitment
only if a patient is an obvious danger to others or to themselves, L.B. has
been released each time. Once off her medicines, she reverts to her bizarre
behavior pattern, wandering the streets, begging for food, until the police
bring her in again.

   You know that this court appearance will be no different. You glance at a
note from L.B.'s mother, who feels helpless in the face of her daughter's
inexplicable behavior and is at her wit's end. "The system is very good at
protecting my daughter's civil rights," she writes in the note. "Who is going
to look out for her human rights?"

What should be done with L.B.? What is your responsibility as an individual
health professional?

(Adapted from a case reported by Jon Rubenstein, M.D. [1978].)    ↓

---

In years past it was often an easy matter to commit a person to a mental    **521**
asylum indefinitely merely on the say-so of a physician. Naturally this in-
vited abuses, especially in totalitarian nations where political dissidents
were often removed from society by being labeled "insane." Recently,
commitment statutes have become much more rigid, and, in the eyes of
many, the pendulum has swung in the other direction. In the old days, a
criminal often had more rights to due process than did the mentally ill; today, according to Curran (1978), the mentally ill must often be treated as
criminals if they are to be taken off the streets at all.    ↓

**522**  As Rubenstein (1978) views L.B.'s case, it is a clear clash of rights — her civil rights to due process in court as opposed to her rights to adequate medical treatment. But our analysis of rights hopefully will lead us to reject this simplistic formula. One's right not to be imprisoned without a hearing — and involuntary mental commitment is imprisonment for all practical purposes — is a well-established legal, constitutional right. On the other hand, the "right to treatment" in this case really amounts to a right to be treated against one's expressed wishes. Maybe it would be better for L.B. if she were treated. But, stated this way, there is no moral basis to call this a right, and there certainly is no legal ground either.

**523**  Instead of a clash of rights, we seem to have an unavoidable tragedy. If we make it too easy to commit a person to a mental asylum, the old abuses rear their heads. If we make it too hard, people like L.B. may suffer. There is no reason to think we could design the ideal commitment law that will avoid making either sort of mistake. We will probably have to live with some cases of either one or the other — or possibly both.

**524**  In this sort of situation, doctors and lawyers are especially likely to disagree. Doctors are oriented toward helping the sick, and cases like L.B. seem to them to be the worst possible state of affairs. But lawyers are trained to be sticklers for rights. Just as the law holds it better that several guilty men should go free rather than have one innocent man imprisoned, it holds it better to uphold civil rights, even if doing so robs us of many opportunities to help those in need. (In technical terms, the law favors deontological over consequentialist ethics — see Appendix I.) But at least mental health professionals have a duty to bring such unfortunate cases as L.B.'s to public attention, in case the law can be modified in the future.

---

## CASE 39

**525**  On this fine day in 1989, T.S., a 31-year-old man, has been incarcerated in a state mental hospital for 5 years. He previously served two short jail terms for aggressive behavior. On his third arrest, a court psychiatrist adjudged T.S. to be suffering from a personality disorder and recommended institutionalization for observation and treatment. The period of institutionalization has been extended since T.S. contended that he was being imprisoned for political reasons and demanded immediate release. He has had several incidents of aggressive and violent behavior toward the staff.

T.S.'s name comes up when a newly developed psychosurgery technique completes the experimental trial period and is approved for therapeutic use. The procedure involves implantation of electrodes into various subcortical areas of the brain. Sensor electrodes are able to detect the discharges that characterize the onset of an aggressive wave. A transducer then directs a microcurrent to other electrodes that stimulate areas that produce a state of passivity until the aggressive wave is past. When the patient has calmed **525** down, the system is turned off. Evidence to date indicates that the surgery cont. is reversible; if the electrodes are removed later, the patient will revert to his preoperative state.

Since T.S.'s parents are his legal guardians, they are approached by a staff psychiatrist and told that if they consent to the surgery and it is successful, T.S. will be released and the "problem" will not recur. Of course, to assure this he must maintain the electrode system and its connections (the transducer is a miniaturized gadget that is worn like a hearing aid), but this would be a condition for his continued freedom. The psychiatrist tells the parents that if they refuse consent, the hospital will be happy to release their son whenever he responds to conventional therapy; but 5 years of such treatment has not made much progress, and the prognosis in that case is considered poor.

The parents are thoroughly confused by all this and turn to you, the family doctor, for advice. What do you tell them?

(Adapted from an unpublished case prepared by Steven Posar.)    ↓

---

We might start our discussion of Case 39 the way we did with some others, **526** by distinguishing the motives involved. But this is not likely to get us anywhere in this case. The physicians will insist that their motives are strictly therapeutic and will support their procedure by pointing to the failure of traditional therapies and the reversibility of the electrode implantation. Critics of the psychiatric establishment will point to the ideological biases that result in a person like T.S. being labeled "antisocial" in the first place and being confined to institutions against their will, and will characterize the psychiatrists' role as merely one of agents for the state. This argument is basically unresolvable, so we might as well try to go directly to the consequences of the proposed course of action and its alternatives.    ↓

One might wish to question whether such surgery would really be revers- **527** ible, given what we know about the complexity of the brain. Wouldn't any such procedure, no matter how small the electrodes, produce some residual permanent damage to brain cells, even though it might be too subtle to measure? The answer is probably yes; we might generalize that any physical or chemical intervention into the brain is irreversible to some degree. However, this applies to externally located stimuli as well; experience is irreversible. If I have an adorable 3-year-old child and I see it run over and killed by a drunken driver, that is an irreversible experience, and the residual damage from that is likely to be significantly greater than from the psychosurgery proposed for T.S. Thus, we cannot build a case against the surgery on the grounds of irreversibility, unless we are prepared to apply it across the board against all forms of conventional therapy as well.    ↓

**528**   This brings us to probably the most significant question about the consequences of the proposed psychosurgery: What is it that constitutes aggression? How the kind of life T.S. would lead with the electrodes measures up against a list of quality-of-life criteria depends strongly on this answer. If it should turn out that the impulses suppressed by the electrodes are restricted simply to those that produce actual violent behavior directed toward the body of some other person, or of T.S. himself, then the quality of life T.S. can enjoy might well be improved by the surgery.

**529**   On the other hand, psychologists are not completely clear to what extent so-called aggressive impulses are responsible for actions that we tend to regard as socially useful and personally fulfilling. Suppose T.S. gets a job after his discharge and decides he wants to work extremely hard in order to get a promotion; would his sensors interpret this as an aggressive impulse and turn on his passivity switch until the thoughts went away? Or suppose T.S. falls in love and, one fine moonlit night, starts to express his passionate desires through word or deed. Would his "electronic conscience" immediately put an end to the performance?

**530**   Note that these considerations apply both to the therapeutic motive and to a narrowly defined social-good motive; in the latter case, we might decide that in our complex and competitive society, an individual who had no aggressive tendencies whatever is a social liability rather than a gain. Two other considerations, however, apply more directly to the therapeutic motive and to the social-good motive if we define it in broad enough terms.

**531**   First, would the electrodes suppress the aggressive behavior only and allow T.S. to retain the awareness that he had had an aggressive impulse, or would the system wipe out both the impulse and all awareness of it? If the former, we might suggest having the surgery as a therapeutic trial: T.S. could go out in the world and see what it would be like to live without acting out his aggressive feelings. If he liked it, it would be all well and good. But he would also have the basis to make an informed choice that he preferred the freedom and dignity of being able to express himself through his actions. If that were the case, he could have the electrodes removed and go back into the institution. But if the electrodes cut out awareness, he would in effect never know that things were different; he could not compare his life after surgery to his previous life. In that case the psychosurgery would be a consciousness-blunting procedure, and would diminish T.S.'s activities as a moral free agent.

Second, would the electrodes be activated by the desire of T.S. to have them removed — that is, if he had a thought that he should have the operation reversed, would the electrodes act to suppress this thought as aggressive? If so, then the procedure clearly has become an irreversible one, even if he would revert back to his "normal" state if the electrodes were to be removed. Again, in this instance, the result of the procedure would have been to limit T.S.'s range of choices, and thus to make him less human in a moral sense. 532

Once we obtain the answers to these questions, we might restate the assumptions upon which we have been basing our inquiry. The major ones might be: 533

1. *In a case such as this, the long-range interests of the individual and of society coincide; that is, it is not in the best interests of society to allow individuals to suffer a lessening in their quality of life.*
2. *While we might not have decided on a definitive list of quality-of-life criteria, our list does include, as a high-priority item, the requirement that a "person" have an awareness of himself and that a "person" be able to make free choices in a moral sense.*

These assumptions, plus the answers to the questions, would point the way to a decision, in our own minds, of what would be in T.S.'s best interests. If his parents overruled this decision, whether we would be justified in ignoring their position would have to be decided along the lines of the determination of ethical participation as described in Chapter 7.

Presumably, if we were in 1989 when this psychosurgery had concluded its experimental stages, we would have answers to the questions that we raised. Right now, we have no answers, because experiments with electrodes of this type have been largely (though not entirely) restricted to animals. 534

This case points up a major problem with all the behavior-control issues: our relative lack of knowledge about how the human mind works. It may be that the acquisition of some of this knowledge in the future will help to clarify our ethical decision making, allowing us to ask the key questions more precisely, where now we tend to get bogged down in side issues. One thing we can predict, however, is that the number of ethical problems related to behavior control will not be diminished by new knowledge. We have had ample demonstration that new knowledge and new technology create new ethical dilemmas even as they make the old ones obsolete.

**535** Before leaving the subject of behavior control, you might want to review Case 14 (Chapter 5), in which part of the question was the effect of behavior-control techniques and mental illness on the patient's ability to give informed consent. You might also want to look ahead to Case 46 (Chapter 11) to see what happens when behavior-control techniques take place within the setting of medical experimentation on human subjects.

**536** ↓ CH. 10

# Control of Reproduction 10

In this chapter we will deal with the topics of contraception, sterilization, **536** artificial insemination, and abortion. There is some overlap between these topics and those treated in Chapter 15. For example, the discussion of test-tube babies (technically, in vitro fertilization) is generally included under the heading of genetic engineering in standard bibliographies and indexes of medical ethics, but this technique does not manipulate the genetic makeup of the embryo and is in many ways much more akin to artificial insemination than to techniques of genetic manipulation. Hence, our division of topics between these two chapters is somewhat arbitrary. ↓

One of the factors lending major importance to the control of reproduction **537** is the age-old human desire to experience sexual intercourse without having to deal with the consequences of pregnancy. There is nothing new or novel about this; contraceptive techniques and potions are described in ancient Egyptian papyri. What is new is the technology that allows "recreation without procreation" to be accomplished with reliability and with minimal discomfort and inconvenience. ↓

Another factor that is a very new issue, however, is the desire to control **538** reproduction in order to slow the rate of population growth. While it was predicted as early as 1800 that population would eventually outstrip food supply, only recently has the immediacy of the population explosion stimulated social planners to advocate widespread and drastic action. The most significant ethical issues are raised by the contention, which is becoming increasingly common, that voluntary measures alone will be insufficient to meet the crisis. ↓

The techniques for control of reproduction are generally put into three cat- **539** egories. Contraception prevents the union of sperm and egg that results in the fertilized zygote. Abortion removes the zygote-embryo-fetus from the mother's uterus and kills it before it is independently viable. Sterilization renders a person incapable of producing gametes and thus unable to conceive children in the future. ↓

**540**  It should be noted that there are gray areas in this categorization, most importantly between contraception and abortion. The intrauterine device (IUD) is generally dispensed and classed as a contraceptive. However, while its precise mode of action is unknown, the best guess is that it acts by preventing the implantation of the fertilized zygote into the uterine wall. Thus, the IUD actually induces an abortion within the first week of pregnancy; since the mother discharges the zygote with her normal menstrual period, she is not aware of ever having been pregnant. The same applies to the "morning after pill" which is now available for limited use.

**541**  Another technique that is presently controversial but growing in usage is that of premenstrual extraction. A woman who has a late menstrual period can have her period induced in the physician's office by means of mechanical suction of the uterine lining with a thin, flexible rubber tube. If the period is late due to pregnancy, the still very tiny fertilized zygote will be removed along with the other material. However, this cannot be labeled an abortion since no tests were done to determine whether the woman was pregnant. If enough doctors are willing to carry out such a procedure, the later abortion in its present form may become unnecessary in many instances. The ethical problems of abortion would still be present, but they would have their emotional impact blunted by the fact that the physician cannot <u>know</u> that he is removing a living embryo.

**542**  Keeping these (somewhat unclear) distinctions in mind, we will deal first with contraception, sterilization, and artificial insemination, where the ethical issues are more circumscribed; we will then tackle the much deeper ethical issue of abortion.

**543**  Contraception has pretty much ceased to be a medical-ethical problem except for certain issues related to religion and to distribution of health care. First of all, very few would attempt to carry their contentions for the fetus as far as the germ cells prior to conception and contend that the prevention of the union of egg and sperm constitutes the killing of a human being. While most of the objections to various forms of contraception have come from religious groups, notably the Roman Catholic church, the Planned Parenthood Association takes pains to point out that <u>some</u> form of birth control is approved by all major religions. (While it is true that the "rhythm method" is the only alternative to abstinence available to pious Catholics, the rhythm method is nevertheless fairly reliable when the menstrual cycle is determined by regular checks of body temperature.) Furthermore, most religions are beginning to temper the Biblical injunction to "be fruitful and multiply" with a realization that parents have an obligation not to have more children than they can care for adequately.

Several religious objections have been lodged against contraceptive tech-   **544**
niques — that they are sinful to use because they are unnatural, that sex
itself is sinful unless aimed directly toward procreation, or that procreation
is so intimately tied to sexuality within the institution of the family that
contraceptives risk interfering with fundamental family values.

Roman Catholics allow periodic abstinence in the form of the rhythm
method. However, Catholic teaching holds that any sex act is sinful if it is
not, at least potentially, directed toward procreation within the family
union. This shows that secular philosophers, who are not bound to adhere
to the teaching of any one religion, often find major inconsistencies within
debates on this topic. (Ashley and O'Rourke [1978] provide a detailed rationale for the Catholic position on the rhythm method.) You may want to
review Appendix II on the role of religious values in ethical decision making.                                                                          ↓

The debate over religious objections to contraception is better left to theo-   **545**
logians. But it is clear, as sociologic investigations have borne out, that the
public at large does not adhere to those religious views, particularly in the
United States. It would not seem to be the role of the health professions to
try to reopen this debate. Rather, our role is to practice good medicine — to
match the right technique with the right patient and to be alert to both the
medical and emotional side effects that contraceptives are likely to produce.                                                                        ↓

If we assume at this point that those people whose religious values allow   **546**
contraception will go to a doctor to request it while those opposed to contraception will stay away, the only ethical problem remaining is the case of
a physician whose own religious views stand in opposition to certain contraceptive techniques that the patient might request. According to our discussion of the contractual model in Chapter 4, this physician cannot be
made to provide information or treatment of this nature if he would violate
his own moral principles by doing so. That is, if he feels that the use of such
contraceptive devices is sinful, and if he feels that to lead others (the patient) into sin is itself sinful, he would be allowed not to provide the treatment.                                                                        ↓
REVIEW DOCTOR–PATIENT CONTRACT ↑ 131

**547**   While up to now we have tended to be uncritical of this "escape clause" in the doctor's side of the contract, we might note two instances in which it would be ethically questionable for the physician to make use of the escape clause in a case regarding contraception. The first would be where the physician only offers to the patient those contraceptive techniques that conform with the doctor's own standards and neglects to mention the existence of alternatives. Recall that the contractual model would suggest that, where no strong medical contraindications exist to any of the contraceptive techniques, the patient should be told about all the alternatives and allowed to choose the one that best suits his or her own values. While many educated people are familiar with the entire range of contraceptive devices simply from reading newspaper articles, many less informed patients will remain ignorant of alternative methods if, for example, a Roman Catholic physician describes the rhythm method as the only form of birth control
↓   available.

**548**   The second questionable practice exists where the patient population is limited in its choice of physicians — a situation that applies to most of the patients in the United States who are members of the lower socioeconomic classes. A physician who, for religious reasons, believes that abstinence is the only acceptable method of birth control presents no problem in an affluent suburb where several other doctors are readily available. This same physician, if he were practicing in an inner-city clinic where he was the sole source of medical care for a certain population, would be guilty of depriving that population of routine medical care if he persisted in allowing his
↓   religious views to influence his practice.

**549**   Given these two examples, it might seem appropriate to amend the escape clause to the following: *The doctor is not obligated to enter into a course of treatment that the patient requests if to do so would violate the doctor's own moral values, except where that doctor represents the patient's only entry into the medical care system, and to deny the treatment would be to deprive the patient of routine and acceptable medical care.* That is, where there is no alternative available for the patient, the obligation to provide medical service takes precedence over the physician's right to protect his
↓   own moral sense when his values conflict with those of the patient.

**550**   This exception seems to be generally tolerable when the value at stake is something on the order of the pros and cons of contraception. Where more important values, such as human life, are at stake, our respect for individual autonomy and self-respect may require that we allow the physician to refuse to participate, even if this robs some people of health services. For a physician who believes that abortion is murder, then, we might be forced
↓   to insist on his right to opt out of the contract.

This exception will not sit too well with physicians with a strong religious     **551**
orientation. After all, if I feel that the birth control pill is sinful, and a patient comes to me requesting contraception, and I tell her that the pill is an
alternative technique which I will not prescribe but which other doctors
will, and she subsequently goes to Dr. X and gets a prescription for birth
control pills — haven't I contributed to her sin just as much as if I had prescribed the pills myself, and am I not just as responsible in the eyes of God?

The counter-argument would be that this is one of the risks a person
takes when he enters a profession that is obligated to provide a service. The
religious physician who cannot accept this kind of moral compromise
seems to have two choices: He may go into a specialty such as radiology
where such moral conflicts are least likely to arise; or he may work in the
political sphere to increase both the number of practitioners and the level
of education of the public, so that in the future patients with different religious values need not come to him.     ↓

One major debate on contraception involves its use by minors. Our society     **552**
has recently become much more tolerant of adolescent sexuality, and even
adolescent pregnancy (the question of how good these social changes are
is beyond our scope here). We are less likely to encounter blanket condemnations of premarital sex, or Puritan ideas that pregnancy is God's punishment for the sinful.     ↓

Legally, the rights of minors to contraceptive counseling and to contracep-     **553**
tive methods have been greatly advanced. The sexually active minor, according to many state laws, is by that fact "emancipated" and can get contraceptives without parental consent, even though parental consent is
required for other types of medical care. Even where the law does not provide for this, many physicians routinely give contraceptives to minors anyway, reasoning that avoidance of an unwanted pregnancy and the resulting
trauma both to the child and to the family is more important than strict
legal observance.

This issue is especially important for the family physician, who may be
treating both the child and the parents and so may feel the pressure of
divided loyalties.     ↓

Another more recent attitude is that all aspects of human reproduction and     **554**
sexuality, including contraception, should be taught in the public schools.
In some states, this requires repeal of laws that forbid this. (In one recent
case, a mother was prosecuted for "contributing to the delinquency of a
minor" for bringing her teenage daughter to a lecture in which population
control was discussed!) Repeal of such laws must overcome the opposition
of those segments of the public mentioned above. In Michigan in 1973, the
state medical society supported the repeal of such a law, but its efforts
were overshadowed by the vocal protestations of public "moralists." This is
an area in which it would seem that the physician in his community could

**554**
**cont.**
↓

do much to increase popular awareness and information on the issues. The decision of the individual as to how much involvement in such political activity is appropriate will be discussed in Chapter 16.

**555**

From an ethical viewpoint, sterilization is irreversible contraception, and the same types of ethical considerations apply. (It should be noted that it is possible to reconnect the cut ends of the males vas or the female oviduct and restore function in a variable percentage of cases of surgical steriliza-tion. However, there is always a significant failure rate, and so most authori-ties hold that the patient should be told to consider the operation of sterili-zation irreversible at the time that he or she is deciding whether to have the
↓ operation.)

**556**

Thus, if we neglect the problem of the physician with religious objections, the ethical problem of sterilization boils down to the problem of informed consent; or, in the case of an incompetent person, the question of who is qualified to give proxy consent. This latter problem has become prominent recently with renewed attempts to sterilize patients in mental institutions. Some civil-rights proponents have apparently taken the position that sterili-zation carried out on a person who cannot give voluntary informed con-sent is intrinsically wrong, since such "treatment" cannot be construed as
↓ doing anything to further the health of the individual.

**557**

One argument in favor of sterilization of mental patients by proxy consent bases its appeal on the idea that such patients will be unable to care for their children in any adequate fashion. The only problem with this is that according to whatever criteria of "adequate" parenthood you might choose, a large number of parents outside of mental institutions would be found unfit, and ethical consistency would demand their sterilization as well (unless they submit to "parenthood training" or some such thing). While we shall return to the question of what to do about incompetent parenthood briefly in Chapter 15, we might note now that the idea of steri-
↓ lization for it would be exceedingly unpopular.

**558**

An argument that sounds a little better would restrict sterilization to those patients in whom the mental illness is known to have a significant heredi-tary component. One could say that if the patient were rational, she would herself desire to be sterilized to avoid passing on the trait to her offspring. Do you think that this is consistent with the criteria for proxy consent we listed in Chapter 7, if the appropriate legal guardian agreed to this? Or do
↓ you regard this argument as a contrived rationalization?

## CASE 40

In your role as a family physician you have been taking care of several of the  **559**
residents of a local facility that provides supervised residential care for
mentally retarded teenagers and adults. One of these is A.P., a 21-year-old
woman with an IQ of about 60, who works in the dishroom of the local hospital. She has been on the birth control pill, and you presume she has been
sexually active (she admits to a boyfriend in the facility, but is very shy as well
as awkward in expressing herself verbally, so you have been unable to elicit
many details).

You now get a call from one of the social workers at the facility. Several
weeks ago, they had had a group presentation for the residents about birth
control, in which tubal ligation as a means of sterilization had been mentioned. Later, A.P. surprised them by requesting that she undergo tubal ligation. They put her off, assuming that she had merely been swayed by the
presentation, but since then she had several times repeated her request.
She stated as her reasons the fact that she would no longer have to be on
the pill; the fact that she was sure she did not want children; and her own
perception of herself as a potentially less than adequate mother due to her
retardation.

You see A.P. for an office visit. After a half hour of detailed conversation,
you have convinced yourself that she fully understands the surgery that will
be necessary, the attendant discomfort, the irreversibility of the procedure,
and that others who have had this done at an early age have regretted the
decision later. You talk to the gynecologist at the hospital clinic. He is willing to do the procedure if he's sure that the patient can give valid consent.

As a rule, you are opposed to sterilization in a woman who is that young
and who has never had children. But you are impressed by A.P.'s persist-
ence, and you have a nagging feeling that refusal to consider her request
seriously would amount to treating her as less than a person.

What do you do?  ↓

---

There are many different values that must be weighed here. Some ethical  **560**
uncertainties hinge on predictions of the future — how likely is A.P. to
change her mind? Would she actually be a poor mother, or is this a negative
self-image imposed on her by her upbringing? Other uncertainties hinge on
the degree to which mental retardation of this degree interferes with the
ability to understand the relevant data and to arrive at a coherent conclusion (and to view that conclusion as one's own).  ↓

In the past, widespread abuses have occurred in the sterilization of the in-  **561**
stitutionalized retarded — in part fueled by eugenics movements, which ig-
norantly assumed that all such retardation was hereditary. This has led to
much more stringent restrictions, including one court decision, reported by
Curran (1974), which prohibited all sterilizations on incompetents.  ↓

**562** Despite the seriousness of abuses, is such a total ban too sweeping? Can sterilization never be in the best interests of an incompetent individual? Recall (in Case 21) that one court has ruled that we can, under the proper circumstances, legally decide on behalf of an incompetent patient that he would be better off without life-prolonging medical treatment. It seems inconsistent to say that we could choose death for an incompetent patient, ↓ but not sterilization.

**563** Talking about sterilization in terms of the best interests of the patient alone is also unsatisfactory in that it leaves out the interests of the children that might be born. This has been viewed as another clash of rights — the rights to privacy and procreation of the retarded individuals vs. the rights of the ↓ children to a decent upbringing.

**564** We could defuse this clash by pointing out that even if the patient is demonstrably unfit as a parent, the rights of the children could still be served by removing them from the parent's custody under the current laws on child abuse and neglect. But this answer is not very satisfactory. Such laws often will not allow removal until major harm has already occurred; and the custody procedure often consigns such children to years in foster homes, which are not necessarily the most healthy environments either. Thus, a strictly legalistic view of the "right to procreate" without any consideration ↓ for the quality of life of the child ought to engender some skepticism.

**565** In point of fact, A.P. was interviewed by a forensic panel including both psychiatrists and lawyers. Their decision was that she was competent to consent to the sterilization. Accordingly, it was performed. A year later, she moved back to her family in another county and so was lost to follow-up by her physician.

We have warned earlier about the error of trying to decide ethics by hindsight. If, 6 years from now, A.P. wants to have children and regrets the operation, that would not <u>necessarily</u> mean the choice to do it was unethical; if she doesn't regret it, that does not <u>necessarily</u> mean it was ethically ↓ sound.

**566** Another category of individuals historically subject to abuses of sterilization includes those who are competent, but who are manipulable by their ↓ social status — particularly the poor and uneducated.

**567** Suppose (as certain politicians apparently would like to have happen) that a black mother on welfare with six children is told that if she does not come to the clinic to be sterilized, her checks will be discontinued. If the mother shows up at the clinic and signs the informed consent form, we can assume that she is informed in that she knows what sterilization will mean for her. But it would take a large stretch of the imagination to call this voluntary consent. Here the coercion is being applied not by the physician actually ↓ doing the procedure, but by external agencies or circumstances.

The problem of what we might call "informed nonconsent" becomes a    **568**
central one as the pressures to limit population growth spawn new social
programs that seek to make people accept contraception or sterilization by
the use of positive or negative reinforcements. Note that while the threat of
punishment if sterilization is not agreed to is a clear case of coercion, the
offer of a significant reward to a poor person also raises the question of just
how voluntary the consent might be — review Case 3 in Chapter 4.

Note that we have not said that informed nonconsent is necessarily
wrong. The person who goes to court to pay for a traffic ticket submits just
as involuntarily as the black woman threatened with loss of her welfare
checks. If society as a whole should decide that the population problem has
reached a crisis stage, it would seem appropriate for society to force individuals to accept sterilization. Our ethical concerns in such a case would be
that the burden is imposed equally over the entire child-bearing population.    ↓

The important point to remember about this is that the doctor who per-    **569**
forms the sterilizations under those circumstances is operating outside of
the doctor–patient relationship as we have defined it. He is a paid agent of
society, and has no special interest in the individual. Therefore, if he has to
justify his actions, he must appeal to social needs rather than to the doctor–
patient contract. This is similar to the observation made in Chapter 9, that
the psychiatrist who treats a psychopath in order to make him less of a danger to society has no business justifying his acts by the therapeutic motive.

There is nothing intrinsically wrong with a doctor operating outside of
the doctor–patient relationship as outlined here. We have already noted
that the nature of this relationship might well change anyway as social
needs become more pressing. The ethical obligation is simply to be honest;
else the ethical decision-making method cannot be applied.    ↓

REVIEW SOCIAL VS. THERAPEUTIC MOTIVES ↑ 455

There is one other problem with sterilization that sometimes is mentioned    **570**
in ethical contexts — should the husband or the wife be sterilized? This
might be strictly a medical decision based on the side effects of the male
and female operations, with the psychologic side effects included. (One
writer on the subject contends that females should be sterilized because
men undergoing vasectomies are much more likely to suffer psychologic
sequelae due to supposed loss of masculinity; if so, he neglects to mention
that this is a treatable, if not a preventable, side effect.) The only reason this
is not strictly a medical decision is because a number of physicians, indoc-
trinated in the male-oriented system that is the medical establishment today, allow their personal and irrational values to interfere with their clinical
judgment. Since we have already shown that this kind of unexamined inser-
tion of values into medical judgments is inconsistent with the ethical
decision-making method, this problem is one of medical sociology more
than one of medical ethics.    ↓

571 Since the ethical considerations regarding contraception and sterilization apply in general to all the various techniques used, we will not bother to list all available kinds of contraceptives and all methods of sterilization. Articles that do list these are given in the references.

572 Artificial insemination is another reproductive issue that is ethically problematic, mainly in connection with particular religious views. Artificial insemination with the husband's sperm (AIH) used in cases such as when the sperm count is low and several ejaculates must be pooled together, tends to be of less concern than insemination with donor sperm (AID) in cases where the husband is completely sterile. However, both AIH and AID are forbidden by some religious groups, including Roman Catholics.

573 In a few cases where the wife has become pregnant by AID without her husband's knowledge (do you feel that performing such a procedure would be sound or ethical medical practice?), the husband has subsequently filed for divorce on the grounds of adultery; such suits have generally been unsuccessful. We will pass over the notion that AID is adultery, along with some other purely religious objections (which are listed in Nelson [1973]) such as the one that artificial insemination is sinful because masturbation is required to collect the specimen.

574 As we suggested with contraception, patients holding such religious objections presumably will not seek the procedure, and physicians with such objections may refuse to do the procedure themselves. Of more concern is the couple seeking to have artificial insemination performed, but where one or both of them is ambivalent and may have psychologic reactions that may be detrimental to the child. Prominent among these reactions might be feelings of loss of masculinity by the husband, and resentment of another man's sperm inside his wife. As with any such procedure, these possible reactions should guide the physician in his interview with the couple and in his discussion of informed consent.

575 Another problem might be a couple in which only one has the religious or emotional objections. Typically the wife might want the baby while the husband is adamantly against artificial insemination. The ethical issue here is more one of an intramarital dispute rather than artificial insemination per se. We should note that the so-called right of a woman to control of her own body (which we will encounter under abortion) might not apply in a case where the husband is responsible for future child support.

## CASE 41

You routinely perform artificial insemination by donor in your gynecology    **576**
clinic, so Wilma and Theresa have sought you out with their problem. They
have been living together as a lesbian couple for 6 years. Both feel that their
relationship is stable and both love children very much, so naturally they
wanted to raise children of their own. Wilma managed to find a man who
would impregnate her 2 years ago. They are very happy with the little girl
that was born, and under their care she is growing and developing well for
her age. They now want another child. It's Theresa's turn this time, but the
other experience with the man was extremely distasteful to both of them.
They have heard about AID and feel it's the obvious solution for them. Incidentally, they also ask whether you can manipulate the sperm sample in
any way so as to increase their chances to have a male child; since they
already have the girl, they want a boy this time if possible.

In answer to your question, they say that they have already considered
adoption, but that no adoption agency would consider them because of
their atypical relationship.

What do you do?    ↓

---

Case 41 is an excellent case for group discussion. It is challenging to sort out    **577**
the different values that one may appeal to in supporting or rejecting the
lesbians' request. It is especially challenging since homosexuality (to say
nothing of AID!) is such a hot topic in our contemporary society. One has
to be alert to two extreme sources of bias. On one side, the die-hard, self-
righteous opponents of homosexuality, who may be motivated by religious
condemnations of "unnatural" sexual acts, want to refuse to homosexuals
the rights and privileges enjoyed by all other members of society. (Psychiatrists can have a field day debating whether these antigay zealots are
motivated by their need to deny latent homosexual tendencies.)    ↓

On the other side, those who are appropriately put off by the fanatical tone    **578**
of the antigays may go too far the other way to show that they are not part
of that crowd. They may idealize homosexuality in subtle ways.

Also, debate on problems by Case 41 may be marred by adherence to
incorrect facts. One who believes wrongly, for instance, that homosexuals
are usually child molesters, or that any child raised by homosexual parents
will grow up to be gay, or that homosexuality is hereditary, will come to
incorrect conclusions about the ethical issues involved.    ↓

**579** Finally, we might touch upon two consequentialist-type objections to artificial insemination: first, that it violates the nature of the marriage bond by separating procreation from the bond of sexual intercourse; and second, that by a domino-type reaction, acceptance of it will justify all sorts of further technological changes in procreation — up to "test-tube babies." The first objection amounts to saying that physical sex is really the key feature of the marriage union; one suspects that this is just a disguised version of the old argument that anything unnatural is unethical (an argument used in the nineteenth century to oppose anesthesia during childbirth). The domino theory argument can best be dealt with in Chapter 15, with regard to objections raised by Paul Ramsey.

↓ We will now turn our attention for the remainder of this chapter to abortion.

**580** As we noted, abortion is an extremely sticky ethical issue. There is no issue so well calculated to cause equally rational, informed, and compassionate people to disagree violently. This means that pat answers and serene assurance that one's own views are infallibly correct are especially out of place here. As one excellent teacher of ethics likes to say, "If you think that the person who disagrees with you on abortion is crazy, then you don't understand the complexity of the abortion issue."

**581** Even if the proponents of the different abortion views are not crazy, however, they can often be heard to make a lot of crazy statements. Perhaps because people despair of ever finding an argument about abortion that will persuade their opponents, ethical "errors" seem to be much more widely tolerated here than elsewhere. These errors may make good slogans for pro- or anti-abortion rallies, but they don't help us with our basic purpose — to achieve a better understanding of ethical issues, and to correct our own views if we find them faulty on critical analysis.

**582** It's not hard to come up with a long list of blatant ethical errors in the abortion debate and to sympathize with McCormick (1978) in wishing that the debate could be carried out under more civilized rules of conversation.

The most obvious errors consist of ethics-by-definition, for example, "abortion is wrong because it's murder," and "abortion is simply an alternative form of planned parenthood." There is no analysis here of what makes murder wrong, or planned parenthood right; so we cannot discuss whether the case of the fetus actually falls under either of those categories.

**583** Other errors involve stating only one aspect of the case and forgetting about other, equally compelling aspects; for example, "How can it be murder if what you're killing is just a mass of cells, growing inside another person's body?" One aspect of a fetus, surely, is that it's a mass of cells growing inside the mother's body; but another aspect, equally important, is that it will, in the normal course of events, become an independent, unique human being.

Errors also arise when one states what on the surface seems to be a reason-   **584**
able ethical position, but fails to carry it to its logical conclusions. Consider:
"It's wrong to cut off public funds for abortion, since the rich can afford
them anyway and so the burden then is borne by the poor." Ordinarily, our
sense of justice is offended if the rich and the poor are treated differently;
but this begs the question about the morality of abortion. Was slavery
wrong <u>because</u> the rich could afford slaves and the poor couldn't — so that
the institution of slavery could have been made morally acceptable by
using public funds to buy slaves for the poor, too?   ↓

Perhaps the most blatant example of this last error is the position: "Okay, so   **585**
the anti-abortionists think abortion is murder; but they should realize that
at least half of the country disagrees with their position, so they have no
business trying to impose their views on others by trying to change the
abortion laws." Superficially this sounds like an appeal for tolerance and
open-mindedness, and so is likely to be an attractive point of view. But, if
you really think that abortion is murder, can you possibly hold to your own
ethical views and not try to make the corresponding changes in the law?
What is the law for, if not to prevent and punish murder? Is murder the sort
of thing we ought to be tolerant and open-minded about? (This assumes
the anti-abortionist has good reasons to equate abortion with murder, of
course, and is not merely engaging in ethics by definition.)
   Consider a high Nazi official testifying at a war crimes trial, "Sure, I personally thought that Jews are human and that it was immoral to kill them.
But many in my party disagreed with me, so I felt that I had no right to
impose my views on them by trying to change party policy." Would we
accept this as a valid defense?   ↓

After we have cleared the air by dismissing these erroneous arguments, we   **586**
are likely to find the remaining arguments stacking up rather evenly on
both sides of the debate.
   For many in medicine, the "liberal" side of the abortion issue is the most
compelling. It follows both the current U.S. law and what appears to be the
majority public opinion. It allows physicians to offer help to a particularly
unfortunate group — women with unwanted pregnancies. It assures that
such women will have access to good medical procedures, rather than do-
it-yourself or back-alley abortions, which cause many deaths. It refuses to
regard the fetus, even though a potential person, as a full-fledged person
with rights; after all, eggs and sperm are in some sense potential people too,
but we do not think that killing them is murder.   ↓

174

**587** Therefore, it is possible to underestimate the force of the "conservative" position on abortion. Consider this way of rendering the conservative point of view:

1. There is no significant moral difference between a human being in the few months prior to birth and one in the few months after birth.
2. It is immoral to kill a newborn baby.
↓ 3. Therefore, it is immoral to kill a human fetus.

**588** There are a number of points worth emphasizing about this rendering of the conservative position. First, it is not crazy. After all, except in size, there is little actual, biologic difference between a 16-week-old fetus and a 2-month-old baby, and those biologic differences that do exist are not clearly morally relevant.

Second, the conservative position is not based on religious teaching and is not restricted to the tenets of any one religion. The reasoning makes no ↓ reference to God or to the Bible, for instance.

**589** Third, this position does not even prohibit all abortions, on further analysis. There may, after all, be some situations in which it is morally acceptable to allow the death of a newborn — under quality-of-life and personhood discussions, we mentioned anencephalic infants and infants with severe congenital defects as possible examples. By statement No. 1, we would then be justified in aborting any such infants, if we could detect the diseases prena-↓ tally.

**590** Fourth, this conservative position throws the ball squarely back into the liberals' court. The liberal, assuming he does not want to endorse baby-killing, can refute the position only by specifying persuasively some way in which fetuses and newborns are different. This can be a tall order. It will not do, for example, to say that a newborn has been born and a fetus hasn't;
**592** ↓ the liberal has to explain <u>why</u> being born is a <u>morally relevant</u> difference.
UNCLEAR * 591

---

**591** * Deciding which differences are morally relevant and which aren't takes us back to the universalizability aspect of ethical statements. A morally relevant difference is one we are willing to universalize — we will accept being treated differently on the basis of that difference, regardless of our individual interests. For example, we would agree that, as far as individual autonomy is concerned, children are different from adults; we could accept as a universal rule treating children differently from adults, even if we ourselves were to become children again. By contrast, we would be unwilling to accept a rule that redheaded people should be denied the right to own property; if we ended up having red hair, we would be unwilling to live with the consequences of this rule. Hence, hair color is an example of a morally irrel-↓ evant difference.

Finally, this conservative argument avoids, or at least evades, a problem that  **592**
has plagued other upholders of the conservative position: specifying a
point in time after which a conceptus becomes a human person with a right
to life. Most anti-abortionists place this point at the time of conception
itself. Ramsey (1973), however, concerned with such theological questions
as when the soul enters the body, prefers the time of individuation — that
time after which it is no longer possible for the embryo to split into twin
embryos. In practice, it makes little difference, since both points are well
before the age when abortion may be considered.                              ↓

Incidentally, most conservatives assume that their job is done when they  **593**
can show that a fetus has a right to life, for whatever reason. Thomson
(1971), however, has argued that abortion may be morally acceptable even
if the fetus is a fully human person with a right to life. In a picturesque
analogy, she asks us to imagine a woman somehow becoming attached to
another adult person, in such a way that the life of that other person was
totally dependent upon remaining connected, and which interfered considerably with that woman's living her own life as she chose. Thomson then
argues that the woman has the right to disconnect herself from such an
encumbrance even if the other person's death results. (This analogy assumes that the <u>primary</u> intent of abortion is "disconnecting" the fetus, and
that its death is an unfortunate but unavoidable sequel.) True, the other
person has a right to life, but that life is <u>overridden</u> by the woman's right
not to be made a prisoner in that manner. It would be praiseworthy, Thomson adds, if the woman accepted this great burden for the sake of the
other's life, but the object of ethics ought to be to require reasonably decent behavior, not great sacrifice.                                          ↓

A possible rebuttal to Thomson is to note that it does not "somehow hap-  **594**
pen" that a woman becomes connected to her fetus (except in a case of
pregnancy resulting from rape); and that even if people in general do not
have the moral duty to preserve other people's lives at the cost of being tied
to them, the special relationship between mother and fetus is different
from the general case of two randomly selected people, and gives rise to
more stringent requirements. Our ethical method would be suspect if the
value system did not allow for the existence of special relationships, such as
those within the family, which have a special value for all of us and hence
entail special obligations.

  We may, therefore, disagree with Thomson, and accept the proposition
that <u>if</u> a fetus can be shown to have a right to life, <u>then</u> abortion is wrong,
unless it is aimed at saving the fetus from some great suffering, such as
might be the case with severe congenital defects. (Such abortions would in
effect be prenatal euthanasia. We saw in Chapter 6 that there is no conflict

**594** between an adult patient having a right to life, and yet being allowed to die
cont. for his own presumed good.) Note that it does not follow from this argument that if a fetus does not have a right to life, abortion is automatically
permissible. There are reasons other than rights (i.e., values) to make an act
↓ ethically acceptable or unacceptable.
REVIEW RIGHTS AND DEATH ↑ 293

**595** Engelhardt (1973) follows this general line of argument. In somewhat the
same way that we argued that Karen Quinlan cannot have rights because
she has no capacity for conscious self-awareness, Engelhardt concludes
that a fetus lacks such capacities and hence cannot be said to have rights.
But then Engelhardt tries to add what the conservative argument demands
— a morally relevant difference between fetuses and newborns. Newborns,
Engelhardt admits, also lack the degree of conscious, rational self-awareness required to be a "person" in the strict sense. But to allow children to
develop properly and eventually to become full-fledged persons, we treat
them as if they were persons from the moment of birth — that is, infants
occupy the social role of persons while fetuses do not.

Nonetheless, fetuses are very close to developing into newborns once
the point of viability (about 28 weeks gestation) is reached; they are able
immediately to assume the social role of a person if born. Engelhardt, therefore, accepts abortion up to the time of viability, and of course is opposed
↓ to later abortion and to infanticide.
REVIEW PERSONHOOD ↑ 280–290

**596** Most of the arguments we have reviewed so far are of the deontological
sort — they refer to acts as intrinsically right or wrong, without looking at
the consequences of those acts. (We will see a little later why this is appropriate in the abortion debate. You can review deontological ethics in Appendix I.) If we are going to take a look at abortion by consideration of its
consequences, we first have to distinguish different reasons we might have
for performing abortions:

1. To end the life of an infant with a known or highly probable congenital
   deformity.
2. To end the life of an infant who, we predict, will suffer from a very bad ·
   family or social environment if born.
3. To save the life of the mother where this is threatened by continuing the
   pregnancy.
4. To eliminate an additional birth in the interests of population control.
5. To remove a pregnancy that the mother does not want due to financial
   or other personal considerations.

Going from the first to the fifth reason, the interests of the fetus are given
progressively less weight while the interests of the mother (or of society)
are given more weight. At the third reason, the mother's and fetus's inter-

ests weigh equally — it is life for one or the other, and we must choose. As    **596**
we noted, abortion in the first reason and perhaps in the second could be    cont.
viewed as in the fetus's best interests and as a form of prenatal euthanasia.    ↓
CAN A FETUS HAVE INTERESTS? * 600

One ethicist who has approached the abortion issue from a consequen-    **597**
tialist viewpoint is Bok (1974). Because she refuses to engage in definitions
of "personhood," an activity which she feels has pernicious consequences,
her arguments have to do with reasons for performing abortion such as in
our list above, and under what circumstances these are strong enough to
outweigh the usual and beneficial social reasons to protect life.    ↓

For one thing, Bok feels that the reasons for protecting life grow relatively    **598**
stronger as the time of viability approaches; thus she sees early abortions as
being ethically preferable to late ones. Also, abortion done by techniques
that simply separate the fetus from the mother ("cessation of life support")
are preferable to techniques that directly damage the fetus. (Unfortunately,
the former may have more medical morbidity associated with them than do
the latter.) Other crucial variables are whether the pregnancy was voluntary
or not, and whether the mother's reasons for wanting to end it are significant or merely capricious.    ↓

Unfortunately Bok does not make quite clear whether she is addressing her    **599**
argument toward the pregnant woman or toward the doctor, as to who
should reason along those lines. If she intends the doctor to do so, is she
more consistent with the contractual or the priestly model of the doctor–
patient relationship? How do you assess her other points?    ↓ **601**

---

\* If you recall our discussion of personhood in Chapter 6, you may have    **600**
thought of a somewhat philosophical point: If a fetus is not a person and
cannot be said to have rights, it ought not be able to have interests attributed to it either. Is this, then, a tacit admission that a fetus is a person, after
all?

It need not be if we remember that a person's interests can be harmed or
helped by events that occur before that person comes into being. If a
mother takes heroin during pregnancy, the baby will be born addicted to
heroin. The mother is harming the rights of the "child-to-be," not of the
fetus, strictly speaking. But those interests come into being when the new
person does; so they cannot be used to oppose abortion. That is, the child-
to-be will have interests if born, but does not have interests that he be
born. If never born, he cannot be said to be either helped or harmed by our
present actions.    ↑ **597**

**601** Do you think that Bok is correct in assuming that she can give good answers to the abortion while avoiding the problem of trying to define personhood? ↓ If not, can you clearly state the flaw in her reasoning?

**602** Of course, this line of ethical justification would be incomplete without consideration of the long-range consequences of adopting a policy of unrestricted abortion. Two places that now provide abortions readily at low cost, on demand, are Japan and Hungary; in both countries the abortion rate is greater than the birth rate. It is clear that in those circumstances the women have adopted abortion as a means of birth control, and have pre- ↓ ferred it, for the most part, above other available means of contraception.

**603** If one considers fetuses as persons, these data seem reprehensible, since fetuses are being killed where the same effect could have been achieved had the women used the standard contraceptive techniques. If one does not consider fetuses as persons, and places a relatively lower value on them as persons-to-be, then the most significant question is the medical one: In terms of harmful side effects, are the women better off undergoing abortions intermittently or using contraceptives such as the pill or an IUD on a ↓ regular basis?

**604** Two sociologic conclusions might be suggested by the experience in the two countries mentioned. One is that if abortion is readily available, the majority of the population do not consider it morally wrong, even in Hungary with its centuries of Catholic tradition. The other is a counterargument to the domino-theory arguments of the Catholics and Ramsey, that abortion-on-demand will necessarily lead to a weakening of the restrictions against infanticide. No such tendency toward infanticide has been observed; clearly the populace can accept abortion while still main- ↓ taining a clear distinction.

**605** I hope these arguments will have increased your respect for the complexity of the abortion issue. Keep the different positions on abortion in mind as ↓ you deal with the next case.

## CASE 42

You are in charge of the obstetric wing of a New York hospital when a 24-year-old woman arrives in labor. You learn that on the previous day an abortion had been induced at a clinic in another part of the city by the saline method (withdrawing amniotic fluid from around the fetus and replacing it with an equal volume of saline). At that time the duration of the pregnancy had been estimated at 22 weeks. From what little you are now able to learn from the mother, she does not want the baby and desires to carry through with the abortion.

A while later the woman delivers a fetus, which you estimate by visual inspection to weigh about 1,700 grams. As you are about to turn away, a nurse suddenly notices that a heartbeat is present in the fetus.

Normal policy in your hospital calls for attempted resuscitation of any child with a birth weight as low as 1,000 grams. There is no policy for attempted abortion resulting in live birth, since this has never happened before in this hospital.

Do you attempt to resuscitate the fetus or not? In either case, what do you tell the mother?

(Adapted from R. M. Veatch, "Case 57." In *Case Studies in Medical Ethics*. Cambridge, Mass.: Harvard University Press, 1977.)    ↓

---

This fetus, while still in the uterus, was defined as a "nonperson" both by the mother, in her desire not to have it, and by the New York law that permits abortion up to the twenty-fourth week of pregnancy. The fetus has now, in effect, put in an application for personhood, and you have the power to reject or accept that application.

Take the last question first. If you elect, no matter what happens, simply to tell the mother that the abortion has been completed (regardless of the ethics of that decision), you still have to decide what to do now. If you tell the mother the truth, she is likely to be equally dissatisfied if you tell her that she had a live baby but that you allowed it to die; or that she has a live baby that you saved for her, and she now has to take it home and care for it; or that she had a live baby which you attempted to resuscitate, but after a few days it died anyway, and she now owes a $4,000 hospital bill for your efforts. None of these later consequences makes any of the immediate decisions more attractive, so you have to decide the immediate question on its own merits.    ↓

**608** From a quality-of-life standpoint, one might frame three arguments. Which do you find most acceptable?

1. The decision as to the child's personhood was already made by the mother when she decided to have an abortion. You have no business interfering at this late time. Let the baby die as planned.       ↓609
2. The original decision of nonperson status was made while the fetus was still in utero and by presumption unable to sustain an independent existence. Thus the mother could bestow nonperson status upon it. Now the situation has changed, and you see that the fetus-child is in fact potentially capable, with your assistance, of a life on its own. Thus earlier decisions do not apply; the fetus has become an individual human being over whose body the mother no longer has any right to pronounce.       ↓611
3. It would be presumptuous for you to make such a complex decision on your own. Assuming that the mother is in good enough shape to give an opinion, you should ask her whether to resuscitate the infant.       ↓610

---

**609** You have made the choice that was actually made by the physician in the real-life case — a choice that has been rejected by a number of other physicians in similar situations. While the act of not resuscitating the fetus might be justifiable, the argument used in No. 1 suggests that once one ethical decision is made, you are bound to carry it out come hell, high water, or new information. This view is a cop-out. We saw in Chapter 2 the various points in which empirical data influence the ethical decision-making process. That carries with it an obligation to reconsider the original ethical decision whenever new data appear that could influence the decision in those ways. If the particular action is already final and irrevocable, the obligation is to reconsider for the benefit of cases you might run into in the future. In this case, however, the decision has not reached the final stage. Since you have new data and you still have a chance to save the fetus, you have an
**611** ↓ obligation to reconsider, even if you have less than a minute to do so.

---

**610** You have tried to duck the decision but you are not going to get away with it. Recall the general principle reached earlier in this chapter — in an emergency situation, when in doubt, treat. A newborn with a heartbeat but no respiration represents a medical emergency. If the idea of resuscitation even crosses your mind, it must mean that you have at least a doubtful opinion that the newborn object might be a person worthy of having its life saved. As long as that degree of doubt exists, you are not justified in delaying treatment even long enough to call the mother's attention to the situation and get a statement from her. This is not even taking into account the shape the mother must be in after just completing labor and being, most

likely, under the influence of various medications that dull her senses —    **610**
under such conditions, how well will any opinion she might give reflect her    cont.
true desires? Go back to the original list and choose another alternative.    ↑ **608**

---

The second choice correctly perceives that the decision on whether or not    **611**
to abort a fetus is different from the decision on whether or not to resuscitate a baby. In point of fact, for this case to have occurred, the original estimate of 22 weeks gestation must have been off by at least 6 weeks.    ↓

If you accept the conservative position, it was wrong to choose abortion in    **612**
the first place and would certainly be wrong to fail to resuscitate now. If
you accept one of the liberal arguments (except Tooley's, perhaps), you
would still conclude that a newborn is different from a fetus, and that its
bid for independent existence places it in a totally different category.    ↓

The only real strategy would be to accept the fetus-equals-newborn prem-    **613**
ise of the conservative argument along with reason No. 2 for abortion, provided you wished to defend a decision not to resuscitate. That is, you
would defend the original abortion decision on the basis of the dismal social outlook for an unwanted baby, given this mother's financial and other
circumstances. You would then argue that the same dismal outlook would
justify denying life to the newborn. But to carry this off you would have to
show that the outlook is <u>so</u> bad that death would be preferable, and it
would seem pretty hard to do this.    ↓

In a rather short space, we have looked at the abortion issue from a number    **614**
of different angles. (We have left out the legal angle for the most part, however; for that, see some of the readings listed in the references for this
chapter.) We are probably no closer to "solving" the problem now than
when we started; but we will have made considerable progress if only we
have put the real issues into sharper focus, and have cleared the stage by
getting rid of the phony issues. If rational and ethically sensitive people are
going to argue, at least they should know what they're arguing about — this
rule seems self-evident, but sadly the history of the abortion dispute shows
how often it has been ignored.    ↓
MAY SKIP TO ↓ 621

- - - - - - - - - - - - - - - - - - - - - - - - - - - - - - - - - - - - - - - -

The abortion issue differs from many of the other ethical arguments we    **615**
have reviewed so far in two ways. First, we have been struck by the apparent deep irreconcilability of the opposing positions; it is much harder to
find any real common ground between the disputing sides. Second, we
noted the difficulties in applying our standard ethical method to the abortion issue. Instead of talking about the consequences of actions, we spent a
lot of time talking in deontological fashion about the intrinsic nature of

**615**
cont.   different things and the intrinsic rightness or wrongness of certain acts, and this deontological argument seemed highly relevant. We could not merely
↓  dismiss it and still deal with the real issues.

**616**   These two puzzling features of abortion make more sense if we see that abortion is a different sort of debate than most others we have considered. To see why this is so, note that any theory of ethics assumes the existence of a community of individuals to which, and among which, its rules and principles are supposed to apply. Different ethical theories will define the community in different ways; but for all the ethical theories we have looked at, adult human beings like you and I are included within the community, and entities like insects, trees, and rocks are outside of the community. Entities that we exclude from the community are those that are so different from us that we cannot see the possibility of relating to them in any moral fashion (since a moral system, as we argued when we were dis-
↓  cussing Skinner's behaviorism, demands a sense of reciprocity of attitudes).
    REVIEW RECIPROCITY ↑ 468–469

**617**   So far, almost all the ethical issues we have raised have been within-the-community types of issues — how members of the moral community ought to act toward each other. We took for granted, in discussing each issue, that we knew who was a member of the community and who wasn't.

    But the debate over the status of the fetus is a different sort of moral question, in which we cannot ignore the problem of defining the boundaries of the moral community. In many important ways, a fetus is like the entities that we all agree are members of the moral community. In other important ways, the fetus is like those entities that we exclude (particularly in terms of its mental capacities, and its lack of memory and self-awareness). The fetus occupies a gray zone at the boundaries of the community, and rational individuals may disagree which side of the boundary it
↓  lies on.

**618**   We encountered one other such boundary dispute earlier — in Chapter 6 when we proposed that Karen Quinlan was no longer a person. We can now see that what we meant by that was that she had ceased irreversibly to be a member of the moral community. Like the abortion debate, this view of the Quinlan case was very controversial, and many serious ethicists would reject our formulating it in those terms.

    Other examples of this boundary dispute occasionally crop up in ethics. If creatures landed from outer space, we would have to decide the question for them — are they enough like us for us to treat them as moral equals, or so different that we should regard them as mere things? (How many science fiction stories have been based on this moral dilemma!) Another example is the current debate about whether animals, while not being full-
↓  fledged persons, might not have some rudimentary rights nevertheless.
    REVIEW PERSONHOOD ↑ 280–290

Serious consequences arise from where we draw the boundary line, so we     **619**
cannot regard this question as one merely of semantics. We have seen sad
historical examples of drawing it too close, when human beings of minority
races or religions were excluded. Drawing the line too widely has its own
consequences. Suppose we decided that the higher animals were sufficiently like us to warrant inclusion as our moral equals. We would then be
prohibited from owning them, killing them for food, and exploiting them
for sport; major changes would have to be made in our social norms.     ↓

*Wherever we draw the boundary line with regard to the fetus, and which-*     **620**
*ever consequences we choose to accept, one thing at least is clear — our*
*action is, in fact, a moral choice based on our basic moral attitudes and*
*values, and is not an empirical decision based on some discovered facts*
*about the fetus.* Both pro- and anti-abortion physicians and scientists often
delight in displaying their knowledge of fetal physiology, but the fact that
the fetus has a heart beat at 6 weeks gestation, or does not have an EEG
until 28 weeks, does not by itself tell us when the fetus becomes a member
of the moral community. The question is still what <u>moral valuation</u> we
place on heartbeat, EEG, and other biologic functions with respect to moral
personhood. No new scientific discoveries can answer that question for us.     ↓

- - - - - - - - - - - - - - - - - - - - - - - - - - - - - - - - - - - - - - - - - - -

This concludes our discussion of control of reproduction. In addition to the     **621**
cases in this chapter, we have already dealt with several cases that involved
abortion and related issues in previous chapters, and will be doing so again
in later chapters. You may have been concerned that in bringing up abortion before (for instance, in Case 32 about the possibility of aborting a fetus
with an XYY chromosome pattern), we did not deal explicitly with it as an
ethical issue; and so hopefully the discussion in this chapter has shown to
your satisfaction how seriously the abortion issue ought to be taken. Still,
there are some sorts of cases in which one must simply take for granted that
abortion is a moot issue, in order to look at some other ethical features of
the case. We will occasionally adopt this strategy elsewhere in this book.

CH. 11 ↓ **622**

# Research on Human Subjects 11

For many years, the fantastic advances made by medical science and technology in the last century — many of which relied heavily on research on human subjects — were accepted without criticism. Recently, however, as nuclear power plants threaten to contaminate the environment and as other undesirable consequences of "progress" multiply, people have become much more skeptical about the benefits offered by science and technology. The public no longer automatically trusts scientists to know what is good for them. In this atmosphere, naturally, the use of human beings as research subjects has been singled out as an area requiring more stringent regulation.    622 ↓

In previous chapters, we have tended to speak with some contempt of attempts to become ethical by following some code of ethics, and of the "Let's form a committee" approach to ethical dilemmas. Human research is interesting in this regard, because the codes of ethics and the committee approach have actually worked well in highlighting the difficult ethical issues and in raising the awareness of those engaged in research. In Chapter 9, we encountered a federal committee, the National Commission for the Protection of Human Subjects of Biomedical and Behavioral Research (hereafter referred to simply as the Commission), made up of 11 members representing medicine, science, ethics, law, and religion. We will have more to say about the various reports of the Commission in this chapter.    623 ↓

To start this chapter, we will depart from the usual format and insert a historical digression. This is appropriate because a few events have had a particular impact upon the ethical thinking in this area. Also, there might be a lesson in the problem of belated awareness, in the fact that problematic research had been going on for so long before anyone called attention to the basic ethical issues — issues that today seem obvious.    624 ↓

The first major dent in the idea that medical science could only be good came with the close of World War II, when the experiments conducted by Nazi doctors upon the concentration camp inmates were revealed to the world. Following the traditional route, the medical profession sought to prevent a recurrence of those horrors by establishing a code of ethics for research on humans. The first such code was the Nuremburg Code of 1949; an updated version is the widely cited Declaration of Helsinki of 1964 (see Appendix IX).    625 ↓

**626**  Despite all this, the general view within the medical profession was that unethical experimentation was carried out only by Nazis or similar degenerates, and so the problem was almost nonexistent in a humane country such as the United States. Thus, an article by Henry Beecher, a respected researcher in anesthesiology, landed like a bombshell when it was published in 1966. Not only did Beecher contend that as many as 12 percent of the studies being conducted by experienced researchers were unethical, but he gave specific examples of unethical research taken directly from scientific journals (with names omitted). Beecher stated: "During ten years of study of these matters it has become apparent that thoughtlessness and carelessness, not a willful disregard of the patient's rights, account for most of the cases encountered." *

↓   It is instructive to look at some typical examples cited by Beecher.

**627**  Example 3. This involved a study of the relapse rate in typhoid fever treated in two ways. In an earlier study by the present investigators, chloramphenicol had been recognized as an effective treatment for typhoid fever, being attended by half the mortality rate that was experienced when this agent was not used. Others had made the same observation, indicating that to withhold this effective remedy can be a life-or-death decision. The present study was carried out to determine the relapse rate under the two methods of treatment; of 408 charity patients, 251 were treated with chloramphenicol, of whom 20, or 7.97 percent, died. Symptomatic treatment was given, but chloramphenicol was withheld, in 157, of whom 36, or 22.9 percent died. According to the data presented, 23 patients died in the course of this study who would not have been expected to succumb if they had received specific ther-
↓  apy.

**628**  Example 12. This investigation was carried out to examine the possible effect of vagal [nerve] stimulation on cardiac arrest. Having been impressed with the number of reports of cardiac arrests that seemed to follow vagal stimulation, [the researchers] tested the effects of intrathoracic vagal stimulation during 30 of their surgical procedures, concluding, from these observations in patients under satisfactory anesthesia, that cardiac irregularities and cardiac arrest due to vagovagal reflex were less common than had previously been supposed.

In the kinds of surgery during which this experiment was carried out, the vagal stimulation was in no way necessary for the success of the therapeu-
↓  tic procedure. No mention of informed consent was made.

**629**  Example 17. Live cancer cells were injected into 22 human subjects as part of a study of immunity to cancer. According to a recent review, the subjects (hospitalized patients) were merely told that they would be receiving "some cells" . . . the word cancer was entirely omitted . . .

While Beecher mentioned no names, this same case was treated in more detail by Katz in his book, *Experimentation with Human Beings* (1972). The case illustrates the attitudes of at least a few medical scientists toward ethi-
↓  cal questions and the rights of patient-subjects.

* Reprinted, by permission. From H. K. Beecher, Ethics and clinical research. *New England Journal of Medicine* 274 : 1354, 1966.

In the early 1960s, a certain Dr. S. was conducting experiments to determine **630** natural immunity to cancer. For this purpose, he had been injecting patients at his hospital, as well as volunteers from prisons, with cancer cells, to see how effectively their bodies would reject the foreign tissue. There was at least some evidence that such injections might result in metastasis with a malignant tumor being formed in the patient's body. Despite this, Dr. S. wanted to do new experiments, in which the response of chronically ill patients (who supposedly had decreased immune response) would be compared with his healthy patients. For this he needed subjects who were chronically ill with diseases other than cancer, and he had no such patients at the two hospitals where he was working.                                            ↓

Dr. S. therefore wrote to a physician at J.C.D. Hospital to get permission to **631** use patients there for his research. He said in his letter:

You asked me if I obtained [written] permission from our patients before doing these studies. We do not do so at M. or J.E. hospitals since we regard this as a routine study, much less dramatic and hazardous than other routine procedures such as bone marrow aspiration and lumbar puncture. We do get signed permits from our volunteers at the Ohio State Penitentiary but this is because of the law-oriented personality of these men, rather than for medical reasons.*

Dr. S. somehow forgot to mention that at least one of these "routine" procedures done previously had produced what seemed to be metastatic cancer.                                            ↓

Dr. S. got permission to use patients at J.C.D. Hospital in New York, and **632** carried out the experiment described by Beecher as "Example 17." However, some of the staff physicians who were involved in the study — and who, unlike Dr. S., had some responsibility for the medical care of the chronically ill patients — raised some objections to the way the research was being conducted. The final result, after a number of months, was that a case against Dr. S. was brought before the New York State Board of Regents, which is responsible for licensing physicians in that state.                                            ↓

At the Board hearings, one doctor testified:                                            **633**

The patient was not told that the injection would contain cancer cells. The reason for this was that we did not wish to stir up any unnecessary anxiety, disturbances, or phobias in our patients. There was no need to tell the patients that the injected material contained cancer cells because it was of no consequence to the patient.*

The patients were asked to sign a consent form before entering the experiment, but the information about the true nature of the experiment was withheld.                                            ↓

* From J. Katz, with A. M. Capron and E. S. Glass, *Experimentation with Human Beings.* New York: Russell Sage Foundation, 1972. Pp. 663–664.

**634** In a news interview during the hearings, one reporter (who was apparently familiar with the ethical decision-making short cut we described in Chapter 2) asked Dr. S. if he would be willing to accept an injection of cancer cells into his own bloodstream. Dr. S. said he would not, because "there are relatively few trained cancer researchers, and it seems stupid to take even that
↓ little risk."

REVIEW SHORT CUT ↑ 45

**635** How did this study stand under the then current (1963) codes of ethics for human experimentation? You can see that it violates several parts of Section III of the Declaration of Helsinki, which was adopted in 1964. It also was in violation of the then current U.S. Public Health Service policy. It was not in violation of the then current AMA code of ethics; that code merely required that the experiment be conducted by skilled medical investigators, be based on animal experimentation, and be conducted with the voluntary consent of the patient (not necessarily informed). In 1966 the AMA updated
↓ its code to conform more with the Declaration of Helsinki.

REVIEW CODES ↑ 67–68

**636** While the provisions of these codes apparently had not been impressed on Dr. S., the Board of Regents was in agreement with them: Dr. S. and a colleague were censured for unethical experimentation. This ruling was not unanimously accepted by the medical profession, as shown by a letter from a physician to the *New York Herald Tribune,* Jan. 26, 1964:

Here, then, we have a wide possibility: If there is such a thing as a biological mechanism as a defense against cancer, then it may be possible to stimulate it either before cancer strikes or perhaps even later when cancer has taken hold. This is the question Dr. S. is trying to pursue. It would be a shame if a squabble over who told
↓ what to whom should destroy a thrilling lead in cancer research.

**637** As for the views of Dr. S.'s colleagues in the research sphere, these were made known quite plainly. The American Association for Cancer Research elected Dr. S. as its vice-president in 1968 and as its president in 1969.

Since that time, the public awareness on the ethics of experimentation has been increasing, culminating with the outcry over the exposure of the U.S. Public Health Tuskegee syphilis study (see Curran, 1973), in which there was evidence that several hundred black males, over a 25-year period, had been deprived of treatment for their disease even after it had become known that penicillin was a highly effective antisyphilitic agent. Given this public mood, it is likely that a scientific body would think twice before be-
↓ stowing public praise on Dr. S. today.

We have now seen the kinds of research that have caused the ethical controversy surrounding research on human subjects and the kinds of attitudes that caused the practices to arise in the first place. However, we would not want to lose sight of the fact that these criticisms are applicable only to <u>some</u> research on humans. For example, soldier volunteers, who certainly knew at first hand what risks they were running, participated in the experiments around 1900 that proved that yellow fever was transmitted by mosquitoes. The research design showed compulsive attention to informed consent and to the continuing welfare of the subjects. Also, as Altman (1972) reminds us, there is a long tradition of scientists using themselves as subjects in some of their riskiest experiments.    ↓

**638**

Before we start discussing appropriate ethical guidelines for medical research, however, it will help to be sure that we know what we're talking about. This has not necessarily been a simple task to accomplish. A lot of the writing on the ethics of research on humans has focused on two potential confusions — between research and practice and between therapeutic and nontherapeutic research.    ↓

**639**

Many physicians have pointed out that, because of the uncertainties that pervade the study of medicine, there is an element of experimentation in all of medical practice. Even when you give a patient penicillin for a strep throat, you cannot be sure that the patient won't have a previously undiscovered allergy to penicillin, or that the patient won't develop a brand new adverse reaction to penicillin that has never been seen before. Therefore, this argument goes, there can be no sharp distinction between research and medical practice, so that we cannot be sure just where the proposed guidelines will apply.    ↓

**640**

Another problem is the distinction between therapeutic research, where the goal is both to benefit the subject and to gain new knowledge, and nontherapeutic research, where new knowledge alone is sought. Various codes of research ethics, such as the Helsinki Declaration, emphasize this distinction, suggesting particularly that nontherapeutic research needs more stringent safeguards to protect the subjects. But here again, the distinction is a fuzzy one. Suppose, as often happens, half the subjects in a study are randomly assigned to get the experimental treatment for their illness, and half to get a placebo (dummy) treatment. Is this experiment therapeutic because each subject has a one-in-two chance of getting the new treatment, or nontherapeutic because he has a one-in-two chance of getting no treatment at all?    ↓

**641**

**642**  As analyzed by Levine (1979), the Commission, in their several reports, had to grapple with these two problems. In doing so, they solicited position papers from many of the most prominent philosophers and medical ethicists in the country. Their final conclusion was that the research vs. practice distinction was more clear than most people thought, and that the therapeutic–nontherapeutic distinction simply didn't have to be made at all.

**643**  The Commission was able to make a clear distinction between research and practice by noting that <u>experimentation</u> may be put both to research and to practical uses. The doctor who juggles the doses of his patient's antihypertensive medications to see if he can get better control of blood pressure without excessive side effects is experimenting, in that he doesn't know beforehand what dose will be best; but he is experimenting within the context of medical practice, as the patient's benefit is the main goal, and any new knowledge gained would be purely coincidental (i.e., knowledge of wider applicability beyond that one patient's case).

**644**  A good example of the research–practice distinction is seen in drugs that have not yet been given approval by the Food and Drug Administration. Trials using these drugs are done to establish their safety and efficacy. Such trials constitute research, since they are done for the primary purpose of gathering new knowledge. The subjects of the research may incidentally improve because of the drug treatment, but this is not the primary aim. At the same time, an individual physician might decide to give one of his patients the same drug — perhaps because he feels the patient would not respond to any of the alternative therapies. (We hope that he gets the patient's informed consent to do this, of course.) This physician is clearly experimenting with the drug, since he doesn't know whether it will work or not, but he is not doing research. His main purpose is to help the patient.

**645**  The Commission took the opposite tack with the therapeutic–nontherapeutic distinction. As they proceeded to their later reports, they concluded that this distinction added nothing to the clarity of their proposals.

One might think that in a nontherapeutic situation one has to safeguard the rights of the subjects more carefully. On the other hand, since a therapeutic experiment holds out more hope of benefit for the subject, there might be more pressure on the subject to volunteer in that case.

In the end, the National Commission decided it was simpler to look at the risk involved in the research, increasing required safeguards in proportion to increasing risk.

The Commission considered various levels of risk. First, being a part of an **646** experiment might involve "mere inconvenience." That is, the risk of harm is no greater than the chances of accidents occurring during normal, daily life. Next, one might distinguish "minimal risk," which is a bit more than the risk of daily activities, but no more than the risks of routine medical examinations — here we might include experiments that require minor interventions, such as drawing blood. Finally, one encounters experiments that entail "more than minimal risk." It is in this last category that it is most important to ask whether the subjects have been adequately protected, and whether there is some benefit to them that counterbalances the increased risks.  ↓

It is also important to put the risk of experimentation into perspective. Be- **647** cause of the publicity given to some particular abuses, it is easy to conclude that being a research subject is a highly dangerous business. But Cardon (1976), in a survey including 133,000 subjects, found 57 injuries resulting in death or permanent disability, all of which occurred during treatment that could have been expected to benefit the patient. Cardon concluded that the risk of nontherapeutic research was no greater than the risks of everyday life, and the risks of therapeutic research were no greater than the risks of medical treatment in other settings.  ↓

Next, we shall consider one approach to determining the ethics of an ex- **648** periment. Recall the praise the *Herald Tribune* letter-writer had for the potential of the line of research Dr. S. was pursuing. The implication was clear that if good results came out of the experiment, it would have been worthwhile, and "squabbles over who told what to whom" would be irrelevant. On the other side of the coin, a speaker at a symposium on the controversial Willowbrook experiment, in which retarded children in a state home were inoculated with hepatitis virus in hopes of eventually developing a vaccine, stated that the experiment was unethical in part because no vaccine had been discovered. (This speaker was premature; the researchers have since published reports of an experimental vaccine.)  ↓

Are the results of an experiment the legitimate guide to whether an experi- **649** ment is ethical or not? *Recall that the purpose of ethical decision making is not to allow us to decide whether to praise or blame other people for what they have done in the past. If ethics is to be of any use, it must be a guide for what we ought to do now.* We can't wait for the results to come in to decide if an experiment we propose is unethical — we must predict as best we can the possible consequences and compare these with our values. What are the consequences of doing an experiment such as Dr. S. did without informed consent, in terms of the future trust of the public in the medical profession? Would people go to doctors if they felt that they could never know if they were being treated or if they were being experimented upon?

**649**
**cont.** How do these risks compare with the slight advantage in terms of convenience of getting subjects by not informing them? Those are the ethical
↓ questions.

**650** While an act is either ethical or unethical at the time it is performed and
does not become one or the other later by virtue of hindsight, the ethical
method makes clear nevertheless that the intended outcomes of the experiment, and their likelihood of achievement, are among the consequences that must be fed into the ethical equation. Specifically, the potential benefits to be gained, both by the individual and by society as a whole,
must be weighed against the risks of untoward side effects to the individ-
↓ ual. This is what is referred to by the common term, "risk–benefit ratio."

**651** However, the innocent-sounding term risk–benefit ratio conceals within it
a major ethical dispute: how risks to one individual are to be weighed
against benefits to others. Although on many ethical issues, different moral
theories give the same answer, on this one the major moral theories are
clearly divided. To a classical utilitarian, people are interchangeable units;
the concern is for the sum total (or the average) of net gain over net loss
(pleasure over pain) that is produced. Thus, research that puts a few individuals at great risk but which produces great benefits for a multitude
↓ would win utilitarian approval.

**652** We saw briefly in Chapter 2 that this feature of utilitarian ethics, which
would permit a few to be sacrificed for the greater good, was often used as
an argument against utilitarian ethics. By contrast, a deontologist, or someone who based ethical decisions on a priori rights and duties, would em-
↓ phasize the need to protect the few who are at risk.
REVIEW RESPECT ↑ 79–84

**653** We have already taken a position in this debate. By accepting autonomy
and respect for the individual as major values in our consequentialist scale,
we agreed with those that weighed the harm to a few as counting more,
morally speaking, than some greater good for the many. We justified this, in
part, by calling attention to the aims of medicine. And a similar argument
applies to research: When we talk of the future benefits to society, it's easy
to forget that the results of research are supposed to contribute to medical
practice, and that medical practice is in the business of aiding individuals
directly, not society. Therefore, any moral approach that justifies harming
some group of individuals now, in order to help another group later, seems
↓ very inconsistent with that argument.

This, in turn, raises a point that might come up from a libertarian perspec-    **654**
tive: It might be argued that the entire ethical problem of research boils
down to informed consent. If an individual freely consents to become involved as a subject, that's all we need to know. The risk–benefit ratio, and
other possible harms, are his lookout, not ours. Then, we can turn our attention to the use of children, the mentally retarded, and other groups that
are incapable of consenting.    ↓

It is certainly true that in groups who are incompetent to give informed    **655**
consent, or whose consent is given with questionable freedom, the ethical
problems of research are multiplied. We will deal with these problems at
some length later. But we can still argue that we have moral obligations to
the normal, competent research subject that go beyond mere informed
consent.    ↓

The argument for protection of the consenting research subject is similar to    **656**
the one we used in describing the doctor–patient contract. We emphasized
that the doctor–patient contract was not one of "let-the-buyer-beware,"
but one in which one party accepted an obligation to look out for the
other's interests — that is, a fiduciary contract. We felt this was appropriate
because of the imbalance of factual knowledge and expertise between the
two parties. We can apply the same perspective here — since the research
investigator is likely to have a much more thorough understanding of the
medical risks and benefits, he has some additional obligation toward the
subject. But this obligation does not replace the need for informed consent,
because only the subject can relate the risks and benefits to his own set of
personal values.    ↓

REVIEW CONTRACT ↑ 131

If the institution of medical science has an obligation to protect its research    **657**
subjects, it also has an obligation to try to maximize the usefulness of the
research results. After all, most people who consent to research do so because they hope to make a contribution to the future. If, because of faulty
experimental design, the resulting information is not useful, we will be
adding, to the harm of whatever risk is included in the experiment, the
harm of having prevented this desired contribution. Therefore, the technical design of experiments becomes a legitimate area for ethical inquiry.    ↓

**658**   Most research reported by physicians before the middle of the twentieth century is of little use — the biases of the observer colored the data in a way that is impossible to detect and allow for. Modern experimental design employs several methods to control observer bias and to assure a high probability that differences observed between treatments are real differences, not due to bias or chance. These devices include:

> The randomized study. A pool of subjects is chosen with the desired characteristics and randomly assigned to receive either the control or the experimental treatment. This prevents, for example, the experimental treatment appearing to work well because the less sick subjects were chosen to receive it.
>
> The controlled study. Some subjects get a control treatment, often a dummy or placebo. If this group does as well as the group getting the experimental treatment, it is then known that the improvement cannot be due to the experimental treatment.
>
> The double-blind study. Neither experimenter nor subject knows who is getting the control and who is getting the experimental treatment, until after the study. This eliminates bias due to unconscious expectations. Many modern studies contain all three of these devices.

**659**   Where no clearly effective standard treatment exists, or where the disease under study is minor, the control group will probably be given an inert placebo (made to resemble the experimental drug, so that the study will be double-blind). But where an effective therapy already exists, the control group may get that therapy, and the experimental treatment will be compared to the standard existing treatment.

**660**   In a therapeutic situation, the ethical question arises of whether a controlled, double-blind study can be undertaken at all. If the two groups are being given drug A and drug B in order to learn which is better and both are known to be somewhat effective against the disease, then the experiment presents minimal ethical problems in that regard. But suppose that you have a new drug that you strongly suspect (but have no proof) is effective against a disease for which there is now no treatment? Is it ethical to deprive half of your sick subjects of this potentially healing drug? And if it is, how would you go about obtaining informed consent for this controlled study?

The dilemma, of course, originates in the uncertainty. If you <u>knew</u> that your    **661**
drug was effective, you would not be doing the experiment. And the his-
tory of medicine is full of highly touted remedies, which upon later
scientific investigation turned out to be worse than the disease. Right now
it looks as if the randomly selected and unknown control subjects are the
unlucky ones. If, on the other hand, the drug later turns out to have a highly
fatal and unanticipated side effect, the control group will have been the
lucky ones. Thus one could just as well argue that it would be unethical <u>not</u>
to have a control group, in order to give at least 50 percent of the patients
the chance to escape any unforeseen side effects.                              ↓

It may be in some cases, however, that in choosing the optimal experimen-    **662**
tal design to generate good data, not enough alternatives are explored.
Weinstein (1974) has criticized the notion that only trials in which subjects
are randomly assigned to the experimental and control groups are statistically valid. Randomization as a strategy has both strong and weak points,
and in some experiments patient self-selection would work as well. Weinstein also encourages more use of adaptive designs: Instead of waiting for
all the data to tabulate results, one feeds in the data as the experiment is
proceeding, so that if one of the two therapies starts to show clear superior-
ity, the minimum number of subjects will have been exposed to the inferior
treatment.                                                                    ↓

---

## CASE 43

You are the chief investigator of the Veterans Administration Cooperative    **663**
Study Group on Antihypertensive Agents. This group was formed because,
while it was known that a number of drugs were effective in reducing the
blood pressure of people with essential hypertension, there has been considerable debate as to whether just reducing the blood pressure is effective
in preventing the sequelae of hypertension — heart attack, stroke, and so
on. To decide this question, it was felt that a controlled study was needed.
In order to get several hundred patients in both the experimental and control groups, a number of hospitals have been enlisted in the study. The
study is planned to last 5½ years and you have received funding for this
period.
     The experiment began in 1963. You are now reviewing some interim re-
ports of data collected after the subjects have been in the study for an average of 16 months. In this particular group, the patients were those who had
a diastolic blood pressure between 115 and 129 mmHg at the beginning.
     In the experimental group, which has been receiving antihypertensive
medication, there has been one stroke and one instance of drug toxicity.
The latter resolved itself without permanent damage when the drug combination was readjusted.

**663**
cont.
In the control group, which has been getting placebos instead of active drugs, four patients have died as a result of conditions attributable to their high blood pressure. An additional 10 patients have developed signs of more severe hypertension and have been removed from the study for treatment. There have also been two heart attacks, two cases of congestive heart failure, and one stroke.

Your statisticians assure you that the differences so far between the control and experimental groups are statistically significant.

↓ What do you do now?

---

**664** The action taken, as a matter of fact, was to discontinue the study. The group felt that the continuation of the study beyond this point would provide no information more convincing than what was already available, and that under such circumstances it would be unethical to go on depriving the control subjects of what you now know is effective treatment. (In the group with blood pressure less than 115 mmHg, the results were more equivocal, and that study was allowed to go the full 5½ years; the end results con-
↓ firmed the effectiveness of antihypertensive treatment in that group also.)

**665** More basic than the question of research design, however, is the question of how the research setting alters the doctor–patient relationship. The usual doctor–patient encounter is characterized by the fact that the doctor's activities are intended for the primary benefit of the patient; the benefit to the doctor, society, and other parties is a secondary matter. But in research (especially if we agree with the definitions proposed by the National Commission), the intended beneficiary is society at large, through the expansion of medical knowledge. In practice, the reputation and fame of the individual investigator is often a major driving force as well. The patient's benefit is a secondary consideration. (In fact, if the research is designed so that the subjects derive major benefits, the motivation is not to help that class of people, but rather to insure that a sufficient number of subjects will volunteer!)

By this analysis, the fact that the researchers wear white coats and stethoscopes, have "M.D." after their names, and demonstrate an unfeigned concern for the well-being of their subjects, is an incidental, not an essential
↓ feature of the relationship between researchers and subjects.

In a nontherapeutic trial, therefore, it seems a gross misuse of words to call **666** the subject the investigator's "patient." The therapeutic trial seems to have some elements of the doctor–patient relationship, but it has other elements that are foreign to it as well. Suppose a patient in the experimental group develops some previously unobserved symptom that might be a side effect of the drug. As a doctor, the researcher's first obligation would be to stop the drug. As a researcher, however, he is strongly tempted to continue the drug in order to get new data about this unexpected discovery. There seems to be a strong conflict of interest here. While in other experimental situations the conflict might be considerably less, it seems that, by the very nature of experimentation, the conflict can never be completely eliminated. ↓

*Awareness of this problem has led many authorities to the conclusion that* **667** *the investigator–subject relationship is inherently different from the doctor–patient relationship; and to place a person into an experiment where he is solely under the care of the investigator is to deprive the person of medical attention. If the patient's own doctor cannot continue his care during the experiment, the investigating group must include a medically competent "patient advocate" distinct from the investigator, who has the power to remove the person from the experiment as soon as it appears to him that continuation would be detrimental to the patient's health.* An institution cannot receive a research grant from the Public Health Service unless it has made provision for safeguarding the rights of the individual subjects in this manner. Other funding agencies are establishing similar policies. ↓

We should note that this distinction, which is so clear to ethicists, may well **668** be unclear to the patient–subject, as John Fletcher (1967) has reported from interviews with experimental subjects. When a person walks up to the bed wearing a white coat and asks them how they feel today, the patients immediately tend to regard this individual as "their doctor" and often do not perceive that he has interests in the matter very different from those of the usual doctor–patient encounter. This problem is especially prominent when, as often happens, a nontherapeutic trial is "piggybacked" on a therapeutic one, and patients already enrolled in the therapeutic study are asked to be subjects for the additional experiment as well. Patients may mistakenly confuse the two studies and feel that if they refuse to join in the nontherapeutic one, they will be excluded from treatment.

This problem of patient misunderstandings has important implications for the next facet of the experimentation issue — informed consent. ↓

## CASE 44

**669** You are the director of a community hospital in Lansing. A Michigan State University faculty member approaches you with the following request.

He is doing research on the laboratory diagnosis of certain infectious diseases, and wants to know how the reactions of blood serum from the general population compare with reactions of serum of individuals with known infectious disease, as far as his new tests are concerned. He requests permission to ask your pathologist for the serum that is left over from the tests that have been run on blood from hospitalized patients. Generally, slightly more blood is drawn from the patient than is required, to guard against spoiling a test, and any excess is just discarded into the sink.

You ask whether he intends to pool the serum or to keep it in individual samples. He says that he intends to keep the samples separate so that, if he should turn up a very abnormal result, he could check the hospital records on that patient to see if any information there might explain the abnormal test.

↓ Would you approve of this request?

---

**670** In your consideration of this request, did you think about the presence or lack of provision to obtain informed consent?

At first glance, this may seem silly. What difference does it make to a patient if you use some of his serum that is already drawn and that would otherwise end up in the sewer?

However, remember what was said in Chapter 5 — that what is routine to you as an expert may not be at all routine from the patient's viewpoint. Suppose you do turn up an abnormal test and want to look into the patient's record to explain it. Does the patient want people who are not directly involved in his medical care snooping into his files? And even if you don't look into the record, many patients might well have had some disease in the past that they do not want others to know about, but which you could detect with your tests. Don't you have an obligation to get the patient's consent before you take a chance on invading his privacy in this
↓ manner? (See the hospital patient's "Bill of Rights" in Appendix III.)

**671** By the levels of risk proposed by the Commission, this experiment would probably fall into the "mere inconvenience" category. This is not to say that our concern over informed consent is misplaced, but rather that our duties to disclose are lessened commensurately with the risk. In this case, a form added to the admission papers informing prospective patients at this hospital that the research is being conducted, and that they may opt to not have their serum used might suffice. If the risk of harm, embarrassment, or loss of privacy were greater, we might be obligated by this principle to go to
↓ greater lengths to inform the prospective subjects.

In Case 44, once the idea of informed consent occurs to you, it is not hard    **672**
to figure out what you would say to the patient in order to obtain his informed consent. But go back to the situation of the double-blind therapeutic trial. The full, morally relevant information is as follows: You are suffering from a disease for which there is now no good treatment; we have a
treatment that might help you but we cannot be sure; we do not know the
risks and the true risks might be very significant, even worse than your disease; if you agree to enter the study you will be randomly assigned to one
of two groups; you have a 50–50 chance of receiving a placebo therapy instead of the real treatment; neither you nor we will know which group you
are in; if, at any point, your life or health seems to be endangered by the
experiment, we will remove you from the study and give you any treatment
necessary. Are you ethically obligated to tell all of this to the patient, or
only some of it? If you tell all of it, how many people will agree to take part
in the experiment? If, as a result of a full disclosure, you have too few subjects to get good results, are you meeting your obligation to society and to
medical science?                                                                  ↓

*Presumably the answer to this problem is clear. If informed consent is to*      **673**
*mean what it says, then a full disclosure of all the relevant information —*
*including admission of uncertainty where it exists and revealing any al-*
*ternative sources of treatment that may be available — would seem to be an*
*absolute requirement. If this procedure leads to too few subjects, this will*
*have social implications, which we will turn to later.*                           ↓

It's worth repeating here that the idea of informed consent is rooted in the    **674**
value of autonomy. The purpose of informed consent, here as well as in
therapeutic medicine, is to allow the patient the opportunity to exercise
individual autonomy. Upon basic, ethical analysis, the purpose of informed
consent in research on human subjects is <u>not</u> any of the following:

1. To get people to volunteer for research that will be of great benefit to
   society.
2. To scare people away from volunteering for experiments that entail
   significant risk.
3. To protect the researcher from possible lawsuits later.
4. To retard the progress of science by multiplying the red tape.
5. To avoid the need to look critically at research design and the risk–
   benefit ratio for the subjects.

Some of these items may be consequences of the informed consent procedure, depending on what procedure is used (and there are many alternative
procedures that may be used for any particular case). But none of these
reasons reveal the basic purpose of informed consent.                             ↓

REVIEW AUTONOMY ↑ 79–84

**675**  Therefore, informed consent, along with protecting the well-being of subjects by concern for proper research design and for the risk–benefit ratio, forms a major issue in deciding whether a particular research proposal is ethically acceptable. It follows that the most difficult ethical decisions in research involve groups who cannot give informed consent in the usual sense. These groups fall into two basic categories:

1. Some groups we have already cited as being unable to give informed consent in any case — research or otherwise. These include children and the mentally retarded.
2. Other groups are competent and can be adequately informed, but their consent may be suspect because of possible coercion. The group most often discussed in this category is prisoners, who in the past have made up a large and available body of potential subjects. (We might also want to include here medical and graduate students.)

**676**  On the question of informed consent, Beecher (1966) is quite dogmatic:

Ordinary patients will not knowingly risk their health or their life for the sake of "science." Every experienced clinical investigator knows this. When such risks are taken and a considerable number of patients are involved, it may be assumed that informed consent has not been obtained in all cases.*

Otherwise, presumably, it was obtained under some sort of duress.

On the issue of prisoner subjects, one extreme point of view states that, in the worst-run prison experiments, the authorities threaten the prisoners with various punishments unless they "volunteer" and often do this behind the back of the researcher. In the best-run trials, the prisoners are either led to believe or allowed to believe that their participation will possibly lead to an earlier parole. In either case, the consent is obtained under a form of duress and cannot be considered voluntary. Therefore all experiments of a nontherapeutic nature involving prisoners is unethical.

**677**  It could be said that no one can ever give consent without being under some form or duress, internal or external. The question therefore boils down to how much duress is tolerable before the consent becomes truly involuntary. For example, we might conclude that a prisoner can give voluntary consent, if he is fully informed, even if the idea of an earlier parole is held out to him. After all, if the risk of the experiment is great, a rational prisoner would decide that an extra year in jail is preferable so long as he emerges in one piece; and if the risk is smaller, who is better qualified than the prisoner to weigh the size of the risk against an earlier opportunity for freedom? On the other hand, we might conclude that the threat of being beaten by the guards would be a clearly unacceptable amount of duress.

* Reprinted, by permission. From H. K. Beecher, Ethics and clinical research. *New England Journal of Medicine* 274 : 1354, 1966.

Another interesting counterview is that a truly repentant prisoner might **677** regret his crime against society and might sincerely wish to try to make cont. amends through some degree of personal sacrifice. Right now, he can do so by volunteering for an experiment. This argument would hold that it would be unethical to deprive him of this opportunity by deciding to discontinue such experiments in the future. (This argument might sound good coming from a prison chaplain. If it came from a researcher, we might suspect some conflict of interest.) ↓

A simplistic debate of the form experiment vs. don't experiment on pris- **678** oners violates our cardinal rule of ethical methodology — first be sure you have looked at all the alternatives. A more useful question might be: Given that certain features of being a prisoner make voluntary consent more problematic and coercion more likely, to what extent can those features be minimized while still allowing the prison to function as a prison?

To take only one example, one feature of prison life that might exert un- due influence on the subject's choice is that being part of an experiment may be the only available way to earn money in the prison or to relieve the boredom of prison existence. This feature could be minimized by refusing to do research in prisons that did not have a variety of other activities avail- able to prisoners and that did not offer other opportunities to earn money. It could be further stipulated that the amounts paid to the experimental subjects should not be out of line with what the prisoner could earn at other prison jobs. (This line of reasoning inevitably involves the ethics-of- research issue with the prison-reform issue and thus quickly runs up against political forces outside of science and medicine.) ↓

The Commission in its report on prison research considered this line of rea- **679** soning, but its studies of actual prison conditions gave it a pessimistic out- look on acceptably reducing the risk of coercion. Its report does not pro- pose total banning of research in prisons, as the one extreme view would call for, but it places severe restrictions that, if implemented, would tend to discourage prison research for the most part. In particular, investigators would be required to show that their study could not be done as well if subjects other than prisoners were used. ↓

Another factor that might be termed duress has been observed to arise from **680** illness itself, not from incarceration. John Fletcher (1967) and others have reported that experimental subjects sometimes seem to have a high level of the guilt that is part of the "sick role" in our society — guilt that comes from perceiving oneself as a burden on others without being able to perform a socially useful function in return. Participating in an experiment for the good of society is an excellent way of assuaging this guilt, and a researcher, deliberately or not, may play upon these guilt feelings (which are often un- recognized by the patient himself, and therefore more easily manipulated) in order to obtain a consent that might otherwise not have been offered. ↓

**681** Problems with the other category of subjects are illustrated by the question of research on children. The report of the Commission on children, as summarized by Jonsen (1978), contains a number of recommendations, most of which are on matters that are open to ready agreement. The Commission agreed that research on children is essential if this group is to continue to receive advanced medical care, since results of drug and other studies in adults cannot necessarily be generalized to children due to basic biologic differences. They approved research on children that did not involve more than minimal risk, and research that involved more than minimal risk but where the child stood to benefit — such as where the experimental treatment was the only effective treatment known for the condition. They required consent of the parents and the "assent" of an older child who could give it ("assent" because it serves to respect the child as an individual but is not legally binding). They also, for reasons we have discussed, rejected the notion of proxy consent to describe the role of the parents in consenting to
↓ research for their children.
REVIEW PARENTAL CONSENT ↑ 383–387

**682** The Commission then had to face the most difficult case — research that could be done only on sick children, which held out the hope of major benefits for later generations of children with those diseases, but which offered little or no chance of benefit for the presently sick children. Research on many of the most serious childhood diseases, now regarded as
↓ incurable, falls into this category.

**683** Again, fairly polarized views have emerged on this issue. Taking one extreme, Ramsey (1976) has suggested that it would be a violation of the child's autonomy and a violation of our duties to protect children, to subject a child to any experiment that entails any significant risk and that cannot benefit the child. Arguing against Ramsey, McCormick (1974) has pointed out a duty to aid the public welfare, which children share along with adults, and which children need to be taught as part of proper child rearing. In some cases, this duty could lead to an ethical requirement to participate in research even if some risk and no benefit for the child were
↓ involved.

**684** The Commission here tried to find a middle ground. There is no denying the clash of values — unfettered research would lead to harming a few children with no corresponding benefit to them, while stopping all such research would deprive future children of new therapies.

The Commission pointed out that there is a large class of experiments that involve no benefit and more than minimal risk to the subjects, but in which the risk is not much greater than that demanded by the routine therapy for that child's illness. Where the benefits of research appear to be great, the Commission endorsed this class of experiments. For example, a spinal tap involves more than minimal risk, while still not being very risky

compared to other medical interventions. If a child's illness demands re-  **684**
peated spinal taps as part of routine treatment, then an additional spinal  cont.
tap for research purposes does not seem morally wrong (provided other
requirements, including consent and assent, are met).  ↓

Some important research on children does not fit into this class. One exam-  **685**
ple would be the initial trials of the Salk polio vaccine, were it to be developed today. The trials would have to be done on healthy children who
would otherwise not have any medical procedures performed on them;
and before the vaccine was tested, no one could say for sure that some of
the children would not contract polio from the vaccine. However, the value
of the perfected vaccine for all children could not be questioned. The Commission left an escape route by suggesting that such research proposals not
falling into its other categories might be reviewed by some national ethics
board. This could be attacked as another example of the "Let's form a committee" syndrome; but on balance, it is probably better than either a blanket ban, or else trying to specify in advance all possible cases that might
arise in the future.  ↓

What ethical principles could justify doing risky research on children who  **686**
will not benefit directly? Ramsey (1976) denies that such a principle exists.
If we do such research because of some overriding public need, Ramsey
argues, we are doing wrong and we simply have to acknowledge that sometimes the practicalities of an imperfect world force us to do wrong. This
argument demands respect as it is certainly superior to facile rationalizations.  ↓

But we might, instead, look at other instances of agreeing to allow a child to  **687**
do something that may be risky, when the child cannot give consent himself. Some such acts are wrong, but others are justified on paternalistic
grounds. One way of justifying paternalism is the notion of restrospective
consent — the child afterwards, now fully competent, would look back and
agree that the action was in his own best interests and would retrospec-
tively approve of the action. (Example: "Now that I've just won the
Tchaikovsky Prize, I'm glad that my mother forced me to practice the piano
every day since I was three, even though I used to hate it.")  ↓ **689**
PATERNALISM WRONG?* 688

---

* In Chapter 4 we spoke disparagingly of paternalism when it arose in the  **688**
form of the priestly model, because it was wrongly applied to competent
adults who could make their own decisions. Children, however, lack the
capacity for meaningful autonomy, and so paternalism is appropriate in
their case.  ↓

**689** With this idea of justifying paternalism in mind, suppose that we have a research project with the following points:

1. Authorities agree that the potential benefits are of great value.
2. The research can only be done on children.
3. Some risk is involved, but the chances that a particular child will be harmed is small.
4. If the research could be done on adults, rational and informed adults would consent to it.
5. We have good reason to believe that children who now become research subjects would, looking back later, approve of this choice on their behalf.
6. The parents, fully informed, do give their consent, and the children, when old enough, assent also.
7. Other requirements for ethical research are met.

We could conclude from all this that it would be ethical to proceed with this research project. A skeptic could argue with us on several points, such as challenging us to say exactly what we mean by "good reason" in the fifth point. But cases such as the polio vaccine trials give us an intuitive idea of ↓ the sort of research project we might have in mind.

---

## CASE 45

**690** Two of the pediatric patients in your practice are sisters, aged 5 years and 18 months, who suffer from hyperargininemia. This hereditary disease, in which cells cannot produce the enzyme arginase, leads to high levels of the amino acid arginine in the blood and spinal fluid and, over a period of time, to severe mental retardation as a result. The older sister is already severely affected and the younger seems to be developing the same way.

You are approached by a scientist who wants to inject Shope papilloma virus into the children. Rabbit experiments have suggested that injection of this virus leads to increased levels of arginase and hence decreased blood levels of arginine. It is hypothesized that the virus carries a gene for its own kind of arginase, and once the viral genes get into the cell, the cell can make this kind of arginase.

The scientist has since observed that 35 percent of lab workers exposed to papilloma virus have lowered serum arginine levels, without showing any signs of disease. Thus, he concludes, there are grounds for believing that injecting the virus into the sisters could lower their arginine levels without harmful side effects. At any rate, he says, considering their quality of life as severely retarded individuals if nothing is done, the experiment is worth a try.

On further questioning he acknowledges that some other experiments suggest that instead of having its own gene, the virus merely stimulates the cell to make more arginase from its own genes. This undermines the rationale for the treatment in the case of these sisters, where there is no cellular gene present at all. Also, he admits that many viruses previously thought to be harmless are now thought to cause serious disease after remaining in the body for a long, dormant period, up to years. The diseases that might be caused this way include a number of different types of cancer. Even considering all these factors, however, he still wants to make the trial.

A week later the parents of the sisters come in and ask, for the umpteenth time, whether anything can be done for their children.

Do you tell them about the scientist's proposal? If so, do you recommend to them that they adopt it or not? If you think the experiment itself is ethical, how do you go about obtaining adequate, voluntary informed consent?

(Adapted from case of the Hastings Center, Ethical issues Hippocrates did not have to face. In *Medical World News*, July 14, 1972. Pp. 39–40.)

---

It is clear that this case fits the category of a therapeutic trial so that, from a legal view, the parents are competent to consent on behalf of the girls. If there is any chance that the treatment might help, would it be ethical for you to withhold information about the possibility of this from the parents? Recalling the doctor–patient contract, we would like to say no immediately. But there might be another consideration here. In this case, the risks are of a fairly sophisticated nature and require a fair amount of biologic knowledge to interpret. If the parents do not appear to be well educated, the physician might think twice about their ability to assimilate the information and weigh it properly to reach a rational decision.

As to how the risks and benefits are to be weighed — what is your opinion of the scientist's reference to the quality of life of the girls? Suppose in addition to the severe mental retardation the older sister also had a heart defect requiring major surgery, and the question arose of whether to do the surgery or allow the girl to die. How would you decide in that instance? Does your willingness or unwillingness to allow the girl to die in that instance suggest how much weight you might give to the risks of the experiment? (That is, if you are prepared to allow the girl to die due to her low quality of life, would it be inconsistent to reject this experiment because it carries an unknown risk of a fatal disease in the future?)

Case 45 illustrates fairly well the kind of risk-benefit ratio calculations that are required in instances of therapeutic experimentation and the problems of informed consent by proxy. Incidentally, this case was based on a real one, which was reported in Germany. The pediatrician did agree to the experiment; but, as of 3 years after the treatment was begun, it has apparently been unsuccessful.

## CASE 46

694  In late March 1973, a three-judge panel of the Wayne County Circuit Court began hearings on the case of "John Doe," who had spent the last 18 of his 35 years in Ionia state mental hospital after confessing to murder and rape. According to hospital authorities, he has been subject to uncontrollable rages and has not responded to any therapy.

John Doe was scheduled to undergo tests to see whether he should have psychosurgery, under a research project financed by the state of Michigan and to be carried out by Wayne State University faculty at Lafayette Clinic in Detroit. However, a suit was filed charging that Doe and other Ionia prisoners were being held unconstitutionally without trials, and that no person so confined could consent voluntarily to become part of such an experiment.

The court is hearing conflicting testimony. The director of the experiment says the operation is to destroy the part of John Doe's brain responsible for his "uncontrollable aggression," and that no surgery would be done unless electrodes implanted into the brain reveal a localized, abnormal brain wave pattern. A psychiatrist on the faculty defends the research protocol as fully adequate and adds that the experiment is not psychosurgery, since the abnormal waves would be indicative of local organic pathology.

A neurologist attacks the view that abnormal brain waves are diagnostic of abnormal behavior, and further notes that implantation of electrodes for such a test is itself a very risky procedure. A second psychiatrist attacks the research protocol as wholly inadequate and states, "If it produced any useful information, it would be almost by accident."

A third psychiatrist who spent 5 hours interviewing John Doe states that he found no evidence for any anger other than a normal and justified response to the poor conditions of the institution. He adds that it cannot be said that John Doe did not respond to conventional therapy, since no adequate therapy exists at Ionia.

John Doe's parents testify that they had signed the consent form for the experiment without reading it, without ever talking to any of the doctors, and without realizing that surgery was involved.

John Doe himself testifies that he gave his consent because he saw it as the only avenue to freedom, and that he has changed his mind after the court suit began, when the testimony indicated that the risk was much greater than he had first realized.

1. Review the discussion on psychosurgery vs. neurosurgery in Chapter 9. Based on your understanding of the testimony, is this a therapeutic, social, or manipulative application of behavior control?
2. Is this a therapeutic or a nontherapeutic experimental situation?
3. Which of the persons mentioned is John Doe's "doctor," if anyone?
4. Was informed consent obtained? If not, what would you have required

to assure that it was obtained, or is informed voluntary consent not ob- **694** tainable at all under such circumstances?    cont.

5. If you were a judge on the panel, what would you order done with John Doe, and what would be your ruling on the continuation of the experiment?

(Adapted from newspaper accounts in the *Detroit Free Press, Detroit News,* and *The New York Times,* March 29 to April 9, 1973.)    ↓

---

John Doe's case combines research problems with some of the issues we    **695** discussed under the topic of behavior control. (You might want to compare Case 46 with Case 39 in that chapter.) Because of this tangle, all three motives we discussed under behavior control — therapeutic, social, and manipulative — are present in a manner that is very hard to sort out.    ↓

In what way does the link between the experiment and his eventual free-    **696** dom raise questions of the voluntary nature of John Doe's consent? If being released is made to depend on John Doe's participation in the experiment, we might conclude that freedom is being used as a pressure to get him into the experiment, and that that constitutes unacceptable coercion. But if release depends on the <u>results</u> of the experiment, then John Doe certainly has strong reasons to participate, but we might not consider that undue coercion. If the experiment works, and thereby removes the cause for John Doe's incarceration in the first place, release is appropriate.    ↓

Incidentally, note that from the brief amount of information we are given in    **697** Case 46, we cannot say that John Doe is mentally incompetent to give informed consent, even if he is constrained by circumstances from giving truly voluntary consent. If anything, he seems more competent than his parents, who signed the form without reading it.

  Also note that if the possibility of freedom might constitute coercion in the case of John Doe's consent, the same thing might act equally as coercion upon the parents, if they see the experiment as the only way to free their son. In such a case, is a proxy consent any better than the subject's own consent, as far as protecting the subject's best interests? How do you feel about requiring the court to appoint a disinterested party to serve as the one who consents or denies consent in such a case?    ↓

It is not possible, from the testimony cited, to reach any firm conclusions    **698** on the design of the experiment from the scientific viewpoint. However, based on the conflicts of testimony and on the scientific credentials (not cited in the case report) of some experts who testified against the experiment, one has some evidence for concluding that there were significant defects in the experimental design. How does this factor influence your decision as to the ethics of the experiment?    ↓

**699**   As a point of fact, the court ordered John Doe freed, because he had originally been sent to Ionia without a trial, and the state law that had allowed this procedure had since been repealed. While the court could then have considered the question of the experiment itself to be a moot point, the judges went on to hear more testimony. They eventually concluded that no prisoners in state mental hospitals could be used as subjects in the experi-
↓  ment.

**700**   Now that we have looked over the primary aspects of the ethical decision on any particular experiment, we might ask what the responsibility of the medical profession and the entire society is regarding human experimentation in general. One question is how to enforce the provisions of ethical codes such as the Declaration of Helsinki. We already noted that some agencies will not grant funds unless the experimental protocol includes ethical safeguards; but in a case such as the Lafayette Clinic psychosurgery, the investigators may have escaped this critical review by getting their funds from the state. Another suggestion is that, since the entire career prestige of a scientist is dependent upon having his works published in a reputable journal, the editors of journals have a responsibility not to pub-
↓  lish the results of unethical research.

**701**   Beecher advocated this view in his 1966 exposé:

> . . . It is not enough to ensure that all investigation is carried out in an ethical manner; it must be made unmistakably clear in the publications that the proprieties have been observed. This implies editorial responsibility in addition to the investigator's. The question arises, then, about valuable data that have been improperly obtained. It is my view that such material should not be published. There is a practical aspect to the matter: Failure to obtain publication would discourage unethical experimentation. How many would carry out such experiments if they *knew* its results would never be published? Even though suppression of such data . . . would constitute a loss to medicine, in a specific, localized sense, this loss, it seems, would be less important than the far reaching moral loss to medicine if the data thus obtained were to be published. Admittedly, there is room for debate.*

Another suggestion is to publish such results with a stern editorial condemnation of the methods; Beecher felt that this was likely to smell too much of
↓  hypocrisy.

**702**   A current suggestion among journal editors favors the publication-with-critical-editorial view. It is suggested that if the editors feel that a piece of scientifically valid research is unethical, they ought to print it with a critical editorial, and ought also to inform the investigator that they intend to do this. The investigator might then either withdraw the article, or make his own written reply if he feels he has been unjustly criticized. Beecher's view, on the other hand, has no provision for redress where a researcher genu-
↓  inely feels that he has taken every necessary ethical precaution.

* Reprinted, by permission. From H. K. Beecher, Ethics and clinical research. *New England Journal of Medicine* 274 : 1354, 1966.

Another question is: Who is to be selected to be the subjects of medical    **703**
research? That is, we do not only have to ask if the burden imposed is worth
the benefits; we also have to ask if the burden is being distributed over
society in an ethical manner. Traditionally this has not been the case, with
the vast bulk of subjects for the higher-risk human experimentation coming
from the prisons, the mental institutions, and the charity wards of hospitals.  ↓

Sullivan (in Barber [1973]) did a survey of experimental subjects, noting the    **704**
relationships between whether the patients were low-income patients
from clinics or high-income patients from private hospitals; whether the
potential benefits outweighed the risks as far as the individual subject was
concerned; and whether the overall benefit to society was great or small as
compared to the risks of the subjects. He found that not only were clinic
patients more likely than private patients to end up in studies with an unfavorable risk–benefit ratio to themselves, but also that the clinic patients
were more likely to be in studies where the overall social benefits were low
in relation to the risks. A traditional justification has held that society has a
need for medical knowledge that only experiments on the poor can provide, and that low-cost or subsidized medical care is society's repayment.
Sullivan's data suggest rather that there are some experiments of potentially
low benefit that might never be done at all, except for the ready availability
of poor bodies to do them on.    ↓

A number of proposals have been made to change the social distribution of    **705**
the burden of being an experimental subject. One, which is easily rejected,
is to halt all human experimentation. This is easily rejected because if one
feels that this experimentation is unethical, in order to be ethically consistent he ought to be willing to refuse for himself all medical treatment that
has been developed in the past through human experimentation − how
many sick people would be willing to do so?

   Another proposal is that since the supposed benefits of these reseaches
fall upon society as a whole (or is it just upon those segments of society
that can afford ready access to medical care?), there ought to be some sort
of national draft or lottery to select subjects, similar to serving on a jury.  ↓

Another question is: What happens if an experimental procedure turns out    **706**
to have severe long-term side effects that had not been anticipated, and the
subjects are left with the need for extensive medical or custodial care? This
problem is analogous to the problem of the children in Europe born with
malformed or absent limbs after their mothers took the drug thalidomide.
This was not an experiment per se, but rather a case of a drug being approved for therapeutic use without adequate testing. In England, after years
of court battles, the company that marketed the drug has finally agreed to
pay the medical bills and damages of these children (which by now has
amounted to many millions of dollars).    ↓

**707**  In a similar manner, it is also being proposed that a drug company, or whoever else sponsors research, should be responsible for paying damages if a similar tragedy should occur. This proposal holds that this is fitting even if it raises the cost of drugs. The suffering and risks undertaken by experimental subjects should be calculated as part of the real cost of the product, and the consumers who benefit from the product should pay the price. If some sort of national subject pool chosen by lottery were to be formed, presumably some sort of national experimentation insurance would be a feature of the plan, unless passage of a comprehensive national health insurance plan rendered this unnecessary.

**708**  We have now seen how human experimentation creates problems in the area of the doctor–patient relationship and in informed consent, and we have touched upon some of the social implications of research in human subjects. To conclude this chapter, we present a case that is complicated by the issues of experimentation, quality of life, and control of reproduction.

---

## CASE 47

**709**  A certain government's Committee on Research Review is meeting to examine the ethical ramifications of a proposal submitted by the prestigious Institute of Embryology at Y University. The Institute has long been concerned with the plight of women who are prone to spontaneous abortions. While new techniques for care of premature newborns allows medicine to save infants born with birth weights as low as 1200 grams, many women cannot carry a baby even that long and thus are deprived of the opportunity to have children. The Institute is therefore interested in the development of an artificial placenta, which might sustain infants as low as 300 grams birth weight. To perfect this technique, it is necessary to use human fetuses; all possible work in animals has already been done.

The Institute proposes to obtain the fetuses voluntarily aborted by hysterotomy (surgical removal of the fetus from the uterus) under the country's abortion laws, which allow abortion up to the twenty-fourth week of gestation. At first, the research team feels that they would be able to maintain vital signs in such fetuses for only a few minutes or hours. As the techniques are gradually perfected, survival time will gradually increase.

Because it cannot be known what types of long-range damage the fetus may suffer as a result of these techniques (e.g., brain damage), the Institute wishes to keep fetuses alive for no longer than a 2-week period at this point. The Institute cannot venture to say what it will do as the techniques are perfected to allow maintaining the fetus to a full-term stage of development, since it has no data at present.

(Adapted from R. M. Veatch, "Case 68." In *Case Studies in Medical Ethics.* Cambridge, Mass.: Harvard University Press, 1977.)

**Questions on Case 39:**

1. Who are the experimental subjects? Are the mothers who abort the fe-     **710**
tuses party to the experiment or not?
2. Is it possible to obtain informed consent for these subjects? If so, from
whom is the consent to be obtained? In what form?
3. Suppose one feels that a woman may abort a fetus because of her right
to control of her own body. Does this right extend also to the right to
allow the fetus to be used as a research subject — or is this an unwarranted additional presumption? How about the right to deny permission
to use the fetus for research?
4. If the fetus is maintained for a week or more beyond the time when, by
law, it has become viable, would "disposal" of it constitute the killing of
a human being? Of a person?
5. Disposal is justified because of possible unforeseen damage, which
would not have occurred had the fetus not been used in research. Does
this disposal then constitute an attempt to rectify one moral wrong by
committing another?
6. Suppose you are now at the point where evidence indicates that the fetus can safely be brought to term without deleterious side effects. Is
there now any justification for disposal? On the other hand, are you
justified in bringing to term an infant that has already been rejected by
its mother?       ↓

The report of the Commission on fetal research (as summarized by Ingel-    **711**
finger [1977]) approved research on fetuses directed toward developing
new therapies for fetuses and pregnant women, so long as there was minimal risk to the fetus used in the experiment. It also approved experiments
done in anticipation of abortion, provided that the fetus was under 20
weeks gestation and that the experiment itself did not alter the fetus's duration of life. It prohibited any inducements to get women to agree to abortions in order to obtain subjects for such research.       ↓

Our discussion of new safeguards for subjects of research shows how far    **712**
we have come on this issue since the days of Dr. S. and of Beecher's original
exposé. Investigators, accustomed to the earlier "almost anything goes" atmosphere, have complained that these new regulations are really an anti-
intellectual reaction against scientific progress. But we have taken pains to
show that most of the new regulations are grounded in basic ethical values
that we have applied to other problems in medical ethics. Time must still
show whether these regulations are workable in practice, and whether the
fears that they will unduly hamper research have solid grounds.

CH. 12 ↓ **713**

# Allocation of Scarce 12
# Resources

The medical resident in the coronary care unit at County Hospital answers **713** the phone call from the emergency room resident. An ambulance is 10 minutes away, carrying a patient with chest pain and a dropping blood pressure. The cardiogram, transmitted over the radio, makes it clear that the patient has suffered a heart attack. But all ten beds in the coronary care unit are full. The resident glances over the chart rack, trying to decide which patient is most stable and can most safely be transferred out of the unit and onto the regular hospital ward, where he will have to do without continuous cardiac monitoring and intensive nursing care. ↓

Meanwhile, in Washington, a U.S. congressman is looking at the latest draft **714** of a bill to appropriate funds for cancer research. The congressman supports such research in principle, and failure to vote for the bill would incur the wrath of many influential citizens and lobbies in his home district. But he also knows that the money appropriated for the bill is that much less money that can be spent on housing, crime control, education, and other pressing national priorities. He scratches his head, trying to figure out the fairest way to divide up the all-too-limited dollars. ↓

Ordinarily the daily lives of a medical resident and of a congressman are **715** very different, but in these two examples both are engaged in making decisions involving the allocation of scarce resources. As the examples illustrate, a wide range of decisions fall under the category of resource allocation. ↓

This spectrum of decisions is nicely outlined by Leon Kass: **716**

Personnel and facilities for medical research and treatment are scarce resources. Is the development of a new technology the best use of the limited resources, given current circumstances? How should we balance efforts aimed at prevention against those aimed at cure, or either of these against efforts to redesign the species? How should we balance the delivery of available levels of care against further basic research? More fundamentally, how should we balance efforts in biology and medicine against efforts to eliminate poverty, pollution, urban decay, discrimination, and poor education? This last question about distribution is perhaps the most profound.* ↓

* From L. R. Kass, "The new biology: What price relieving man's estate?" *Science* 174 : 779, 1971. Copyright 1971 by the American Association for the Advancement of Science.

**717** To be a little more specific we can look at some decisions related to artificial kidney machines, one of the most widely discussed examples of expensive, life-saving, and sometimes scarce medical technologies. These decisions include the following:

1. Which of two patients should get access to a kidney machine when only one is available.
2. Whether more kidney machines should be produced, or whether that same money should go into better prevention of kidney disease, based on our existing medical technology.
3. Whether we should spend money to support treatment and prevention of kidney disease based on current knowledge, or should try to expand that knowledge by funding expanded kidney research.
4. Whether we should fund kidney research, or fund research into some other category of disease or handicap like heart disease or stroke.
5. Whether we should try to improve people's lives by funding medical care and research, or by funding other social programs such as education, food, and housing.

↓

**718** *We can use the useful economic terms* microallocation *to describe decisions about which individuals should get available goods, and* macroallocation *to describe decisions about which goods society ought to make available.* In the kidney machine example, the first decision is the "micro" end of the scale and the decisions get increasingly more "macro" moving from
↓ the second decision through the fifth.

**719** In general, practitioners of the health professions become involved in resource-allocation decisions only at the micro end of the spectrum. But any micro decision presupposes that the more macro decisions have already been made in a certain way. For example, if there are enough kidney machines to go around, so that one does not have to make the tough choice in the first decision, this means that the second through the fifth decisions have already been made in favor of making more machines (and training the skilled technicians to run them) instead of using the money for prevention, research, other diseases, or other social needs. Therefore, a thorough ethical analysis of the resource-allocation issue requires attention
↓ to both microallocation and macroallocation.

**720** Before we look at some features of macroallocation, it may be worth reminding ourselves that you don't have to be director of a renal dialysis program to be involved in making microallocation decisions. Consider the resource allocation decisions made by a doctor in family practice. He or she has to decide how many patients to admit to their practice, how much time to spend with each, and how much time to spend working instead of with his or her family. Along with time, the doctor's compassion and empathy is

another scarce medical resource, and many decisions on how emotionally    **720**
involved to get with one's patients are really types of resource-allocation    cont.
decisions.    ↓

Discussions of macroallocation in medical ethics books and courses tend to    **721**
be rather unsatisfactory. This isn't because people discussing medical ethics are stupid, but rather because ethical theories and principles are tools
that are good for some jobs but not for others. Resource decisions prove
Clouser's point (1975): "[E]thics is a fairly blunt instrument; it does not cut
finely. It can be precise and rigorous, but it does not determine one and
only one action that receives the moral seal of approval."
  If our congressman in the original example studied ethics, he might learn
some general theories of social justice, but he would not learn a formula to
determine exactly how much federal money should go to the various competing social programs, and that's what he really wants to know.    ↓

Because ethics "does not cut finely" on these matters, many have turned to    **722**
economics for an answer to macroallocation dilemmas. There is an increasing interest in cost-benefit analyses and other economic tools for dealing
with this type of problem. And economic analysis is certainly a necessary
ingredient in any macroallocation decision — before making our choice, we
would want to know if a more efficient alternative is available, and that our
choice will not have unforeseen economic consequences.    ↓

But economic analysis, at its best, is only a way of showing how our value    **723**
judgments can be put into operation, and at its worst, it is a way of concealing value judgments so that we do not realize that they're being made.
  For example, a decision to avoid policy choices on the distribution of
health care, and instead to let the free marketplace determine the allocation, might at first seem like a purely economic solution. But as a practical
matter, in any given society, a certain group will have more power in the
marketplace than other groups, and that dominant group will have its own
peculiar interests and values. While in theory other groups have the opportunity to achieve dominance in time, in practice the dominant group can
use its power to maintain its position. Therefore, a decision to let the market decide is really a decision to favor some social groups and some social
values instead of others.    ↓

In addition to the inherent limitations of ethical theory and economic anal-    **724**
ysis, there are some other practical limitations that need to be taken into
account in studying the macroallocation issue. Some of these limitations
have come into focus only recently and they are often neglected in popular
discussions of medical resources, so we should look at them in some detail.    ↓

**725**    First, we should underline the obvious — scarce-resources decisions are difficult decisions precisely because the resources are scarce. In reply to the view that "there cannot be sufficient resources to allow maximal social application of current scientific technology (medical or otherwise), much less an unfettered expansion of that technology," Leibel (1977) writes, "Despite the rantings of various 'zero-growth' factions, . . . there is no a priori limit on the ability of the human mind and its societies to expand." But Leibel's view reflects more wishful thinking than clear perception of the escalating spiral of population growth and food and energy shortages that characterize the modern world. Authorities are virtually unanimous in declaring that the problem of scarcity will get worse rather than better with time.

**726**    A few figures illustrate the extent of this problem on a national level in the United States. In 1975, the Congress elected to underwrite the costs of kidney machines for all Americans with end-stage renal failure, to insure that no citizen did without this medical technology because of financial barriers. Partly as a result, there is currently no major shortage of kidney machines in the United States. But the cost of the program, estimated at first to reach $1 billion annually by 1985, in fact hit the $1 billion mark in 1976. Revised estimates held that the program (which serves about 50,000 people, less than 0.02 percent of the U.S. population) would cost $1.9 billion by 1984, and $3 billion by 1989.

**727**    Another life-saving but high-cost technology currently under development is the totally implantable artificial heart, which could avoid the rejection problem encountered with heart transplants. Current projections indicate that such a device could be ready for use by 1990. The number of people who could benefit is roughly equivalent to that who now benefit from kidney machines. But the annual cost of an artificial-heart program is estimated at $20 billion. By contrast, the total U.S. health budget in 1977 was $104 billion.

**728**    These figures tell part of the story of the financial burden of medical technology, but so far we have only looked at the story from the perspective of one country, a very privileged one by world standards. A few years ago, the United States was very worried about a doctor shortage, and took vigorous measures to increase medical school class sizes in order to ward off this danger. At the time that this "threat" was being dealt with, the United States had about one doctor for every 600 people. By contrast, there was one doctor for every 5,000 to 40,000 people in various countries in Africa, and per capita health expenditures were minuscule compared to those of the developed nations.

    Clearly, if a worldwide government were to come into power under a benevolent dictator committed to equalizing health care, the dictator would have little patience with the debate over whether to manufacture artificial hearts. He would be too busy shipping United States doctors and dollars overseas to fight malnutrition, parasitic infestations, and malaria.

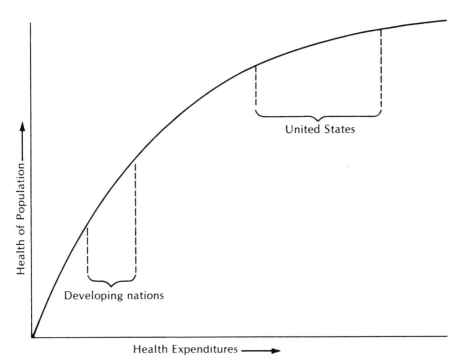

**Figure 3.** *Relationship of increased health-care expenditures to actual increase in the health of the population in the United States and in developing nations.*

Figure 3 gives us another angle on the worldwide distribution problem. If you start with a population getting no health care, just a little money invested will greatly improve the overall health standard. At this stage one is treating mostly infectious and parasitic diseases and malnutrition, for which low-cost, effective cures are often available. But as you steadily improve the medical care, you eliminate these easy-to-treat conditions and are left with the chronic diseases such as cancer and cardiovascular diseases, for which cure is often impossible and for which even palliative treatment can be very expensive. At this point on the curve, a very large increase in the health budget may yield only a very minor improvement in the overall health standard. The United States has now clearly reached the flattened part of this curve. **729**

But this does not mean that the public demand for new and more expensive health-care technology has fallen off along with the proportional benefits. If anything, the spectacular advances made on the steep part of the curve have produced unrealistic expectations and demands for our health-care system. But how are we to weigh the demands of an American cancer patient for expensive chemotherapy that will extend his life by 3 months against the needs of children in developing countries for the most basic vaccinations and food supplements? **730**

**731** While our own internal resource-allocation problems seem perplexing enough, especially in light of the huge and rapidly growing sums of money involved, they quickly pale by comparison to the worldwide problem. But we must now add yet another wrinkle. So far, we have assumed two things: (1) that the best way to improve people's health is to provide more health and medical care and, (2) that health and medical care actually do make people healthy and are a social good. Recent critics of the medical establishment have set out to challenge these assumptions.

**732** We are becoming more and more aware of the extent to which many diseases — especially the costly chronic diseases that plague advanced societies — are produced by certain life styles and behaviors, such as smoking, overeating, not getting enough exercise, and so on. Furthermore, the diseases that affect the poor often go hand in hand with poor housing, shortages of food, and lack of education. Attempts to ameliorate these conditions, or to change unhealthy behaviors, may pay off better than improved health care.

**733** For example, the government of Canada decided some years ago to try to get a handle on its national health policy — in effect, to come up with the "formula" that our congressman seemed to want in the example at the beginning of this chapter. Lalonde (1974) describes the way that this problem was tackled.

**734** A problem in macroallocation, which we have ignored so far, is specifying the "health" that you are trying to achieve. (We will deal in detail with the problem of defining "health" and "disease" in Chapter 17.) The Canadians settled on what seemed to be a reasonable life expectancy, and then ranked diseases and accidental causes of death in order of "life-years lost." That is, the "worst" diseases were those that killed the most people, or that killed them the earliest in advance of their expected age of death. This way of assigning priorities meant that auto accidents and heart disease became high-priority problems, while cancer, which affects mostly the elderly, assumed somewhat lower priority. (What value judgments are hidden in the decision to use "life-years lost" as the major determinant? How might the priority ranking be different if other measures of health were used — for instance, days lost from work?)

**735** Next, the Canadians looked at various strategies to deal with these high-priority causes of death, trying to estimate how many life-years would be saved and at what cost. By this approach, a program that might help only a few people, but at a cost of just a few cents per capita, might be given higher priority over a program that could help many people, but at a cost of hundreds of dollars per capita.

The final conclusion (and here we are, of course, oversimplifying a very    **736**
complex and sophisticated analysis) was not to train more doctors, build
more medical equipment, or improve hospitals. Instead the Canadian government decided it could promote the better health of its citizens, in the
most cost-effective way, by instituting programs to require drivers to wear
seat belts and to get smokers to stop smoking.    ↓

We might think that the role of nonmedical programs in improving health    **737**
is a special feature and is a peculiarity of our modern culture, but this turns
out not to be true. Powles (1973), for example, has argued persuasively that
we have given medicine too much credit for past improvements in health.  ↓

Let's look at one instance: The biggest drop in the infant mortality rate in    **738**
urban America in this century began around 1910, following two major social changes — chlorination of drinking water and pasteurization of milk.
These were public health measures, which most of the medical establishment either ignored or derided at the time. By contrast, when antibiotics
first came into use in the 1930s, the effect on the mortality rate was much
less.

Going back even farther in history, we learn that the mortality from infectious diseases in Britain began to drop off fully 100 years before the antibiotic era. Changes in housing, plumbing, and urban garbage disposal seem
to have been most responsible — again social changes that had no relation,
at the time, to medical policy.    ↓

The lesson is clear: If we spend all of our resources on health care, we may    **739**
be neglecting other social changes that, by themselves, could have an even
greater impact on the public health standard.

Some critics, notably Illich (1976), have gone even farther and argued that
we may be promoting ill health by our continued support of the medical
establishment. By "medicalizing" society, and placing all health concerns in
the hands of experts, we may be destroying the sense of individual responsibility, which in the long run, may be the most important factor in keeping
us healthy. It is not necessary to agree with these more extreme criticisms in
order to realize that we ought to be much more critical of "more medicine
is better" than we have in the past.    ↓

**740** Finally, we have to realize that health is only one of a variety of important primary goods, and that a life governed only by pursuit of health, without concern for the other things that make life worth living, would be a rather empty life. Engelhardt (1979) notes that a society that elected to take its chances with disease, and instead devoted its public resources to creating elegant gardens and other things of beauty, would be odd by our standards, but this use of resources would not be obviously unjust or incoherent. (Health professionals often talk to patients as if health were something to be valued over all else, no matter what sacrifices are necessary. But how many
↓ health professionals actually do that in their own lives?)
REVIEW PRIMARY GOODS ↑ 383

**741** Having now listed some of the difficulties in discussing macroallocation, we might ask what help we can get from ethical theory. In looking at ethical questions of resource allocation, we encounter many of the same issues we will be discussing in Chapter 16, especially the right to health care. You will recall that a certain claim or demand has much greater moral weight if we can establish it as a "right." Therefore, if certain sorts of health care for certain people really counts as a right, it follows that an ethical policy of resource allocation will give the highest priority to those elements of health care. For this reason, a full ethical discussion of the macroallocation issue
↓ requires some of the considerations we will be postponing until Chapter 16.

**742** The simpler sorts of allocation decisions are closest to the micro level — where one can identify the proposed beneficiaries of the distribution as individuals or as groups, and where what is to be distributed among them is roughly the same. Decisions become harder when one has to allocate among very different sorts of things, such as between treatment and basic
↓ research.

**743** Several principles for ideal distribution of social goods have been proposed, and Outka (1974) nicely summarizes them as they apply to health care. One could distribute health care resources according to the following:

1. Who merits or deserves it the most.
2. Who has contributed the most to society.
3. Who has the greatest ability to pay — in money or in other goods desired in the marketplace.
4. Who needs it the most.
↓ 5. Similar treatment for similar cases.

The fifth principle specifies a general condition for a <u>just</u> program of distri-    **744**
bution. If A and B both demand health care and are in similar circum-
stances, and we fulfill A's demand while refusing B because of B's race,
where he lives, or our dislike for him, B has good grounds to claim that he
was treated unjustly. But this holds true regardless of which of the principles, the first through the fourth, we choose; so we must still deal with that
question. The fifth principle does serve to remind us that we cannot create
a privileged class to receive our resources while others get the short end of
the stick. (What would the fifth principle say about the present distribution
of health resources between the United States and the poorer countries of
the world?)
                                                                                    ↓

We now have to choose among the first through the fourth principles or    **745**
suggest alternative principles if we do not find these satisfactory. The first
impulse of many health professionals would be immediately to reject the
first, second, and third principles in favor of the fourth. Is this just because
we are emotionally conditioned to help those in need? Or is there an underlying ethical justification for this choice?
                                                                                    ↓

One way of justifying the "need" principle is to look back at the basic value    **746**
we chose earlier — respect for the individual and for individual autonomy.
If we distribute an important social good because of one's past contributions, or because of how much money one has, we pervert this value —
regarding individuals not as valuable as individuals, but as valuable because
of what they do or what they have. If we distribute it based on merit or
desert, we must provide value judgments to determine who is more deserving. Invariably, in a pluralistic society, there will be disagreement about this.
Some will have chosen to live their lives according to different values, and it
would seem unfair to let them suffer because of this autonomous choice.    ↓
   REVIEW INDIVIDUAL ↑ 79–84

The need for health care is likely to arise among all classes of people — rich    **747**
and poor, social contributors and hermits, the upright and the sinful. If we
distribute health resources on the basis of need alone, we avoid those sorts
of judgments that threaten the dignity of the individual and instead recognize the equal worth of all individuals. Thus, the need principle has at least
some initial support as an ethically sound principle of resource distribution.    ↓

However, before the need principle can be adopted as the ultimate deci-    **748**
sion principle, a number of problems must be worked out. The first is the
one suggested by the figures we studied for the cost of new medical technologies. For instance, right now there is a group of people who will die of
irreversible heart failure and who could be saved if we had an artificial
heart. We saw how costly such a device could be, but there is an undeni-
able need for it. If we allowed needs alone to govern allocation of resources, the needs would quickly outstrip the available funds.    ↓

**749** Second, there is a problem in defining when a need has been met. Suppose, as might seem reasonable, we try to designate a level of acceptable health; when a person has been brought up to that level of health, we will consider his needs to have been met. But many individuals, suffering from congenital handicaps or chronic debilitating diseases, will never be brought up to that minimum level no matter how much of the available resources we devote to their care. These people could then go on making demands on the health system indefinitely. Again, it seems that we would quickly break the bank if we used need as a criterion.

**750** Third, a problem arises if we learn our lesson from the first two problems and decide to develop a priority of needs. Inevitably we will have to make value judgments about which there will be disagreement, and which run the risk of trampling on individual dignity. Recall our choice between giving chemotherapy to a cancer victim to extend his life by a few months, and using the money to vaccinate school children in a poor area against infectious disease. We might want to say that here is a clear ranking of need and that the children have priority. But the extra months of life may still be extremely important to the cancer victim, and refusing treatment may make him feel just as abandoned, devalued, and embittered as would the parents of the poor children if they had to do without vaccinations.

This does not mean, however, that an appropriate way of choosing among competing needs could not be developed, which would win a sufficient degree of public acceptance to be politically feasible.

**751** We will not now consider any cases that feature macroallocation issues; many of the cases we will look at in Chapter 16 will have resource-allocation elements. Instead we will go on to consider the ethics of microallocation.

**752** The most commonly cited microallocation problem in medical ethics is how to distribute a number of kidney machines among a larger number of patients with end-stage renal failure. This problem was a very practical one for a number of years after kidney dialysis was first introduced, when demand far exceeded the supply. (As we saw, this problem was partly eliminated when the federal government decided to make kidney machines available to everyone regardless of ability to pay — thereby exchanging a microallocation problem for a macroallocation one.)

**753** But microallocation problems are hardly new to professors of ethics. One sort of case that has been discussed for many years is the lifeboat case: An overcrowded lifeboat will sink in heavy seas unless the load is lightened; either all aboard will die, or some way must be selected to choose who will be allowed to stay in the boat. As Childress (1970) notes, one such case, U.S. v. Holmes, was actually adjudicated in the courts in 1841.

In the lifeboat case, fate has determined who will be in the lifeboat, and therefore who will be subject to the final selection. But in the kidney machine cases, a prior selection process is necessary, to decide who are the potential recipients who can be helped by kidney machines. This prior selection process has been characterized as the application of "medical criteria," which must then be followed by selection of the actual recipients by some other criteria.                                            ↓

754

Some of the medical criteria used by the early renal programs included age less than 55 and absence of other medical complications, such as diabetes. But a little consideration will show that these criteria are not strictly "medical" in the sense intended. People who are older than 55, or who have other serious diseases, can still live longer if their renal failure is treated with dialysis. A decision to eliminate them from consideration in favor of younger or more healthy renal-failure victims is a clear-cut value judgment.

755

The only truly medical criteria than can be used to exclude potential dialysis patients are making sure that the diagnosis of end-stage renal failure is correct and that the patient really can benefit from dialysis (e.g., excluding patients who have such poor blood vessels that they cannot be hooked up to the machine).                                            ↓

Next, one has to choose from that pool the patients who will get the machines, assuming that there are not enough to go around and that those patients turned down will, if a machine does not become available in the near future, die of end-stage uremic poisoning. Here the groups have tended to go in one of two directions. One was the phenomenon referred to in Chapter 7 as the "Let's form a committee syndrome." In this case it was assumed that, if the committee was given the right composition from the start, with the proper mix of clergy, laymen, physicians, and so on, ethical decisions would magically arise from the subsequent deliberations. Hence, the attention was directed to the criteria to select members of the committee instead of the criteria that the committee was to use to actually select patients for the kidney machines.                                            ↓

756

Once these committees were formed (and immediately dubbed "God committees" by the cynics), the members belatedly came to the problem that those dialysis groups who took the second direction came to in the first place: by what kind of criteria do you select the patients who will live and who will die? The way in which the committees handled this problem provided a field day for medical sociologists, but the results represented less than a bumper crop of ethical insights.

757

(For instance, one conclusion the sociologists reached was that physicians tended to make poor members of the committee as far as the actual decision making was concerned. It seemed that their prior training made it

**757**
cont.
nearly impossible for a physician to say "no" to putting anyone on a life-saving machine. Eventually the lay members had to step in to take the burden of the final decision off the doctor's shoulders.)

**758**
The most basic way of approaching the problem of criteria is to decide to have none at all. Everyone will be chosen by purely random procedures, so that there can be no question of favoritism or unfairness. This sounds attractive in its simplicity. How does it measure up when one is faced with a specific case?

---

### CASE 48

**759**
You are a one-man God committee (all the others called in sick today) who has two kidney machines and five patients who are about to die of renal failure if they do not get a machine. The information you have been given on them is as follows:

| Patient | Sex | Marital Status | Age | Number of Children | Occupation |
|---------|--------|----------------|-----|--------------------|------------|
| A | male | married | 35 | 2 | ? |
| B | female | single | 28 | 0 | ? |
| C | male | married | 38 | 3 | ? |
| D | female | married | 32 | 1 | ? |
| E | male | married | 30 | 0 | ? |

Are you going to select your two lucky winners at random? If not, what criteria are you going to use? What further information would you need to apply those criteria? How can you obtain that information in a way that will not bias your results?

---

**760**
One interesting feature that the medical sociologists have observed is that given the amount of information presented in Case 48, the majority opinion tends to favor a random selection. However, as more information is added, people want to start to apply specific criteria. For example:

## CASE 49

At your next meeting you are still alone, and again five patients are vying for two machines. This time, however, you have an additional item of information for each.    **761**

| Patient | Sex | Marital Status | Age | Number of Children | Occupation |
|---------|-----|----------------|-----|--------------------|------------|
| A | male | married | 35 | 2 | Mafia hit man |
| B | female | single | 28 | 0 | Concert violinist |
| C | male | married | 38 | 3 | Accountant (currently unemployed while on trial for embezzlement) |
| D | female | married | 32 | 1 | Manager of house of prostitution |
| E | male | married | 30 | 0 | Researcher on kidney physiology; last year became youngest man to win Nobel Prize for his role in developing the kidney machine |

Are you going to select the two at random? If not, by what criteria? Are these criteria different from those you adopted in Case 48?    ↓

---

Unlike most of the other cases we have presented, we cannot claim that    **762**
Case 49 is a true situation. However, it illustrates the way that emotional components are bound to enter into the decisions of such a committee. If the committee operates on an ad hoc basis, the emotionalism will influence the decisions directly. If the committee operates by criteria, the emotionalism will influence the choice of the criteria.

One observer, noting the tendency of the committees to emphasize middle-class, church-going virtues in their criteria for selection, commented that Henry David Thoreau with bad kidneys would never stand a chance.    ↓

A model committee made up of medical students chose as its criteria the    **763**
number of years of biologic survival that the patient could expect. It might have been only a coincidence that since medical students are uniformly young, they would have been at the top of the list according to their own criteria.

On the other hand, when dialysis machines were first introduced into use in Sweden — a culture with a long heritage of respecting older persons as valuable members of society — preference was uniformly given to older patients over young ones.    ↓

**764** Possibly the most bizarre, while still entirely rational, criteria are recounted in this anecdote. One committee had continually given preference to men who were happily married and who had children dependent upon them. The crunch came when the committee had to choose between two men about the same age, both married, and with the identical number of young children. After deliberation, the committee decided to proceed by figuring out which of the two wives, by virtue of good looks, bank account, or whatever, would have the easiest time getting another husband and remarrying. The decision was then to give the access to the dialysis machine to the husband of the other wife.

**765** These illustrations may help to explain why, in those situations in which it is still necessary to select patients for life-or-death matters, the idea of forming God committees to do the job is losing popularity. But is anything gained by this? An individual still has to choose, either at random or by some set of criteria similar to the ones discussed. The only gain is that these decisions are more private than committee meetings, so that if a complete lack of ethical consistency and a mockery of distributive justice is what is actually taking place, at least one is not making a public spectacle of it.

**766** However, as we said at the beginning of Chapter 7, it is important not to let the committee syndrome distract attention from the actual features of decision making. If committees use social-worth criteria, what are the implications of this choice?

---

## CASE 50

**767** At long last another member of the committee has shown up for work. In the last case, you elected to employ a set of social-worth criteria (since the five candidates had already been chosen by virtue of the fact that medical criteria had been met). As a result, patients B and E are receiving renal dialysis, and you have sent flowers to patients A, C, and D. At this meeting, however, two new candidates have applied. Both are reasonably upstanding individuals. One meets the medical criteria better than either B or E, in that she has fewer medical complications outside of the primary renal problem. The other is a highly placed politician whose particular interest has been to get additional government funds for research and development of dialysis programs. Since you can always train more physiologists, while enlightened politicians are hard to come by, you conclude that this candidate meets the social-worth criteria better than either B or E.

You state that it is indeed a pity that no opening in the program exists for either of these two individuals; but your fellow committee member says that this is no problem — you will simply put B and E off the machines to allow these new candidates to have them. When you object that it is improper to stop treatment on people once they have been accepted, he replies that if one takes the medical and social-worth criteria seriously (i.e., **767** that certain individuals are more worthy of being saved) his proposal is the cont. logical conclusion. If not, in actuality you are simply allocating resources on a first-come, first-served basis; and this is random allocation and not allocation by medical and social-worth criteria.

Do you accept this argument? What do you do with the new patients?   ↓

---

A policy that would allow dropping one patient from treatment because a **768** more promising one came along violates what Fried (1974) calls the "right to personal care," which is closely linked to the notion of the dignity of the individual coupled with our contractual model of the doctor–patient relationship. The patient has a right to expect that having been started on a course of treatment involves a commitment to continue through completion. This expectation forms a fundamental part of the trust that ought to characterize the doctor–patient relationship. How many would consent to being put under anesthesia for surgery if they could not be sure that the physician might not leave them lying cut open on the operating table, in order to take care of a more deserving patient who suddenly appeared? Therefore, if the situation envisioned in Case 50 is actually a consequence of choosing according to social-worth criteria, we have good grounds for rejecting these criteria.   ↓

Rejection of social-worth criteria leaves us with random selection again **769** (unless we are willing to let everyone die, on the grounds that any choice on our part would involve an immoral action). While it may initially seem callous and arbitrary, random selection actually embodies the fifth principle of a just scheme of allocation: similar cases should be treated similarly. It also seems to embody our value of the dignity of the individual, since anyone who is rejected can blame chance alone and not any negative judgment made about him by some other party. These reasons, as Childress (1970) notes, give strong support to random selection.   ↓

But random selection has the negative consequence noted in Case 49. It **770** would seem to most people very unfair if a skid row bum were selected over the President of the United States for some scarce life-saving medical care. Even if we find social-worth criteria distasteful in the vast majority of cases, there still seems to be a small number of cases where the social-worth judgment is clear-cut and should be given preference over random selection.   ↓

771    Is this appeal to social-worth criteria in special cases an emotional reaction that has no firm ethical base? Or is it a real flaw in the random-allocation theory?

There are at least some cases in which special dispensation can be allowed without overturning the theory on which random allocation rests. Suppose, in the classic lifeboat case, there is only one person aboard with the experience to steer the boat in heavy seas. All the rest might rationally agree to exempt that person from the drawing of lots. The justification for this is that even those who are losers in the drawing might reflect that they would be just as bad off had the seaman been thrown overboard in their place, only to leave the boat foundering for want of a competent helmsman.

772    This justification would seem to allow us to make exceptions to the random-allocation scheme for certain individuals who possess knowledge or skills upon which our entire society depends.

But note that this justification does not go very far. It might exempt the President of the United States in wartime, if a change in leadership at that crucial time might spell the destruction of our society. But it is not clear that this justification would exempt the President in a peacetime situation, provided that the Vice President appeared roughly as competent to take over. Thus people like Rescher (1969), who support a social-worth scheme, are not likely to be satisfied with it.

773    We have now reviewed some of the ethical issues involved in both macro-allocation and microallocation decisions. In conclusion, consider this case.

---

## CASE 51

774    Mrs. Smith is one of the saddest cases you have had to deal with in a long time. This unfortunate mother of three young children has been diagnosed as having acute myelogenous leukemia. Two courses of intensive chemotherapy have made her quite sick but have not arrested the disease. Despite the likelihood that death is only months away, both Mrs. Smith and her family continue to cling to any hope that is offered and to ask repeatedly whether there isn't some "miracle cure" not yet tried.

You are discussing her case with Dr. Jones and happen to mention that the thought of bone marrow transplantation has crossed your mind. This would involve transferring Mrs. Smith to one of the special centers where this procedure is carried out, assuming that an appropriate tissue match could be found among the family. Her old marrow, containing the leukemia cells, would then be killed by high-dose radiation, and the new marrow injected by intravenous transfusion. The procedure would have a very small chance of success. Mrs. Smith might die in great suffering from the effects of radiation, from infection while her body was without its normal immune defenses, or from "great-versus-host disease" if the new marrow attempted

to reject her normal body tissue. Still, you add, in their present state of des- **774**
peration, she and the family might agree to anything.  cont.

Dr. Jones puts in, "I don't think you ought even to mention to the Smiths
the possibility of marrow transplant." He recites the same figures we have
looked at about the spiralling costs of medical care and the duty of all physicians to help keep costs down. "Here you have a very expensive procedure
with a very small chance of success. You'd be socially irresponsible to
offer it to your patient."

Do you agree with Dr. Jones's assessment? What do you say to the Smiths
regarding marrow transplantation?  ↓

---

While there might be other reasons not to tell the Smiths about marrow **775**
transplantation, let's stick with the reason offered by Dr. Jones. From what
we have seen so far in this chapter, it seems safe to say that a physician has
some responsibility in the allocation of scarce medical resources. But what
is that responsibility, and how far does it go?  ↓

To begin with, it seems inarguable that physicians should avoid any medi- **776**
cal costs that, in fact, offer no benefit to their patients. Included here are
tests, x-rays, and drugs that are not really needed for diagnosis or treatment,
but that are ordered for completeness — to rule out a diagnosis that is very
unlikely to begin with, or to protect the doctor from an imagined threat of
lawsuit. These costs fall into the category of mere waste and cannot be
justified on any ethical grounds.  ↓

But Mrs. Smith's case does not quite fit here. The chance of benefit is small, **777**
and the cost is high. But (as we argued on informed consent) only Mrs.
Smith is in a position to say whether the chance of benefit is worth the cost
to her. The doctor–patient relationship, as we have been viewing it, would
require that you offer to Mrs. Smith this possible benefit.  ↓

Does this obligation to Mrs. Smith conflict with an obligation to preserve **778**
scarce resources? Fried (1974) has argued that we can best view these two
obligations as belonging to different levels of the medical decision-making
hierarchy. For the individual physician, the main obligation is to help the
patient. For decision makers in government, who do not bear responsibility
to individual patients but who are instead servants of the public at large,
the main obligation is to conserve resources.  ↓

**779**  Clearly this course would involve physicians in direct conflict with government decision makers (as we are seeing today). The doctor wants to offer his patient the latest technology and cost be damned; and the bureaucrat wants to hold costs down even if individual patients have to suffer along the line. Fried suggests that this conflict between levels of the social hierarchy is more desirable than internal conflict within the physician were he to try to follow both obligations at once. In trying to cut costs and preserve resources, he might be led to violate his duties within the doctor–patient relationship. On the other hand, if bureaucrats, following guidelines laid down by our democratic lawmaking processes, prohibit certain uses of resources (for example, prohibiting marrow transplants for patients with acute myelogenous leukemia), the doctor is "off the hook." He may fume at being unable to help his patient in that way, but as a member of our society he is bound to respect lawful social decisions.

**780**  In Case 51, then, your obligation is clear. You must decide whether telling the Smiths about marrow transplantation would be to Mrs. Smith's benefit and would be required under your contract in the doctor–patient relationship. You are not obligated to consider the resource-allocation aspects of your decision in your role as Mrs. Smith's doctor. (In other roles, such as member of your local medical society, you may be obligated to consider those issues.)

**781**  This two-level approach may seem too easy a way out of the dilemma, especially to those who wish physicians would more readily take the broader social viewpoint on issues of public concern. But it seems to provide a handy way to view the conflicting obligations in a way that does not deny the importance of either obligation. It also suggests that if physicians and government bureaucrats find themselves at loggerheads over cost-containment policies, it is not a cause for dismay; it merely shows that both physicians and bureaucrats are doing their jobs.

**782**  Naturally, in this brief chapter, it is difficult to do full justice to the difficult subject of resource allocation. We have indicated the spectrum of decisions that fall into this category, mentioned some of the most important ethical principles that apply, and clarified the responsibility of the individual health professional in resource-allocation decisions. As we noted before, we will be dealing with a number of related issues in Chapter 16.

**783** ↓ CH. 13

# Active and Passive Euthanasia 13

## CASE 52

G.W., a 67-year-old farmer and former military officer, had developed a severe upper respiratory infection, which had spread to involve the windpipe, and the swelling now threatened to block the air passages entirely. The best physicians in the neighborhood were consulted, and the most advanced treatments were applied but without success.

Despite the difficulty in making himself understood, G.W. appeared to remain in full control of his faculties throughout this illness. He finally succeeded in communicating to his doctors (as one recalled later) "a desire that he be permitted to die without interruption."

There are still a number of treatments that the doctors have not yet tried.

Should G.W.'s desire be honored? Or are the physicians obligated to go on treating as long as any hope is left?  ↓

**783**

---

Case 52 presents a commonly encountered case in which the issue of passive euthanasia, or allowing to die, might arise. It is often said that this ethical dilemma is a result of the successes of modern medicine. Now that we can keep people alive with respirators and other exotic equipment, it is said, ethical dilemmas arise which did not trouble physicians in earlier times.

With this in mind, it might interest you to know that in Case 52 G.W. is George Washington. The facts of the case are substantiated in a letter published by his physicians early in 1800. (It is not clear from the published account whether his desire was honored or not.)  ↓

**784**

The issue of euthanasia grows out of our discussion of terminal-care decisions in Chapter 6. Recall our three categories of cases. The first category involved brain death and the second category involved patients in a chronic vegetative state. We argued that in these categories, while there were good ethical reasons to support various terminal-care decisions, we could not speak of those decisions being "in the best interest of" or "on behalf of" the patients themselves.  ↓

REVIEW CATEGORIES ↑ 299

**785**

**786** In the third category, the patients are persons, and their interests must be taken into account — they must also be allowed to participate to the extent they are capable. In such cases, based on the quality-of-life assessment we discussed, it is conceivable that a quicker end to their lives could be in their best interests, if prolonged life would lead to greater pain or suffering with no compensating benefits. In this category of cases the question of euthanasia arises.

**787** The origin of the word "euthanasia" is from the Greek, meaning simply "a good death." But in modern usage the word has lost its etymologic meaning and has been applied only to cases in which deliberate actions are taken to change the normal course of dying. Thus, euthanasia is no longer applied to activities such as giving comfort and supportive care to the dying.

**788** Arguments about euthanasia have sometimes suffered from confusions of definitions, particularly of the terms used for what we will be calling "passive euthanasia" and "active euthanasia." Some authors use the term euthanasia strictly for active measures to terminate life and refer to passive measures as "allowing to die." Others use euthanasia as synonymous with allowing to die, and instead use the term "mercy killing" to denote active intervention.

**789** There is nothing wrong with any of these definitions as long as they are used consistently. To try to avoid confusion and emotionally laden terms, we will be using the following definitions in this chapter, based partly on the analysis of Beauchamp and Davidson (1979):

> Euthanasia. Intentionally expediting the death of an individual for that individual's own benefit, because of suffering that individual is undergoing or will undergo
> Passive euthanasia. Euthanasia performed by means of withholding or withdrawing life-prolonging therapy (e.g., turning off a respirator or not treating a pneumonia with antibiotics)
> Active euthanasia. Euthanasia performed by means of active interventions designed to cause death directly (e.g., injecting an overdose of morphine or potassium chloride)

**790** The main thing to remember about all these definitions is the inclusion of the qualifier, "for that individual's own benefit." These definitions explicitly exclude killing or allowing to die to get rid of unwanted members of society, or so that the next of kin can inherit the estate, or to cut costs of medical care. Therefore, arguments against the ethics of these sorts of actions will not count as arguments against the ethics of euthanasia. (We will see later whether such arguments apply to the question of the legality of euthanasia.)

With these definitions in mind, we can turn our attention in this chapter to   **791**
the following questions:

1. Is there a morally relevant difference between passive and active euthanasia?
2. How does one decide whether or not euthanasia is appropriate in
   specific cases?
3. If active euthanasia is ethically acceptable in some cases, ought the laws
   be revised to include this course of action as a legal alternative?   ↓

Notice one question we did <u>not</u> include: Is euthanasia (active <u>or</u> passive)   **792**
ever ethically justifiable? We answered this question in Chapter 6, when we
argued that a sanctity-of-life view (which would prohibit any kind of euthanasia) cannot be ethically supported. In actual practice almost every religious and secular philosophical view will support some type of euthanasia
in some circumstances — for example, a Catholic theologian would endorse
passive euthanasia for a dying individual who requests it, when the treatment that is withheld or withdrawn is "extraordinary" treatment by his criteria.   ↓

REVIEW SANCTITY ↑ 249–262
REVIEW EXTRAORDINARY ↑ 312–318

---

## CASE 53

You had thought that being a pediatric intern for 6 months had prepared   **793**
you for any shock, but you are still jolted when the frantic nurse calls you
into Janie's room. Janie, a healthy 10-year-old, had been admitted for routine, overnight hospitalization and observation after she fell and hit her
head on the corner of the fireplace at home. The wound was superficial and
no fracture was found on x-ray. Janie looked fine earlier in the evening with
no sign of concussion. Now, on the routine 2:00 A.M. bed check, the nurse
has discovered Janie still in bed, blue, and not breathing. It's anybody's
guess how long she's been like that, you think, as you go in to find the
nurses doing cardiopulmonary resuscitation. You find that Janie's pupils are
fixed and dilated.

With your resident's help, you intubate Janie, hook her to a cardiac monitor, and continue resuscitation with drugs. After ½ hour a heartbeat is re-
stored; pupils are still fixed and dilated. Everything points to a prolonged
period of brain anoxia with irreversible damage, but you cannot be sure.
You propose to the resident that Janie be placed on a respirator in the intensive care unit and have the various tests performed to determine brain
death or irreversible loss of conscious function. If those turn out the way
you expect, the respirator can then be turned off, and you will be much
more certain of the diagnosis.

**793**
**cont.** The resident objects, "If you put her on the respirator, you're stuck. You can't stop a treatment once it's started; you'll have to continue it come hell or high water. It'll be much easier on the family and on us not to get started down that road."

↓ What do you do?

---

**794** Let's focus on the specific ethical proposition in Case 53 that seems to be implied in the resident's position: Once you begin a treatment, you are morally committed to its continuance in a way you would not be commit-
↓ ted had you not started it in the first place.

**795** This position reflects a frequently encountered emotional reaction of physicians and health professionals to terminal-care decisions. One often sees a spectrum of actions in hospital settings — ranging from a crude sanctity-of-life view to endorsement of euthanasia, even without the direct request or consent of the patient. (One generally does not see active euthanasia performed, since it is clearly murder under the law, but physicians may practice it in rare instances and may endorse it even when they feel con-
↓ strained from actually doing so.)

**796** This spectrum of actions might include:

*Antieuthanasia*
1. Treat vigorously.
2. Treat with ordinary means but withhold extraordinary measures.
*Passive Euthanasia*
3. Decline to initiate treatment.
4. Stop ongoing treatment, having obtained consent of patient beforehand.
5. Stop treatment without consent of patient.
*Active Euthanasia*
6. Give patient means to kill himself.
7. Directly bring about death with patient's consent beforehand.
↓ 8. Directly bring about death without patient's consent.

**797** Physicians generally will pick a place along the spectrum and be willing to go that far, but no farther. This seems to be the case with the resident in Case 53: He will accept the third action but would balk at the fourth or fifth. The questions then arise: Is this "drawing the line" based on valid ethical grounds? Or is it an emotional reaction without an ethical basis, simply reflecting the fact that physicians find some acts psychologically harder to
↓ perform than others?

While emotions always play a role in our decisions and deserve careful **798**
scrutiny, the distinction between ethical argument and emotion should always be kept in mind. For example, it is easy to imagine a physician who
agrees with the argument that a fetus is not a person and that abortion is
therefore acceptable, but he might be emotionally unable to perform abortions and watch the fetus being killed or dismembered. If this physician
refers women to other doctors for abortions, he is not being a hypocrite or
being ethically inconsistent. From his emotional reaction, it doesn't follow
that abortion for him is morally wrong — any more than it would follow that
for the hardened criminal who can kill without a flicker of an eyelash, murder is morally right.                                                       ↓

Once we make this distinction, it's easy to find the mistake in the resident's **799**
position in Case 53. Ethical decisions are based on the best available data at
the time; if the data change in the future, the correct course of action may
change as well. If you begin administering penicillin for a patient's sore
throat, and the culture turns out to be negative for strep, you are not obligated to treat the patient with a full course of penicillin therapy just because you started it and are therefore committed.                           ↓

From an ethical standpoint, the decision is whether or not to treat a particu- **800**
lar patient at a particular time. It is ethically neutral whether treating means
starting a new treatment or continuing an old one.
   Interestingly, this is not necessarily the legal state of affairs. Failure to
start a respirator is not homicide under the law, but turning off a respirator
is a definite act that can be linked causally to a patient's death and hence is
homicide (except in cases of legally recognized brain death, of course).
Still, courts have never applied this strict definition; no doctor has been
prosecuted for turning off a respirator on a hopelessly ill patient.         ↓

There is another ethical issue involved in Case 53 — a general policy ques- **801**
tion of whether we want our health professionals to err on the side of treating or not treating. If physicians approach cases of this sort the way the
resident does, it seems probable that a few patients who might have recovered, given intensive treatment, might be denied care because all the facts
were not available at the time of initial judgment. A general policy of starting treatment and then withdrawing it as soon as the prognosis is clearly
shown to be hopeless, seems a much wiser policy.                             ↓

**802**    So far we have been arguing that "stopping treatment" and "not starting treatment" may be ethically identical actions, even if the emotional reaction to them is different. Here, at least, an act of commission and an act of omission turn out to be morally equivalent. Can we generalize this to the difference between passive and active euthanasia? Since the goal in both is the same, that is, shortening the patient's life for his own benefit, aren't the
↓    exact means used relatively immaterial?

UNCLEAR* 805

**803**    We might go even further and claim that in some instances active euthanasia would be <u>more</u> ethical than passive euthanasia. We mentioned in Chapter 7 a case of an infant born with Down's syndrome and duodenal atresia, in which the parents refused surgery for the bowel blockage. The child, unable to absorb nutrients, gradually starved to death over many days.

We objected to the choice made in this case. But, assuming that it is ever acceptable to allow such an infant to die (perhaps if the defect is much more severe than Down's syndrome), wouldn't it be kinder in such a case
↓    to kill the infant quickly, instead of allowing it to starve slowly?

**804**    The standard medical judgment in such cases, which has been stated by many doctors and enshrined in the code of ethics of the American Medical Association, is that passive euthanasia is acceptable in some cases — especially when the terminal prognosis is clear and the physician has the agreement of the family, but active euthanasia is always contrary to the tenets of medical ethics. This judgment, however, belongs to Aiken's "level of moral rules" and not to the "ethical level." That is, it is a statement of right conduct unaccompanied by any clear analysis of possible objections that might be raised. And, in recent years, many philosophers have raised cogent ob-
**806** ↓    jections to challenge this view.

REVIEW LEVELS ↑ 61–66

---

**805**    It may not be obvious just what we mean by saying that two actions are "morally equivalent." Surely, stopping treatment and not starting treatment, or active and passive euthanasia, are not <u>identical</u> actions from a descriptive or empirical standpoint. Moral equivalence refers instead to the amount of personal responsibility and the extent of praise or blame that we attribute to the actions. If a patient is likely to recover fully with treatment, stopping that treatment is a blameworthy action, and it would be <u>just as</u> blameworthy not to start treatment in the first place. Alternatively, if a patient is suffering terribly from a terminal illness and requests that treatment be withheld, it would be praiseworthy not to start treatment; and it would be <u>just as</u> praiseworthy to stop the treatment if it had already been started
**803** ↑    against the patient's wishes.

The attention paid by philosophers to the active–passive euthanasia debate is instructive in showing medical people the value of philosophical analysis in grappling with a medical-ethics problem. If the philosophers are right in criticizing the standard view on euthanasia, it follows that some things that physicians have taken for granted are actually problematic and need to be discussed further, while other issues that physicians have been debating at length are really side issues and should be dropped. These are useful things to know if one is trying to arrive at valid ethical guidelines.

806

One way to start a criticism of the standard medical view is to observe that we can easily be biased on a general issue by familiarity with specific cases. We might base our judgment on those cases, forgetting that they do not accurately reflect the issue as a whole.

807

Often the distinction, "active vs. passive euthanasia," is construed as "active killing vs. allowing to die." This terminology tends to make us think of cases such as the following:

The Godfather. A hired Mafia killer wipes out an enemy with a submachine gun.

Marcus Welby. A kindly but realistic family doctor decides to withhold aggressive therapy to let a terminally ill patient die with dignity.

Clearly, the Godfather is a case of active killing, while Marcus Welby is a case of allowing to die. If we had those two cases in mind as our prototypes, we might well conclude: "Allowing to die might be all right in some cases, but active killing is definitely wrong."

808

Now think about these two cases:

The Green Berets. A soldier, fleeing with his buddies from the Viet Cong, is wounded in the leg and cannot go on. If captured, he is well aware that he will be tortured mercilessly, then put to death after he has given all the information he knows — information that could jeopardize the secret base camp. He begs his friend to put a bullet into his head.

The Jealous Lifeguard. A lifeguard hears a call for help and sees a man drowning — a man he recognizes as his mistress's husband. He pretends that he has something in his eye. By the time he gets out to where the man is, the man has drowned.

These examples put a different light on the matter. If we had only those cases to go by, we might conclude: "Active killing might be all right in some cases, but allowing to die is always wrong."

809

Notice, in passing, that we have included both Marcus Welby and the jealous lifeguard as "allowing to die" cases. These can be distinguished from a much larger group of "not saving" cases. For example, right now we are

810

**810
cont.** reading this book, and so we are not saving starving children in Biafra. Normally we do not hold an individual morally to blame for this type of "not saving."

The Marcus Welby and the jealous lifeguard cases are different from those not saving cases, however. Doctors and lifeguards have some sort of presumed duty to save those people who fall within their purview. Both Marcus Welby and the jealous lifeguard knew that the particular person was dying at that time. Both Welby and the lifeguard possessed the necessary skills to save the person, had they chosen to do so. And neither Welby nor the lifeguard were restrained by special circumstances, such as being tied to their chairs. These factors make their actions a true case of allowing to die, not just a case of not saving (although we tend to praise Welby and
↓ blame the lifeguard for their choices).

**811** In conclusion, these four cases have clouded the issue by bringing in a number of extraneous points to bias our judgment. One philosopher, Rachels (1975), felt that he could get to the heart of the issue if he could design two cases that were identical in every respect save one — that one was a case of killing while the other was a case of allowing to die. If we judged the characters in the two cases to be equally praiseworthy or equally blameworthy, Rachels felt we would prove that killing and allowing to die
↓ were morally equivalent actions.

**812** Here are Rachels' two cases:

Smith. Smith has a 6-year-old nephew who stands between Smith and a large inheritance. Smith decides to get the inheritance by killing the child. One day, while the child is taking a bath, Smith sneaks in and holds the child's head under water until he drowns.

Jones. Jones, like Smith, has an inheritance problem because of a nephew, and decides on just the same action. He also sneaks into the bathroom, fully intending to drown the nephew just as Smith did. But, just as Jones enters the room, the nephew falls, hits his head on the tub, and slips unconscious with his face under water. Jones could easily save the child merely by holding his head out of the water, but instead he stands by, doing nothing, and the child drowns.
↓

**813** There is no question of giving either Smith or Jones the Uncle of the Year award; clearly they are both disgusting, immoral people. The question is: Do we find that Smith is any more or less blameworthy than Jones, because Smith killed the child while Jones merely allowed him to die? Rachels concludes (as seems perfectly reasonable) that we find the two actions equally
↓ blameworthy and hence morally equivalent.

Obviously, Rachels would not say that all cases of killing are morally    **814**
equivalent to all cases of allowing to die. What he <u>is</u> concluding from the
Smith-Jones example is: If you decide that a case of killing is wrong and a
case of allowing to die is right, you must be deciding on the basis of the
motives of the people involved, the consequences of the actions, or the
special circumstances of the two cases. You cannot be deciding on the basis of the "bare difference" between killing and allowing to die, because
that difference, taken by itself, makes no moral difference — as the Smith-
Jones example proves.    ↓

Rachels' intriguing example makes us rethink the active–passive euthana-    **815**
sia distinction and suggests that it carries a lot less moral weight than we
might originally have thought. But, as we would guess, others have not
been content to let Rachels have the last word in the argument. Of all the
objections raised against Rachels's argument, many are erroneous or miss
the point Rachels is trying to make. But there are several telling objections.    ↓

Trammell (1979) objects that Rachels cannot use the Smith-Jones example    **816**
to show that the active–passive euthanasia distinction is <u>never</u> morally relevant <u>in any context</u>. In the particular context of that case, we can base our
moral judgment on obvious features — the evil intentions of both Smith
and Jones, for example — so the active–passive distinction need not enter in.
In another context, however, that distinction may make all the difference.    ↓

Beauchamp and Childress (1979), on the other hand, object that even if Ra-    **817**
chels has proved what he set out to prove, that isn't really very much. Rachels, after all, says that instead of the bare difference between active and
passive euthanasia, we should be looking at the intentions of the parties
involved, the consequences of the various acts, and the special situation
that exists. But since, in making ethical decisions, the motives, consequences, and circumstances are exactly what we are interested in, Rachels
has not brought us much closer to an answer.    ↓

Looking at all these different arguments and counterarguments, what can    **818**
we conclude about the role of the active–passive euthanasia distinction in
reaching decisions about particular cases? Menzel (1979) has given us the
most useful synthesis of all the arguments touched on above.    ↓

Basically, Menzel feels that the active–passive euthanasia distinction has    **819**
moral weight, but primarily because the distinction calls our attention to
the <u>general</u> reasons that make allowing to die preferable to active killing.
But these reasons may be absent in a <u>specific</u> case. If we can show for a
specific case that these general reasons are absent and, in addition, that
there would be important benefits from killing rather than allowing to die
(e.g., if the resulting death would be quicker and less painful), we might
conclude that active euthanasia is morally preferable in that specific instance.    ↓

**820** Some general reasons to prefer passive euthanasia to active euthanasia (always assuming that we have already decided that euthanasia itself is morally appropriate) are:

1. If we have mistakenly diagnosed a terminal illness, the patient allowed to die without treatment may recover spontaneously; the person we kill cannot recover.
2. If we have been mistaken about an individual's true desire to die, withholding treatment may allow time for the patient to set us straight; killing eliminates this chance.
3. If what we sometimes consider the patient's suffering is actually our own discomfort at his plight; active killing seems more likely than allowing to die to be open to the abuse of "disposing of" the uncomfortable patient, ostensibly for his benefit but really for our own.

↓

**821** By this list, we see the value of Rachels' analysis: while these reasons may be more likely to occur in cases of active euthanasia, they may still occur in cases of passive euthanasia as well. Therefore the rule, "Always avoid active euthanasia but don't hesitate to perform passive euthanasia" is just as likely to lead us into serious ethical errors as is acceptance of active euthanasia.

↓

**822** Consider three patients on respirators in an intensive care unit; none are irreversibly comatose but all will die immediately if the respirator is unhooked. The first patient has a diagnosis of terminal cancer, but the diagnosis is wrong and the patient could actually recover over a period of time. The second patient really wants to be kept alive as long as possible, but has never communicated this desire. The third patient is not suffering, but has infected bedsores that make him distasteful to the hospital staff. In all three caes, we might unplug the respirator, thinking we were doing the right thing, and yet be mistaken. Therefore, the three reasons we considered to avoid active euthanasia may in some cases count just as strongly against passive euthanasia.

↓

**823** Ten years ago, the most common ethical mistake made in terminal-care cases appeared to be the continuation of life support to the bitter end — long after cure was impossible and even contrary to the expressed wishes of patient and family. As a result of the "death-with-dignity" movement and public awareness of famous cases such as the Quinlan case, this attitude appears to be changing, and physicians are now much more willing to allow a patient to die. Still, too often this decision is based on the physician's own views on the value of continued life for that patient. The family may be consulted but, even when the patient is alert, many physicians are unwilling to deal openly with the death issue and to elicit the patient's views directly.

In such instances, one might wonder if a false emphasis on the active–

passive distinction ("After all, I'm not killing the patient, I'm merely allowing him to die") has not made physicians less sensitive to their true duty under the doctor–patient contract, which would demand that the patient be involved in such a decision if possible.

**823 cont.**

↓

---

## CASE 54

A child has been born with meningomyelocele, a congenital defect of the spinal cord and its coverings. The indicators for this child are poor — the defect is large, located high on the spinal cord (auguring for paralysis of the whole body below that point), and the baby already has signs of hydrocephalus (fluid accumulation around the brain from an associated defect). Surgical correction can help children with milder meningomyelocele lead lives marred only by the physical handicap, but surgery cannot help this child much and a severe degree of retardation is also likely to occur.

**824**

A pediatrician argues that since the child is likely to have a very poor quality of life in any event, surgery should not be attempted. But if no surgery is done, the child can survive for weeks or months until it dies from infection or some other complication. Therefore, this pediatrician argues, active euthanasia would be preferable: "Having seen such children lying around the wards waiting to die, I can't help feeling that the highest form of medical ethic would be to end the pain and suffering now, rather than to wish the patient would go away."

The chief of pediatrics retorts that our attribution of suffering to such infants reflects our own discomfort; there are no objective signs that the infant is in any pain, and it doesn't have enough awareness of self and future for us to say that it is lying around waiting to die. He adds, "The parents, not the children, may be the ones to suffer. But haven't we also seen love and devotion, not just misery, come to families who have to care for a handicapped child? Surely every pediatrician has seen a case where a handicapped child, even one who lived for a brief time, brought a lot of joy to the family." He favors surgery to provide for whatever brief survival is possible.

Assuming that the child's parents will agree with the course, do you favor:

| | |
|---|---|
| Surgical treatment | ↓ 825 |
| No surgery, with death by passive euthanasia | ↓ 833 |
| Active euthanasia | ↓ 834 |

(Adapted from a case described by J. M. Freeman, Is there a right to die — quickly? With rebuttal by R. E. Cooke, Whose suffering? *Journal of Pediatrics* 80 : 904–7, 1972.)

825 One might choose surgery because of an unwillingness to extend one's own ideas of quality of life to this infant, whose experiences none of us can share. One might also be reluctant to choose euthanasia of any sort for someone who cannot voluntarily consent. But what about choosing surgery because "handicapped children often bring joy to the family"? First, this may be true for some families, and not this one; and second, is it justified to make the child a <u>means</u> to bring joy to the family, if life is really an unacceptable burden for this child? Also, are you willing to consider this
↓ sort of care a valid use of scarce medical resources?

---

826 Case 54 is an especially difficult context in which to discuss euthanasia. For one thing, the patient is an infant who cannot now, and never could in the past, make known its own wishes or its own assessment of its quality of life. For another, the illness discussed is not necessarily terminal; the proposed euthanasia will prevent the possibility of many years of life, even if it is a lesser quality of life. Therefore, the fact that it is very difficult to agree on judgments about Case 54 should not lead us to conclude that there are not
↓ other cases that are more clear-cut.

827 But even when one is dealing with adults and terminal-illness situations, careful medical judgment must be used to avoid serious errors. Euthanasia, either active or passive, is an irreversible step, and it stands to reason that great care should be exercised in all such decisions. Jackson and Youngner (1979), by means of some sample cases, suggest useful categories of
↓ mistake-prone cases for which health professionals can be on the lookout.

828 Jackson and Youngner correctly point out that patient autonomy is the underlying value that ought to guide the medical team in terminal-care decisions. Their categories are useful because they illustrate types of cases in
↓ which patient autonomy may be difficult to define.

829 Their categories include the following:

   1. Ambivalence. The patient may first refuse treatment, then later beg for it as his condition worsens and may continue changing his mind over time.
   2. Depression. The desire to terminate treatment may reflect a psychiatric depression. When the depression is properly treated, the patient may become more hopeful and may then request that treatment be continued.
   3. Hidden message. The patient asking to be allowed to die may really be expressing reactions to other emotional issues, such as a feeling of abandonment by family. If these issues are addressed, the request for euthanasia may be withdrawn.

4. Fear. Patients may refuse treatment based on unreasonable fears of the treatment itself.

5. Family disagreement. The patient may give one message to the health team while the family requests another course of action.

829 cont. ↓

*All of these categories suggest that a request for euthanasia from either patient or family cannot be accepted at face value; there must be a good deal of inquiry to establish its basis.* The second and third categories suggest that psychiatric consultation may be an important part of this process. *Where doubt remains, continuation of life-prolonging treatment seems necessary until the doubt can be resolved (if ever). This assumes that the medical team is actively working to resolve the doubt by gathering whatever data are necessary. That is different from using the possibility of doubt as an argument to prohibit euthanasia across the board.*

830

↓ 832

The fact that mistakes of this sort can be made in practice has led some to conclude that euthanasia simply ought not to be practiced. Kamisar (1976), for example, has offered an argument that goes something like this: The only legitimate use of active euthanasia would be in the case of a patient with severe, intractable pain. But such a patient could never give a fully rational consent for euthanasia. Therefore, there is no legitimate use for active euthanasia.

831

↓

Several rebuttals to this argument arise from our discussion so far. First, there may be other types of suffering besides pain that give rise to a lowered quality of life and hence justify euthanasia. For example, most patients can be made reasonably pain-free with appropriate drug treatment, but this may be at the expense of their mental alertness and their awareness of surroundings. For some patients with certain personal values, such a trade-off may not be worth it, and a speedy end would be preferable to a pain-free but drugged state.

832

↓ 835

---

If you have already decided that surgery is inappropriate, is passive euthanasia the best alternative? You may be shrinking from active euthanasia because it is illegal, which is a reasonable view to take. But we have argued that passive euthanasia cannot be preferable <u>just because</u> it is passive and not active. Furthermore, it seems that some reasons for preferring passive to active euthanasia, such as possibly mistaken diagnosis and uncertainty as to what the patient wants, do not or cannot apply to this case. On the other hand, if the second pediatrician is correct in that it is us and not the infant who is benefitted by its death, active euthanasia might be a way of dodging this issue and thus might be less ethically acceptable.

833

↑ 826

**834** If you choose active euthanasia here, you have company. We noted that this type of case seems to be the prototype of cases in which active euthanasia is to be preferred to passive, if any such cases exist at all. Still, active euthanasia may be a quick way out compared to reevaluating the original decision not to do surgery. If these particular parents do not want the burden of raising a child with this severe handicap, does it automatically follow that the child would be better off dead than in a foster home or an institution? We might think more carefully about this if we had to face the prospect of caring for the child for weeks or months while waiting for it to

**826** ↑ die.

---

**835** Second, Kamisar's argument makes no allowance for instruments such as "living wills," which might allow a fully rational and competent individual to give consent to euthanasia before the fact. And finally, this argument neglects the fact we stressed — that any mistake that can be made in applying active euthanasia can also be made in applying passive euthanasia. But to prohibit both kinds of euthanasia would amount to support for a
↓ sanctity-of-life ethic, which few ethicists would support.

**836** However, in talking so far about possible mistakes, we have been talking about the ethics of euthanasia. But euthanasia is a legal issue as well as an ethical one. If, as we have argued, we have no ethical grounds to prohibit totally the practice of active euthanasia, and if active euthanasia may be the preferable mode of treatment for a small but distinct class of terminally ill patients, isn't it a legal outrage that such a practice should be considered murder in the eyes of the law? Shouldn't the statutes be revised to make
↓ allowances for active euthanasia, with the proper safeguards?

**837** It is too simplistic to assume that just because active euthanasia is ethically justifiable, it should be made legal. We are all aware of the fallacy of assuming that just because something is held to be immoral it ought to be made illegal. We now have to look at the flip side of that coin — whether it should ever be the case that an action may be ethically justifiable but ought to
↓ remain legally impermissible.

**838** The legal status of active euthanasia is rather intriguing. It is unquestionably a felony, yet the people who are proved to have committed this felony are uniformly acquitted. In the United States, during the last 30 years, at least two physicians and a number of patient's relatives have gone on trial for "mercy killings." In one of the more dramatic cases, a man walked into an intensive care unit and blew off his brother's head with a shotgun, at his brother's request, following paralysis in a motorcycle accident. The juries have uniformly accepted pleas such as, "not guilty by reason of temporary
↓ insanity," and have let the defendants go free.

On May 18, 1979, in Washington, D.C., a woman entered the hospital room **839** where her father lay dying of esophageal cancer, snipped the intravenous lines with a scissors, unplugged the respirator from the wall, and sat by while he expired. The woman even signed a statement of her intent to end her father's life peacefully; but a grand jury, despite this evidence, refused to return an indictment charging her with a crime. (It is interesting that this woman was held to be committing a mercy killing, or active euthanasia. Had her father's physician written orders on the chart to disconnect the IVs and the respirator, the act would have amounted to precisely the same thing, and the case would have been viewed as a typical example of passive euthanasia.) ↓

To some, this inconsistent legal status of active euthanasia amounts to an **840** unacceptable hypocrisy. If, in a carefully selected class of cases, active euthanasia is the more kind and hence the ethically preferable approach, it seems insufferable that the physician who elects to perform this final service for his patient should run the risk of criminal prosecution. Legalization of this activity should be much more straightforward than resorting to a fictitious temporary insanity. ↓

Naturally, this argument in favor of legalized active euthanasia comes from **841** physicians who believe that active euthanasia is ethically justifiable. Just as naturally, those physicians and ethicists who feel that active euthanasia can never be justified totally oppose legalization. ↓

We might add here that there is an interesting compromise position fa- **842** vored by a few physicians — that physicians themselves be prohibited from active euthanasia, but that this be permitted to family members or other lay people. The argument is that active euthanasia is justifiable, but that active killing is so contrary to the usual values of the medical profession that any involvement of physicians in such activities would inevitably lead to a decay in the moral fiber of the profession.

This position seems to rest on questionable psychological assumptions. Surely a physician who "euthanized" dozens of people daily would soon become hardened to his role and would tend, perhaps, to lose respect for human life in general. But it is probable that any single physician will have to face in his career only a few cases in which active euthanasia seems to be the best ethical alternative. It seems very unlikely that these tragic cases, few and far between, will lead to any major loss of sensitivity. (Certainly the individual physician may always refuse to participate, just as he may refuse to do abortions or sterilizations.) ↓

REVIEW REFUSAL ↑ 546–551

**843** So far all these positions on the legalization of active euthanasia are readily understandable. But the most interesting position is that taken by a number of physicians, ethicists, and lawyers — that active euthanasia is acceptable in a few cases, but that it should never be legalized and should remain always an extralegal activity. In general, those holding this position base their arguments on the possible abuses of any law allowing active euthanasia and on the difficulty to write such a law without leaving unintended loop- ↓ holes.

**844** This argument, which does not attack at all the morality of active euthanasia, reminds us of the domino-theory arguments we discussed earlier. It relates to the second kind of domino-theory argument — that even though we can distinguish in principle between the good and the bad uses of euthanasia, in practice people will fail to make this distinction and so will be ↓ led by the new law to commit unethical actions.
REVIEW DOMINO THEORY ↑ 258–261

**845** We argued before that this sort of domino-theory argument had limited application in ethical debates. Ethics should be based on the appeal to rational arguments and to the good intentions of the parties. While any realistic ethical analysis will allow for the fact that we do not always live up to our goals of rationality and benevolence, we must still conduct ethical debates on a relatively high plane; just because some people prefer to murder, rape, and steal does not mean that we should debase all ethical discussion ↓ to their level.

**846** But in the law, and generally in public policy debates, the second form of the domino-theory argument carries much greater weight. By its nature, the law must look at the worst possible cases, not the best; and it must be designed with one eye toward the attempts that the unscrupulous will make to misuse it in the future. When we make an ethical judgment, we can hedge by restricting our decision to a very narrow class of cases and to situations as they presently exist. But a law, once passed, may be used in the ↓ future to decide cases that we cannot currently anticipate.
REVIEW LAW VS. ETHICS ↑ 69–71

**847** Obviously the major loophole we will be concerned with is the use of a euthanasia law to justify removing a sick relative for monetary gain, or liquidating whole classes of the infirm or retarded as supposedly useless to society. In our ethical discussion, we simply removed any such cases from consideration by our definition of "euthanasia" — that it was necessarily an act intended for the good of the individual himself. This is a legitimate move in ethical discussion, but it holds very little water when it comes to designing a sufficiently stringent law. Any such appeal to motives, as op- ↓ posed to overt behavior, will be very difficult to apply or prove in practice.

Furthermore, appeals to overt behavior instead will not eliminate all problems. We could, for example, restrict active euthanasia to those individuals who had previously signed a document requesting it, but we would then have to take into account the possibility of forging documents or of coercing signature. We could enact stiff penalties for such forgery or coercion, but these penalties would be of little use after the fact to the person who had been wrongly killed.   **848**

It would be an instructive group exercise to try to draft such a law. After getting the best possible set of safeguards, the group should then take the opposite point of view and try to imagine ways to get around the safeguards.   **849**

Of course, having safeguards that are too loose is only one way that such a law could prove defective. The safeguards could also be made so stringent that patients who can be helped by active euthanasia might be denied this aid. Although the California Natural Death Act of 1976 dealt with passive euthanasia under a living will document, and not active euthanasia, many critics felt that it committed this second sort of error — that its restrictions were so tight that it could benefit only a small minority of those patients who are candidates for passive euthanasia. (See the California living will in Appendix VII.)

Some authorities assume that it will be almost impossible to draft an active euthanasia statute in which provisions will not be either too loose or too tight (or, for that matter, both at once). They conclude then that since, of all the patients who are candidates for euthanasia, active euthanasia will be preferable for only a few, and active killing of anyone for any motive is a very momentous undertaking, it is better in the long run that any physician who undertakes such an action does so with a healthy respect for the possible legal consequences. One might predict that, if this policy is followed, a few patients will suffer because their physicians will be too scared to institute active euthanasia even when morally indicated; but if a law were passed, even more would suffer due to the possible abuses of the law. This, by a consequentialist approach, favors the present policy.   **850**

Many physicians, who are already paranoid about their possible legal liabilities anyway, would find such an argument insufferable. But it seems that the only effective rebuttal is to propose a draft statute for active euthanasia that persuasively avoids the various pitfalls we have mentioned. So far, no proposed legislation has quite met these standards. (Baruch Brody has argued, however, that there is no fundamental problem with such legislation; see his essay in the collection by Kohl [1975].)   **851**

**852**    We should not leave the legal arena without pointing out one feature of our earlier argument about the lack of a sharp moral distinction between active and passive euthanasia. If legalized active euthanasia is open to these sorts of abuses, then legalized passive euthanasia should be open to the same sorts of abuses — and indeed, arguments like those we have just reviewed have been lodged against a Michigan bill that would formalize procedures for making medical decisions, including passive euthanasia, on behalf of incompetent patients (see Relman [1979]). The major difference is that most acts of passive euthanasia are legal, so the potential for such
↓   abuses already exists.

**853**    We have now touched upon the important features of the euthanasia debate. As we saw in Case 52, it is not a new debate, but it has gathered greater urgency with the development of new technology and the removal of the death setting from the privacy of the home into the relative publicity of the hospital. *We have seen that acts of euthanasia, both active and passive, may be ethically justifiable, but that all such acts require, in addition to a full understanding of the values of personal autonomy and quality of life developed in Chapter 6, impeccable medical judgment to assess prognosis accurately and to rule out any condition, such as depression, which might interfere with the patient's ability to make a truly autonomous decision.*

**854** ↓  CH. 14

# Mass Screening Programs 14

Most of the ethical issues we have looked at so far could be viewed on the **854** basis of the contractual model of the doctor– (or health professional– ) patient relationship that we developed in Chapter 4. In this chapter we will look at one set of problems to which this model does not apply very well. These problems arise in mass screening programs, such as screening for communicable diseases, undiscovered hypertension, or carriers of genetic diseases. Of all these screening programs, genetic screening has received the lion's share of attention from writers on medical ethics. We will discuss genetic screening a good deal, thereby setting the stage for our discussion of genetic engineering in the next chapter, but our major concern will be with the problems of mass screening programs in general. ↓

At first glance, it might seem that these programs are sufficiently like the **855** usual doctor–patient relationship to fall under the same ethical model. After all, the services are delivered by doctors or other health professionals. Individual patients are involved and, in many cases, their health is improved by this involvement. The aim of such programs is to prevent or cure major diseases.

Despite these similarities, there are important differences between the usual doctor–patient encounter and at least some of the many sorts of mass screening programs. These differences have enough ethical implications to make it worthwhile for us to consider a different model for them, the "public health model," as opposed to the contractual model we have used for the more usual doctor–patient relationship. Table 4 illustrates several key differences between the two models. ↓

Glancing over Table 4, we immediately see several potential ethical prob- **856** lems. In the contractual model, the free entry of the patient into the relationship, the role of the patient in defining the goals of the relationship, and the focus on the patient as an individual, all combine to place great stress on the value of individual autonomy (and to lead, in turn, to the importance of truth-telling and informed consent). In the absence of these considerations in the public health model, there seems to be much more allowance for coercion or manipulation. This denial of autonomy may be appropriate in some contexts — other, overriding values may take precedence over autonomy. On the other hand, it may slip in unnoticed. Traditionally, authorities who have good intentions and who are seeking worthwhile goals have been slow to notice when their activities violate some of the rights of those they are trying to help. ↓

**Table 4.** *Comparison of the Contractual Model of the Doctor–Patient Relationship with the Public Health Model*

| Contractual Model | Public Health Model |
|---|---|
| Generally involves the individual patient | Generally involves a group or population of patients |
| Patient initiates the relationship by seeking care | Individual patients in the group usually do not initiate the encounter |
| Patient has a large role in defining and negotiating the goals of treatment | Authorities in charge of the program usually determine goals (although involvement by lay and community representatives is increasing) |
| Patient's own good is of paramount importance | Good of individual patients is important, but other important values may compete for priority |
| Patient is viewed as free party to the contract | Individuals may be manipulated or even coerced to promote the chosen goals of the program |

**857**  Another set of ethical concerns arises from the focus on knowledge that is often a feature of mass screening programs. In the usual doctor–patient relationship, the doctor is always seeking new knowledge about the patient and is trying to pass important knowledge along to the patient, but this takes place in a trusting environment. The patient has reason to believe that this knowledge is ultimately for his own good and is directly connected with his medical treatment. In the public health model, though, the knowledge may be collected and disseminated in a setting more suggestive of an impersonal bureaucracy. The program may be designed solely to generate knowledge of disease, and the patient may be forced to go elsewhere for treatment if disease is found. Finally, the knowledge may be of the sort that does not lead directly to assistance, or at least not the sort of assistance that fits into one's life values. The knowledge that one is the carrier of a genetic disease, where the only possible action is to choose not to have children, could be an example of burdensome and possibly undesired knowledge.

**858**  Which of these ethical problems will arise, and how serious they will be, depends in part on the type of screening program and its goals or intentions. We can distinguish several sorts of programs that are commonly encountered:

1. Screening for communicable diseases, where the public health agency has a legal mandate to discover and treat cases to prevent epidemics.
2. Screening for environmental health hazards, such as air and water pollution, either routinely or in the wake of a known or suspected accidental contamination.

3. Screening for treatable diseases that generally do not produce symptoms in their early, treatable stages (such as hypertension or early cancer).
4. Screening for genetic carriers, or for risk factors leading to the increased likelihood that one will have children with severe genetic disease.
5. Screening for a wide variety of diseases or risk factors as part of epidemiologic research. (We can dismiss this topic for this chapter, as it falls under the problems of human experimentation, which we discussed in Chapter 11.)

**858 cont.**

↓

We can also list several possible motives or intentions for embarking upon a screening program, such as the following.

**859**

1. A view of the right to health care (which we discuss at length in Chapter 16) may suggest that the population in question deserves such services.
2. A paternalistic desire to help the members of the population may promote a program, based on the supposition that the members, if left to themselves, would be too uninformed (or lazy) to seek help.
3. An efficiency analysis may suggest that it would be much cheaper to provide these services on a mass scale, despite the fact that the services could be provided by individual physicians or other health professionals.
4. The condition being screened for may constitute so great a public danger that aggressive measures to detect and treat it are warranted (as with virulent, epidemic infectious diseases).
5. Society may elect to save money by detecting and treating disease early by aggressive screening, instead of waiting for later stages of disease where treatment and rehabilitation may be more expensive.
6. Society may want to keep its work force at peak productivity by eliminating morbidity. (This argument is seldom expressed in this country, but forms a major justification of the health practices in socialist countries.)

↓

We can now imagine several possible sources of ethical errors that we will need to look for in evaluating specific screening proposals. We can particularly watch for three general sorts of errors.

**860**

↓

The first sort of error is to argue from the wrong model — to act as if the contractual model is in use when in fact the public health model is applicable. This can cause us to wrongly condemn some practices. For example, communicable disease–reporting laws require physicians to report cases of gonorrhea, and the patients are then questioned about their sexual contacts. Viewed solely from the perspective of the doctor–patient relationship, this would seem to be an unethical invasion of privacy and violation of confidentiality. But, within the public health model, the greater public good of controlling contagious diseases may be invoked to justify these practices. The question then becomes: How great an invasion of privacy can be justified, given the severity, communicability, and so on of the disease in question?

**861**

↓

**862** Another example of this sort of error is to argue in justification of various invasive screening practices based on the fact that, after all, it is for the good of the patient. This argument has some force (although limited) under the contractual model, since the patient entered into the contract voluntarily and has some say in deciding what his own good is. But these factors are not present under the public health model; where the patient is stripped of some of the safeguards he enjoys under the usual doctor–patient relationship, we cannot base our argument on features of that relationship.

**863** The second sort of error we might envision involves confusing different sorts of screening programs. We have already suggested that the public menace of communicable disease may justify a certain level of coercion — for example, forcing people to be immunized if an epidemic threatens. Arguing that genetic diseases are "communicable" in the sense that they are passed from parents to children, some have tried to justify forced participation in genetic screening programs by analogy to the communicable-disease case. But genetic disease, however serious and costly, does not present the same sort of immediate threat to the public welfare that an epidemic would, so this analogy is a flawed basis for ethical argument.

**864** Finally, the third sort of error is to miscalculate the actual risks or benefits of a screening program. We might easily endorse a questionable program if we judged either that the degree of coercion or of invasion of privacy was less than it really was, or that the health benefits to the patients were much greater than they really were. Usually we will have to look at specific cases to see whether this sort of error exists.

**865** Avoidance of these errors requires that those planning a screening program be able to share the point of view of the population to be screened. This may be made more difficult when the population (as is often the case) represents a different economic, cultural, or racial group. Difficulties with sickle-cell anemia screening in the black community illustrate the point all too well. For decades, black, inner-city communities received adequate medical care only when it served the purposes of the white community — such as when poor patients were needed as "teaching material" for medical schools or as subjects for research. So now, when the people in the white coats march in and explain that the screening program is strictly for the greater good of the black community, that community can be excused for excessive suspicion. The suspicion is also bound to be fueled by some of the provisions of hastily enacted sickle-cell screening laws, such as the mandatory screening of grade school children. One would have to ask whether, if a cheap and reliable means were available to detect carriers of some genetic disease present only in whites, legislators would have been willing to enact laws with some of the same provisions.

Public ignorance, especially about genetic disease, can exacerbate the con-   **866**
sequences of hastily enacted screening programs. The name "sickle-cell
trait" applied to carriers of sickle-cell anemia genes has suggested to many
that the carriers themselves are the victims of a disease. In fact, sickle-cell
trait can affect one's health only under very unusual circumstances (such as
very high altitudes). But this has not prevented some blacks from being denied jobs, refused military service, or having their insurance canceled, just
because the label "sickle-cell trait" had been applied to them as a consequence of some screening program.                                             ↓

Furthermore, in genetic screening programs, the intended outcome of the   **867**
screening involves changes in the reproductive practices of the people
screened — in particular, it is assumed that those found to be carriers of a
genetic disease will either refrain from marrying other carriers or, if already
married, will elect not to have natural children (or to have amniocentesis to
detect the diseased fetus and then to abort that fetus). It may be difficult for
those running the screening program to envision the impact of this information and these recommendations on the people involved, especially in
cultures where fertility and child-rearing play a large role in the individual's
self-esteem and community standing.                                       ↓

---

## CASE 55

As director of the county health department, you are approached by an offi-   **868**
cial from the United States government's food stamp distribution program.
The food stamp people are concerned about the high incidence of iron
deficiency anemia among children in lower socioeconomic groups in this
country, as revealed by national surveys. It has also been feared that, because of their cultural patterns and inadequate knowledge of nutrition,
food stamp users might purchase foods that are not the most nutritious and
therefore the children might be exposed to dietary deficiencies.

The program proposes to have public health nurses at the distribution
center to take finger-prick blood samples from the children of food stamp
recipients to test for anemia by hematocrit — the same procedure that you
routinely carry out in the well-baby clinic. To assure compliance, the blood
test would be made a requirement for the mother's obtaining food stamps.
Since your department already has provisions for treating anemia with free
iron supplements, immediate therapy would be made available whenever a
case of anemia were found.

You are in agreement with the objectives of the idea, and you acknowledge that since many mothers do not bring their children in, your existing
facilities are not detecting all the iron deficiency cases in the community.
However, you are concerned about the compulsory nature of this screening proposal.

**868**
**cont.**
The official replies that since the amount of blood drawn is minuscule, the deficiency disease may have few outward symptoms, the disease is perfectly treatable by oral supplementation, and free therapy will be provided, no reasonable mother could refuse to have her child tested. Even if the mother were unreasonable, the child has a right to good health care. Anyway, just to make it all officially proper, each mother will be asked to sign a consent form for the testing.

The food stamp program has no trained personnel to do the blood tests and thus is dependent on your providing nurses for the proposal. Do you agree
↓ to the proposal as it now stands?

---

**869**
The proposal in Case 55 meets one of the requirements for screening programs that was just hinted at — providing treatment along with the knowledge. The hangup, obviously, is the question of compulsion. First, it ought to be clear that making the test a condition for obtaining food stamps represents coercion, regardless of how many forms may be signed. The question is then: On what grounds might such coercion be justified?

Is a child's right to good health care adequate justification? In addition to the problems we mentioned before when there is no specification as to who is obligated to fulfill a right, we have a problem in that we usually assume that a right will be asserted by the party whose interest is actually involved, and that that party may choose to waive the right. We assume, therefore, that a right to health care, if it exists, can be met by providing opportunities for care. We do not think of this right as requiring us to sally
↓ forth into the streets to recruit patients actively.

**870**
However, an exception might have to be made here, as in the case of the presumed right to life of the unborn, where the party to whom we attribute the right is unable to claim it himself; under such circumstances it does not seem so odd to appoint ourselves as stand-ins.

We can suppose, also, that if the program were established at the food stamp distribution center on a voluntary rather than a compulsory basis, some children with anemia would be missed in the screening. (Just how many would be missed might be information that would be of value in making this ethical decision. Therefore, an alternative proposal might be setting up a voluntary testing program to see how high compliance is, with
↓ the option of altering the program later if expectations are not met.)

Presumably we know the consequences of a compulsory program — ill feel-    **871**
ings on the part of the "patients," increased distrust of governmental agencies with a possible carryover against the health professions because of
their participation in the program, and so on. We put a minus weight on
these consequences in our ethical calculations. Now, we have to decide:
How many anemic children put on the other side of the balance would
outweigh these consequences? There could be wide disagreement here.
Some who are particularly sensitive to the social discontent of the under-
privileged citizens might say that no matter how many anemic children are
missed, the social ills would not be outweighed. (Note that while moderate
anemia in children may slightly retard physical and intellectual development and may help predispose toward infection — the results of research
are unclear — it is hardly a life-threatening illness.) On the other side, someone who is gung-ho for the right to adequate health care may insist that
these social consequences are of minor impact if even a single anemic child
is missed in screening.    ↓

There is one flaw in the latter view that might indicate that the ill feelings    **872**
generated by such a program have to be taken more seriously. The idea that
it would be bad to miss some anemic children supposes that identification
will automatically lead to treatment and cure. Treatment does not take
place when you give the mother the bottle of iron syrup, but rather when
the mother actually gives it to the child. A mother who is upset by the element of coercion in the program, and who therefore cannot identify with
the program's goals seems much more likely to forget or neglect to give the
child his medicine. A voluntary program, on the other hand, if it is combined with a genuine attempt at education, might miss some children but
increase the long-range benefits of those who are identified.    ↓

The point underlying all this is that in the absence of an intensive public-    **873**
education campaign, which might or might not be successful if attempted,
the attitudes of the food-stamp mothers toward asymptomatic iron deficiency anemia is probably very different from the attitudes of the health
authorities. It is easy for us, as health professionals, to think that health
ought to be everybody's primary concern (even if we don't live our own
lives that way). On the other hand, given their limited resources of money
and energy, the mothers might be much more worried about other things in
their environment — such as whether their apartment will be heated in the
winter. As a general rule, the views of the program planners about the
severity of the disease and even the nature of the disease, or whether it is a
disease at all, are likely to be different from the views of the target population. As a practical, political matter, this divergence of views is an important
feature to consider in designing screening programs. (We'll take up the
problems related to differing concepts of health and disease again in Chapter 17.)    ↓

**874** Concepts of disease, and the degree of negative value placed on specific diseases, are therefore culturally relative phenomena and will differ among various populations and subcultures in our society. Another culturally relative value is the degree of coercion that people will accept as a matter of course. In many countries with a long history of government regimentation, people would accept without a murmur a much more coercive public health program than that envisioned in Case 55. In the United States, people have regularly disconnected various seat-belt reminder devices in autos; in many other countries, mandatory seat belt laws have been passed and have successfully reduced traffic-accident fatalities. This may mean that people in other cultures value individual freedom less than we do, or that they value it every bit as much but regard certain activities as irrelevant
↓ to true freedom and so not worth bothering about.

---

### CASE 56

**875** Now that Congress has just passed a comprehensive and compulsory national health insurance act, you have been appointed to the panel of experts who are determining just what the provisions of national insurance coverage shall be. You have come to the question of screening for genetic disease, and it has been generally agreed that if the physician feels that a patient is at risk to have a child with a diagnosable and untreatable genetic defect, the insurance ought to pay for amniocentesis or other diagnostic procedures as well as for an abortion carried out as a result of the findings.

The panel has now turned to the question of paying for the institutional care of mentally retarded individuals with genetic defects. This is a controversial issue because of the large sums of money involved. One panel member, M., states that a provision should be added to the program that would deny reimbursement to parents who received prenatal diagnosis of the defect or of the strong likelihood of a defect and failed to abort the fetus. He argues that if one has the means to prevent the birth of such an individual and chooses not to, one should pay for the consequences and not expect society to pick up the tab. To have society pay for such children, argues M., is simply an encouragement of "irresponsible parenthood."

The debate continues:

R.: What if the parents' religious beliefs forbid an abortion?

M.: If your religious beliefs say your kids should go to a parochial school, you pay for it yourself. Either you give up your religious beliefs or you pay for them. You are free to have the beliefs but not at the expense of taxpayers who do not share them.

L.: What if the person had normal diagnostic results but an error was made, and a deformed child was born anyway?

M.: We ought to pay for that. It wasn't the parents' fault; they took every reasonable precaution.

*T.:* It seems that then you ought not to pay for amniocentesis unless the  **875**
parents sign a form or something to say that they will abort if the child  **cont.**
is abnormal.

*M.:* I agree, that sounds logical.

*R.:* It seems that if you are going to be consistent, you have to provide for
the killing of these "mistaken diagnoses" that L. was talking about,
since you were prepared to abort them had the diagnosis been correct
rather than have the taxpayers foot the bill.

*M.:* You're twisting what I said. Once they are born they are citizens and
you're stuck. All I'm saying is that we should provide for reasonable
precautions and preventive action, before you get to that stage.

*B.:* I don't see how your proposal would work. If parents thought they
might not want to have an abortion, they would avoid having any prenatal diagnosis in order to protect their insurance payments.

*M.:* I would propose that the failure to have prenatal testing, when the
doctor had recommended it and it was available, would also constitute
grounds for nonpayment of costs of institutionalization, just as would
be the case if they had the tests but ignored the results.

Do you accept M.'s proposal or not?  ↓

---

Case 56, like the previous case, presents the prospect of using economic  **876**
compulsion to get individuals to submit to screening, and also to get individuals to have abortions if the screening test shows a genetic defect. We
could approach this case in accordance with our ethical decision-making
method. By taking the form of administrative regulation, the proposal is already expressed as a general rule and not as an ad hoc decision applying to
a particular case. We simply need to list all the consequences of this general rule and assign positive and negative value assessments.  ↓

But, on further analysis, this case presents some basic challenges to a con-  **877**
sequentialist mode of ethical decision making. In particular, until we add
some notions of personhood and of individual rights of the sort we dealt
with in Chapter 6, we will be unable even to begin assigning value weights
to the various consequences. For example, by some sorts of crude utilitarian
thinking, the continued existence of seriously retarded children is a drain
on social resources and hence a strongly negative value. By a view that
takes cognizance of the personhood and of the basic rights of these individuals, their continued existence is consistent with our most basic positive
values.  ↓

REVIEW PERSONHOOD ↑ 280–290

**878** In the same vein, one's reaction to the proposal is bound to be colored by one's assessment of the morality of abortion. To one who feels that abortion is murder, the proposal is simply wrong, and nothing more can possibly be said in terms of positive and negative value weightings. To one who accepts abortion as a morally neutral act, it is necessary to look at the other consequences to decide whether the proposal is acceptable or not. And, as we saw in Chapter 10, the abortion debate is not one that is likely to be ↓ decided on the basis of good or bad consequences.

REVIEW ABORTION ↑ 585

**879** Suppose, for the purposes of argument, that one adopts this stand on these key questions: (1) fetuses are not persons and so abortion is morally permissible in such a case; and (2) severely retarded children are persons and so, once born, have a right to life and deserve at least minimal provisions of food and shelter, regardless of who has to pay. (We have outlined in Chapters 6 and 10 the sorts of arguments that would support this stand.) On this basis it seems initially plausible to say that the fact that the society will have to foot the bill justifies a fairly high degree of social involvement in the decision on whether or not to abort. After all, it might be argued, no one is being forced to have an abortion, but only to pay for the results of not having one. If this results in the rich being able to maintain their retarded and deformed babies in institutions while the poor are forced financially to have abortions, this is merely to place the having of such children in the same "luxury" category as owning three Cadillacs; no one argues that the ↓ poor ought to be able to do everything the rich do.

**880** Balanced against this argument are two other considerations. The first is the suggestion that the institutionalized individuals do contribute something of value to society (or that they embody something of value), which helps to "reimburse" the cost of their upkeep. If we cannot imagine such a compensating value, it may be due to our poverty of imagination in having to think of such a value only in dollars-and-cents terms. (How many of us could calculate monetarily what we are really worth to society, if any- ↓ thing?)

**881** The second consideration has to do with the degree of intervention and coercion involved in implementing this program. While it is all very well to argue that a person whose religious (or other) values prohibit abortion should be made to pay for the consequences of his or her beliefs, the fact remains that such a person, perhaps forced by financial considerations into having an abortion, will feel resentment toward the social order that forced this predicament. A feeling of resentment, ill will, and injustice among the members of a society lessens social harmony and stability and needs to be viewed as a negative consequence for society, affecting even those mem- ↓ bers who are not directly involved in the coerced activity.

A decision on Case 56 would then involve weighing the cost to society of     882
maintaining the incapacitated individuals against the two other considerations — the negative effect of coercion and the value to society represented by those individuals. A full-scale analysis would involve comparing
alternative uses of the social resources (reminding us of the allocation of
resources issues raised in Chapter 12). You might want to use this case as
the basis for a small group discussion of these various issues.                     ↓

The last two cases have dealt with coercion in a screening program result-     883
ing from factors independent of the screening itself. However, is screening
intrinsically a coercive activity in a more subtle sense? From the point of
view of the individual tested, the major or the only "product" of a screening program is knowledge. And knowledge may not only be extremely burdensome, but may also profoundly affect the life of the person later. A person going to a program to be tested may come out with reassuring good
news or with crushing bad news, and the odds of the two depend on the
type of disorder being tested for. If no outside coercion is present, it is very
likely a weighing between the reassurance and the crush that leads an individual to decide whether or not to be tested. What would people do if the
chances were exactly equal?                                                                 ↓

---

## CASE 57

Huntington's chorea is an inherited disease of the nervous system in which     884
symptoms usually develop in an affected individual at age 35 to 45. The
disease leads to progressive mental and physical deterioration with death
occurring 10 to 15 years after first onset. The final stage of the disease has
been described as, "the pitiful picture of the complete ruin of a human being." The inheritance is autosomal dominant with complete penetrance —
therefore, one-half the offspring of an affected individual will carry the
gene, and all who carry the gene will develop the disease ultimately. There
is no treatment. Because of the late age of onset, most patients have had
several children before they become aware that they have the gene.

   One of the patients in your practice is a 42-year-old man who has shown
Huntington's symptoms for a little over a year. He has two sons, aged 19
and 17. The fact that each has a 50 percent chance of carrying the gene
weighs heavily on their minds, since each hopes to start a family and have
children soon. Each would have serious reservations about having children
if they knew they carried the gene.

   You are aware that a new experimental test is available in which a patient
at risk may be given a drug, levodopa, for a period of time. If the patient
carries the gene, he will develop symptoms — facial grimaces, tics, or other
involuntary movements — typical of the early stages of the disease itself,
and these symptoms will disappear with withdrawal of the drug. If the person is not a carrier, no symptoms will appear.

**884**
**cont.**
↓

Do you inform the sons of your affected patient about the existence of this test? If you do, and they seem uncertain about what to do, do you encourage them to have the test, or not?

---

**885**

In an article on this subject, Hemphill (1973) assumed that the test had been fully developed experimentally and then listed what he felt to be the major positive consequences of adopting the ethical proposition, "All people with a known family incidence of the disease should be tested before childbearing if possible":

1. If all those with positive tests refrained from having children by natural means, the level of the gene in the population would be significantly reduced.
2. Those with positive tests would know the approximate span of their active years and could plan their lives accordingly, without engaging in false hopes.
3. The knowledge of the disease per se could be considered good in that it increases the humanity of the individual who knows — it allows him to make a wider range of informed choices.

As a supplement to the first consequence we would add:

4. By not having children, the person would avoid the bad consequences of knowing that he had passed the gene on to his children, with the feelings of guilt, resentment, and so on, that would be bound to develop within the family in that case.

↓

**886**

Hemphill also considers the following negative consequences:

1. Early diagnosis of Huntington's chorea can make no difference in the terminal course of the disease, since there is no treatment.
2. By doing the test, one gives the patient a "sneak preview" of the actual symptoms that fate has in store for him. Thus, his feelings of anguish and dread, that he is bound to carry with him for 10 or 20 years, will be heightened.
3. While the option is supposedly "free," the psychological factors that determine acceding to the test or not must be powerful. A patient may take the test in an unrealistic hope of being reassured by a negative result and then be totally crushed when a positive result occurs.
4. Given social demands, there is no reason to believe that a test that starts out free of coercion will remain so. Life insurance companies may de-

mand that individuals at risk take the test before a policy will be sold; **886**
employers may follow suit.                                                      cont.

On the basis of these consequences, Hemphill concludes that the negative
consequences are weighty enough to force "careful scrutiny" before giving
the test. Do you agree?                                                          ↓

The test for Huntington's chorea on which Hemphill based his discussion    **887**
has proved with time not to be as accurate as originally predicted and is not
currently in regular use. The issues raised in the debate over Case 57, however, are important, since the likelihood of similar tests for this and other
diseases is increasing. We may, for instance, soon be able to predict which
individuals are at high risk for having cancer later in life, without having a
corresponding ability to treat the cancer when it appears. Such information
would be an emotional burden, but would also be useful in allowing the
individual to avoid known environmental contributors to cancer, such as
cigarettes. We will have to decide for such tests whether the negative emotional consequences outweigh the value of the information in deciding
whether to offer the test to individuals on a wide basis.                        ↓

How do you weigh Hemphill's social consequence — that coercion may be    **888**
applied by insurance companies, employers, and so on? It seems this cannot be dismissed lightly. If medicine provides a test knowing that other social institutions may react in a certain way, and they subsequently do, medicine can hardly wash its hands of the affair and deny any share in the
responsibility. Therefore these social consequences must be weighed in
the equation, but it is not at all clear that they outweigh, all by themselves,
the good consequences of providing the knowledge to the individual.             ↓

Huntington's chorea is atypical among those genetic diseases for which    **889**
screening tests have been proposed. It is inherited by the autosomal-
dominant pattern, which means that the only parents that can pass the disease to their children are those who will develop the disease. The more
usual situation is the autosomal-recessive pattern, typified by sickle-cell
anemia, Tay-Sachs disease, and cystic fibrosis (seen most commonly in
blacks, Ashkenazi Jews, and caucasians, respectively). In these diseases, carriers of a single gene will show no outward signs of disease; but if two carriers marry, each child has a 25 percent chance of being afflicted. Hence,
where relatively simple screening tests for carrier status have been developed, the emphasis has been on detection of carriers before they marry or
bear children.                                                                   ↓

**890**  Screening for sickle-cell anemia has aroused the most ethical interest, both because it was one of the first types of screening to be administered on a widespread basis, and because of the sociocultural factors mentioned at the beginning of the chapter.

Currently there is no effective treatment for sickle-cell disease other than medical management for the periodic sickle-cell crises, and blood transfusions for anemia. While the severity of the disease varies markedly among afflicted individuals, generally life span is reduced. At some centers, doctors can make the diagnosis of sickle cell disease during pregnancy and abort the affected fetus, but such prenatal diagnosis is quite complicated and is ↓ not widely available.

**891**  We have already alluded to several of the questionable practices associated with sickle-cell screening — compulsory screening mandated by law, required testing of children entering school (where the association with reproduction is stretched very thin), failure of confidentiality, and subsequent damage to those diagnosed as being carriers. Such abuses led various groups to recommend guidelines for ethically sound screening programs. The most widely cited guidelines are those proposed by a research group of ↓ the Institute for Society, Ethics and the Life Sciences (Hastings Center).

**892**  The Hastings group recommended that all genetic screening should be voluntary and free of compulsion or stigmatization for those who choose not to be screened or, having been screened and found to be carriers, choose to have children. They recommended informed consent prior to screening, which would include information about available treatment or the lack of it. Individual privacy should be preserved, but information about the policies and practices of the program should be freely available to the community, and community participation and overview should be encouraged. No screening test should be used unless it is sufficiently accurate to guarantee a ↓ very low level of mistaken results.

**893**  This concern over the accuracy of the testing method is not misplaced. Any screening test (or diagnostic test, for that matter) has a fixed percentage of mistaken results ("false-positive" if the results mistakenly show a normal individual to be diseased, "false-negative" if they show a diseased individual to be normal). Therefore, the more widely the test is used, the greater the number of false results that will be generated. An example is the widely used test for phenylketonuria (PKU); children with this disorder will develop mental retardation unless begun on a special diet soon after birth. This test was enthusiastically received and was made compulsory in most states; it was discovered later that the test has had many false-positive results, and some of these normal infants may even have been harmed developmentally by being placed on the special diet. (In many cases, the diagnosis suggested by the screening test can be confirmed by more expensive and more precise follow-up tests, which helps solve the false-positive prob- ↓ lem but not the false-negative problem.)

In addition, in some cases a test with a high rate of mistaken results may **894** seem better than having no information at all. What are the ethical implications of acting upon the results of such a test?

$\downarrow$

---

## CASE 58

You are having lunch with two of your obstetrical colleagues and mention **895** one of your patients who is now about 8 weeks pregnant. She has one son with classic hemophilia who has had a number of serious medical problems due to his bleeding disorder. Your statements about the many hemophiliacs who lead almost normal lives have been to no avail — she does not want to have another child with hemophilia, and she came to you because she read in a woman's magazine about amniocentesis to detect some disorders in utero. She is likewise adamant in wanting more children if she can possibly have them. She has an appointment this afternoon at which you are to give her your answer and advice.

One colleague, Dr. M., points out what you already know — since hemophilia is sex-linked, and the mother is now proven to be a carrier, 50 percent of her male children will be expected to have it and none of the female children (though 50 percent of them will be carriers). There is no prenatal diagnosis for hemophilia per se. However, Dr. M. goes on, some centers have adopted the strategy of doing amniocentesis to determine the sex of the baby by karyotype, and then aborting all male fetuses. While the mother can have only female children, she is assured of having children free of the disease.

At this point Dr. D. chokes on his sandwich and begins to object strenuously. An opponent of abortion on demand, Dr. D. can accept abortion when the baby is known to have a genetic defect. But here, he says, you are aborting a perfectly normal fetus 50 percent of the time. "Since when in medicine do we treat an individual for a disease we think his brother has?" demands Dr. D. "Especially when the treatment is death." He feels that it would be immoral even to mention this possibility to the patient.

You disagree with Dr. D., since you have read the section above about withholding information from patients due to one's own moral values. But, if the patient has amniocentesis done, you, as her obstetrician, will be the one to do the abortion.

Are you prepared to abort a male fetus if she requests it? $\downarrow$

**896** Case 58 is another example of a dilemma caused by a half-way technology — the case would not exist, in its present form, if there were a reliable means of diagnosing hemophilia, not just male sex, by amniocentesis. Better tests of this sort are currently being developed; meanwhile, a number of abortions have in fact been performed for the reasons mentioned in Case 58.

**897** One justification offered by physicians doing these abortions is that they are protecting the right of the mother to bear a normal child. Is this a legitimate right, or an ad hoc right trumped up to end ethical discussion of a particular issue? If such a right were to be decided upon, what would our obligations be? One obvious problem is that we have no way to guarantee such a right. About 1 in every 65 births currently results in a child with a genetic defect, although many are more mild than the illnesses we have been discussing. There are 100 or so defects that can be diagnosed in the uterus by amniocentesis — but generally only one or two tests are done on a specific woman because she is known to be at risk for those conditions. It would be utterly impractical, to say nothing of enormously expensive, to screen for all 100 defects in a given woman, and even then normality could not be assured, as the fetus may have a defect that could not be detected by known tests.

**898** On the other side of the issue is Dr. D., using arguments that have been put forth most forcefully by Ramsey (1973). Again, anyone who is anti-abortion will condemn the proposed "treatment" in Case 58, while anyone who favors abortion on demand is unlikely to be squeamish about the 50 percent of normal male fetuses that will be aborted. But Ramsey's argument goes beyond the abortion issue itself.

**899** Ramsey opposes all ethics based on consequentialist theories of the "greatest net good," which he condemns under the title of "statistical morality."

> To screen by means of sex determination and to catch a normal male fetus in a statistical net is in no instance to deliver medical care in his case. Such mistaken identification is rather like operating on the wrong patient — which no one would excuse by saying that the condition to be remedied was graver than the operation.

**900** Ramsey's argument seems to have force in Case 58 where the chances of error are 50 percent. But, in principle, the argument could be extended to cases where there is even a 5 percent or a 1 percent chance of mistake. Ramsey does not shrink from such an extension, but for many, it makes his arguments much less plausible.

It is easy, however, to misunderstand what may be involved in statistical **901**
morality. Genetic counselors have great difficulty trying to explain that
"each child will have a 50 percent chance of having the defect" does <u>not</u>
mean the same as "50 percent of your children will have the defect." As all
of us learn in math class, but tend to forget in our daily lives, this family
could have ten children and all of them (or none of them) might have the
defect.

This makes the "killing his brother" analogy inapplicable. It suggests that
we could know in advance which half of this class of fetuses are hemophiliacs and which are normal, and we choose callously to wipe them all out
just because we are too lazy to select beforehand. But, in fact, we cannot
know this; we can only know that a particular male fetus has a 50 percent
chance of being affected. Assuming we have not ruled out abortion on
other grounds, we must next ask whether this knowledge in itself justifies
abortion.                                                                    ↓

We use statistical morality very widely in medicine because our knowledge **902**
is very seldom certain. For example, consider screening for hypertension. If
we discover a 47-year-old male with a blood pressure of 165/110, there is a
certain statistical chance that, by treating him, we can prevent a later heart
attack or stroke. There is also a lesser statistical chance that he will become
ill from the side effects of the treatment, and a much lesser but nonzero
chance that the treatment will actually kill him. Is the decision to treat him
statistical morality?                                                        ↓

If we asked Ramsey why statistical morality would be all right in the hyper- **903**
tension case but wrong in the hemophilia case, he is most likely to reply
that the 47-year-old male is a competent adult and can choose on his own
whether to accept the risks. The fetus, on the other hand, is at our mercy
and relies on us to choose in its best interests, so no possible source of
error, however small, is admissible.                                         ↓

But this reply makes two assumptions — first, that the fetus is the sort of **904**
being that has such claims upon our protection, which some theories of the
personhood of the fetus would deny; and second, that our duties toward
incompetent patients entail prolonging life if there is any uncertainty at all.
This is what Ramsey argued in connection with the *Saikewicz* court ruling,
and we saw reasons in Chapter 6 to refute this position. In conclusion, then,
this argument about statistical morality is reduced to an argument for the
personhood of the fetus and for an unqualified duty to prolong the lives of
the incompetent.                                                             ↓

REVIEW SAIKEWICZ ↑ 319–321

**905** Even if we dismiss the argument of statistical morality, we are left with at least two pressing questions. The first is the one we raised ourselves: Does our knowledge of the chance that the fetus may have hemophilia justify the rather extreme course of abortion? Is the seriousness of hemophilia the deciding factor? If not, what other factors will be relevant in our decision?

↓

**906** The second question is raised by Ramsey, independent of our duties to this particular fetus. Ramsey asks: To what extent is our present willingness as a society to care for the sick, the handicapped, and the deformed an outgrowth of assumptions that many, if not most, such conditions are inevitable and are outside of human control? If this changes in the future, and we adopt a more aggressive attitude toward screening, eliminating the "abnormals" and the "defectives," our willingness to care humanely for the defectives that slip through our screening net may lessen proportionately. Some commentators would point to our willingness to consider euthanasia for defective newborns as an example that this hardening of public sensibility is already occurring.

↓

**907** While we could, of course, argue over just what constitutes the most "humane" care for severely defective newborns, the basic point remains — *a policy of genetic control is not just a way of deciding how to handle individual cases. It is also an expression of some of our most basic social values; and changes in such policies may reflect — and, indeed, may actually cause — changes in what we hold to be most important as civilized people.* These questions, then, lead us naturally into the discussion of genetic engineering in the next chapter.

**908** ↓ CH. 15

# Genetic Engineering 15

On July 25, 1978, at 11:47 P.M. Louise Brown was born to overjoyed parents in Manchester, England, amid great media hoopla over the world's first "test-tube baby." Unable to conceive naturally because of blocked fallopian tubes, Mrs. Brown sought the help of Drs. Patrick Steptoe and Robert Edwards, who had been experimenting for years with the technique known as in vitro fertilization.

After hormone treatment to stimulate egg production, Steptoe removed an egg from her ovary through a laparoscope, which was inserted through a small abdominal incision. This egg was then fertilized in a Petri dish (not a test tube!) with sperm from Mr. Brown. While the egg divided over a period of 2½ days, Mrs. Brown received other hormones to prepare the uterine lining to receive the egg. Finally, the egg was inserted into the uterus through a plastic tube, where it attached and continued to develop normally. Birth would have been uneventful except for a blood pressure problem in Mrs. Brown, which necessitated a cesarean section to deliver the 5-pound, 12-ounce baby girl.

For years, the medical ethics community had debated the issue of in vitro fertilization. Ethicists such as Paul Ramsey, a teacher of Protestant ethics, had expressed grave doubts about "manufacturing" babies artificially, and feared that in vitro fertilization would open the door to much greater manipulations and abuses in the future. Ramsey (1972) went so far as to go on record as <u>almost</u> wishing that the first baby born by this technique would be a monstrosity, so as to dampen enthusiasm for further developments of the technology. (He could not <u>really</u> wish for this because, in his deontological approach to ethics, this terrible harm visited upon one baby could not be justified, however great was the good that might result for others.)

Unfortunately, from this viewpoint, Louise Brown, in her first year of life, appeared to be a completely normal baby.

Some who rejected the arguments about the artificiality or the abuses of in vitro fertilization still opposed the method on resource allocation grounds. Especially with overpopulation plaguing the world economy, it seemed strange to devote so much money and effort to allowing a few women who could not conceive on their own to bear children.

But even here the events seemed to defuse the argument. Once worked out, in vitro fertilization held the promise of being a rather simple and inexpensive procedure — certainly cheaper, for example, than microsurgery to repair Mrs. Brown's scarred fallopian tubes, an operation that few medical-care systems in developed countries would have denied her.

**912**   In the final analysis, many ethicists wondered what all the fuss had been about for so many years. In retrospect, the debate over in vitro fertilization looked like a tempest in a teapot. Infertile couples greeted the news with appropriate satisfaction, and there was no rush on the part of fertile couples to forego old-fashioned sex in order to have babies by this new technology.

Is the entire debate over genetic engineering a similarly misplaced concern? Or is there more to the conservative arguments than that, at least when applied to more radical technologies instead of in vitro fertilization? We will take up those questions in this chapter.

**913**   As a start, we might list some of the specific technologies we might want to consider under the general title of "genetic engineering." A list of some of the technologies often discussed in this context is provided in Table 5. Louise Brown's case, for example, would be included under II-C-1. (Lest we think that this entire issue has newly sprung upon us as a result of ultra-modern technology, we should recall that avoidance of inbreeding [I-C] has been a social practice since prehistoric times. The first recorded pregnancy by artificial insemination in humans [I-A-3] occurred in the 1780's, and transplantation of fertilized eggs from one animal to another was accomplished in 1893.)

**914**   New technology does, however, add an urgency to our consideration of these issues. If the techniques listed in Table 5 have not yet been performed, it is not (in most cases) because of any theoretical barrier to their development. Most of the techniques could be developed for general use within a relatively short period — given some additional applied research and, of course, the decision by society to go ahead and develop them.

**915**   Before going any further, we ought to make note of some terms used in this context. An individual's *genotype* is the complete set of genes that he carries, as determined (normally) at the time of conception, while his *phenotype* is the observable set of traits of the individual, as determined by the constant interaction between his genes and his environment. *Eugenics* is the practice of genetic engineering by selecting which genes are to be allowed to combine to form the genotype. One might distinguish *positive* eugenics as selective breeding in hopes of producing superior individuals, and *negative* eugenics as the avoidance of the production of inferior individuals. *Euphenics* does not change the genotype; rather it alters the inner environment of the somatic cells so that either bad genes are not expressed in the phenotype, or good genes are expressed more fully. *Euthenics* also leaves the genotype alone, but instead alters the outer environment, so that what might have been a bad trait in the old environment is turned into a neutral one. The meanings of these terms can best be clarified by applying the terms to specific examples, as we shall do in the course of this chapter.

**Table 5.** *Some Possible Technologies for Human Genetic Engineering.*

I. Selective Mating
   A. By phenotype of parents
      1. Sterilization of "unfit"
      2. Encourage mating of selected pairs
      3. Artificial insemination with selected sperm donor
   B. By genotype of parents, as in A., but with specific knowledge of parental genotype
   C. By relationship of parents − avoidance of inbreeding, incest, etc.
   D. By age of parents − encouraging earlier pregnancy when incidence of chromosomal defects is less
   E. By genotype of gametes
      1. Differentiation of sperm carrying "normal" gene from those carrying defective genes, followed by artificial insemination with "good" sperm
      2. "Vaccination" of mother so that defective sperm will be rejected by immune mechanisms
II. Technologies Involving Developing Zygote
   A. Parthenogenesis − development of unfertilized egg (genotypically identical to mother)
   B. Cloning − development of multiple individuals, all with same genotype, by separating cells at early embryo stage
   C. Extracorporeal gestation or test-tube baby
      1. Egg fertilized outside body, implanted in mother's uterus as treatment for infertility
      2. Egg or embryo already fertilized, removed and developed to term in artificial placenta, as treatment for tendency to abort spontaneously
      3. Development of individual completely outside of body from conception to birth
III. Technologies Involving Somatic Cell Gentoype
   A. Directed alterations of genes
      1. Using viruses as DNA transmitters − naturally occurring viruses, or viruses modified specifically to replace missing genes
      2. Specifically induced mutations − no good approach now known
   B. Random mutation with selection of cells with altered properties, followed by refusion of selected cells to host

These definitions give us a clue to why the in vitro fertilization case might seem, in retrospect, to be much ethical ado about nothing. Our major concern would seem to be the issue of eugenics. Positive eugenics would seem to be more problematic than negative eugenics, since we can at least agree in large part on what constitutes genetic diseases to be avoided, but we might disagree totally on what constitutes the genetic "ideal" to be sought after in a positive-eugenics program. However, in vitro fertilization is neither of these − it is eugenically neutral. The baby born by in vitro fertilization is genetically no better and no worse than the one that would have been born to these same parents, had the mother been able to conceive normally (although, once in the Petri dish, the fertilized eggs can be examined and any eggs that are subject to obvious malformations can be discarded). ↓

**917** The list of different technologies in Table 5, and the various definitions in Frame 915, suggest the complexity of the genetic-engineering debate. Clearly, what counts as a good reason against one genetic-engineering practice may not count at all against another practice. Despite this complexity, however, a number of arguments, pro and con, are encountered quite frequently. It is worth going over some of the most common arguments. A few of the worst arguments can be dismissed right away, while some of the better arguments should be kept in mind throughout our dis-
↓ cussion.

**918** We can start with the following arguments that are sometimes raised in favor of genetic engineering:

Utilitarian. Certainly genetic engineering entails some risks, but the potential benefits to mankind through the lessening of genetic disease, and possibly by improving the human race and other species in the long run, far outweigh these risks.

Rationality. Our rationality is what makes us human compared to other animals. Where advanced technology makes this possible, then, it would be immoral not to use the opportunity to choose the genetic makeup of our offspring in a rational way, instead of abandoning our fate to chance.

Genetic decay. We have already, willy-nilly, engaged in genetic engineering, but in a negative way. By keeping people with inherited diseases (such as diabetes) alive, and allowing them to reproduce, we are gradually polluting our gene pool. We need to take active measures to
↓ counteract this genetic deterioration of the species.

**919** And then we must consider the following arguments sometimes raised against genetic engineering:

Unnatural. Genetic manipulation attempts to replace our natural procreation, in the context of marriage and the family, with an artificial manufacturing process in the laboratory.

Uncertainty. We can never be sure of the outcome of genetic engineering, and so we can never rule out disastrous consequences.

Ignorance. We remain largely ignorant about the long-range consequences of altering the basic genetic makeup of a species. Other recent experience in meddling with complex systems suggests that unanticipated but dangerous consequences may be likely. Hence we should go slowly with this new technology.

Bad values. The desire to change the genetic makeup of our offspring may represent or reinforce social values that have undesirable consequences.

Future abuse. Just as the Nazis tried to practice positive eugenics to create a "master race," genetic engineering technologies across the board

are open to exploitation by tyrants that may come to power in the fu-  **919**
ture.                                                                    cont.

Resource allocation. While genetic engineering may be good on other
grounds, our scarce resources can best be devoted to other technologies that are more developed.

Unethical means. Even if the ends of genetic engineering are ethically
sound, it must be prohibited because the means are immoral. These
include such things as killing the fertilized eggs that are discarded during in vitro fertilization and the experimentation on the children-to-be
who are born as a result of a genetic-engineering technique, while that
technique is still in the experimental phase.                    ↓

Some of these arguments, as they are stated, are simply misguided or fail to  **920**
take into account relevant facts. One such argument is the "genetic-decay"
argument, which makes some unsupportable assumptions about the actual
impact on the gene pool — for example, keeping diabetics alive and able to
reproduce by giving them insulin, whereas formerly they died before reproducing so that their genes were eliminated.                           ↓

The scientific evidence for and against the idea of genetic deterioration re-  **921**
quires some sophisticated genetics knowledge to evaluate, so we cannot
do justice to the issue here. One geneticist, Crow (1968, 1971), estimates
that relaxation of natural selection by allowing individuals with bad genes
to survive will, as a net result, produce very little change in average gene
frequency. In the case of a sickle-cell gene, where the selection pressures
are different for the heterozygous and the homozygous states, the frequency of the gene might go up or down depending on which selection
pressure predominates. A similar process occurs where selection works on
groups of genes instead of on a single gene, as with diabetes. Even in the
case of a single recessive gene, Crow estimates that if the original frequency
of the gene in the population is 0.5 percent, and the gene did cause total
sterility but with new medical treatment has no effect on the individual,
with random mating it would still take 70 generations for the incidence of
the gene to double to 1 percent.                                      ↓

Because of all these factors, Crow estimates that the rate of new mutations  **922**
to form harmful genes might be much more important in determining genetic deterioration than the problem of relaxed selection. Since we know of
a number of environmental hazards, notably radiation and certain chemicals, which can increase the mutation rate, our efforts to prevent genetic
deterioration ought to be directed against those hazards instead of trying to
manipulate the genes directly.                                        ↓

**923**  It is also important, with regard to the question of relaxed selection, that humans do not randomly mate and have children, and social factors can have more influence on the gene pool than strictly medical ones. These social factors are reflected in the "Selective Mating" types of genetic engineering listed in Table 4, which, as we have seen, have been in use for long periods and thus are known to be relatively free of side effects. Lappé (1972) notes that when Japan passed a law that did no more than introduce legal abortion and encourage earlier marriages, the number of births of Down's syndrome children was reduced by one-third, and the births of children with all other congenital defects dropped by one-tenth. Therefore, these kinds of social factors may be keeping up with or even surpassing ↓ medical advances in their effects on the gene pool.

**924**  Another argument, which is sometimes uncritically applied, is the "future-abuse" argument. While some sorts of abuse are real possibilities, several of the "scare scenarios" are ludicrous when examined in a calm manner. We can look at the fears regarding cloning as one example, since it seems to be ↓ a perennial favorite with newspaper columnists and lay writers.

**925**  Cloning involves taking a cell from one organism and causing its nucleus to begin dividing as an embryonic cell would, eventually creating a second organism with the same genotype as the first. This possible mode of bypassing sexual reproduction (and so far used successfully only in more primitive animals) has given rise to two common fantasies — first, people making "Xerox copies" of themselves to use as "spare parts" banks in case they need organ transplants (being of identical genotype, the organs would not be rejected); and second, future Hitlers producing whole armies of uniform ↓ clones for nefarious uses.

**926**  The writers who cite these fantasies seldom go on to point out that a human being produced from a cloned cell would be a human being, and presumably would have the same rights as other human beings. Your Xerox copy would stand in the same moral relation to you as an identical twin would, since identical twins presumably have the same genotype. This does not give the twin born first any automatic demand on the other twin's organs. Indeed, if you produced a clone and your clone happened to suffer kidney failure before you did, it would have as much right to one of your ↓ kidneys as you would to one of its.

Also, a future Hitler breeding, say, clones of Einstein would be forgetting   **927**
the heavy impact of environment on human personality. Genetically identical Einsteins raised in different environments would be quite different people and would certainly not constitute an army of identical automatons.
We should remember that the worst dictators in human history were able
to bend masses of people to do their will by purely environmental manipulation. We have every reason to believe that tomorrow's despots will follow
suit, instead of opting for the difficult, expensive, and uncertain techniques
of genetic engineering.

In conclusion, there are real abuses to be feared from genetic engineering, but the ludicrous clone scenarios are not among them.   ↓

Let's look next at a pair of arguments — the "rationality" argument in favor   **928**
of genetic engineering, and the "unnatural" argument against it. The main
exponent of the former argument has been Joseph Fletcher (1974). However, even if we accept the gambit about rationality being the highest human virtue — it seems rather to be only one of a number of important human characteristics — it is not necessarily a clear answer to any dilemma to
say that the more rational course of action should be followed. Usually, the
point in dispute is precisely <u>which</u> of the alternatives <u>is</u> the most rational.
However, we have learned recently at least a couple of things — just because a new technology becomes available, it is not necessarily the most
rational course to use it; and just because we embark on a course of action
with clear, rational goals, we are not protected from encountering unanticipated and dangerous consequences.   ↓

On the other side of the coin, to condemn something as unnatural is just as   **929**
vague as to praise something as rational. Just about every scientific advance, from anesthesia in childbirth to air travel, was originally attacked by
moralists as unnatural. Certainly the vast majority of medical practices are,
strictly speaking, unnatural and would be condemned if this argument
were taken to its logical conclusion. In actual practice, "Don't do what's
unnatural" seems to boil down to "Don't do what I happen to disapprove
of."   ↓

Further, anyone who finds the artificial manufacturing of babies morally   **930**
repugnant would seem obligated to condemn artificial insemination. This is
at least one technology from Table 5 with which we have had a good deal
of experience. That experience would suggest that anyone saying (1) that
parents desiring artificial insemination to allow them to have a child are
deficient in the best marital and family values, (2) that artificial insemination renders the pregnancy and childbirth a sterile, emotionally hollow experience for the parents, or (3) that the baby born as a result of artificial
insemination is somehow not "fully" a human being, is ignorant at best,
and cruel and heartless at worst.   ↓

REVIEW INSEMINATION ↑ 571–579

**931** The rationality and unnatural arguments, then, seem to cancel each other out from opposite extremes. Where it has some good points to make, the rationality argument would probably better be expressed as a form of the "utilitarian" argument. Similarly, where the unnatural argument has some valid concerns, these concerns would usually fall under the "bad values" argument.

**932** What can we say about the "uncertainty" argument? This argument also seems to go overboard in demanding too much. We are never, in practical matters, in possession of full certainty, so this argument would condemn us to inaction.

By contrast, the "ignorance" argument (which at first glance might seem very similar to the uncertainty argument) is a more modest and hence more reasonable one. Surely ignorance about possible consequences is generally a good reason to be very cautious about the action in question. The ignorance argument also allows for a gradual increase in the degree of genetic-engineering technology we would support, if in the future this ignorance about its effects were to be lessened.

**933** A good example of the ignorance argument, as expressed by two scientists, is the following:

In our view, gene therapy may ameliorate some human genetic diseases in the future. For this reason, we believe that research directed at the development of techniques for gene therapy should continue. For the foreseeable future, however, we oppose any further attempts at gene therapy in human patients because (1) our understanding of such basic processes as gene regulation and genetic recombination in human cells is inadequate; (2) our understanding of the details of the relation between molecular defect and the disease state is rudimentary for essentially all genetic diseases; and (3) we have no information on the short-range and long-term side effects of gene therapy. We therefore propose that a sustained effort be made to formulate a complete set of ethicoscientific criteria to guide the development and clinical application of gene therapy techniques.*

**934** Another argument that does not seem to be easily dismissible is the "unethical means" argument. One manifestation of this argument is the condemnation of in vitro fertilization because a number of eggs are commonly fertilized in the Petri dish; only one is inserted into the uterus and the rest are discarded. Clearly, the moral condemnation of this practice depends upon attributing personal life — with a right to life — to the egg immediately following fertilization; anyone disagreeing with this view will not find this argument persuasive.

* T. Friedmann and R. Roblin, Gene therapy for human genetic disease. *Science* 174(3) : 949, 1972. Copyright 1972 by the American Association for the Advancement of Science.

A counterargument frequently offered is that "disposing of the extras" and,   **935**
particularly, "disposing of the mistakes" is the rule in nature, whether or
not we adopt it in the genetics laboratory. It is likely that at least one-
quarter of all fertilized eggs either fail to implant in the uterus, are shed
with the next menstrual cycle, or eventually undergo miscarriage; and many
of the eggs that are lost in this way can be shown to be genetically defective. By this argument, our lack of concern for these lost conceptuses
should be carried over to the in vitro fertilization case — especially since the
entire purpose of the process is the creation of a baby that otherwise would
never have been born. (For a related moral problem, see Case 47 in Chapter
11.)

But Ramsey (1972) has emphasized an unethical means argument that does   **936**
not depend on attributing rights to embryos. Ramsey focuses on the possible harm to the child-to-be after birth, if the genetic technology turns out
to have unanticipated risks. Even if we test the technology on many fetuses
without allowing them to progress to full term, and tests on those fetuses
show them to be normal, there has to be a first time that we allow a baby to
come to term and be born. If that baby turns out to have a defect due to the
artificial technology, however minor (perhaps his IQ is 5 points lower than
it would have been if he had been born "normally"), we will have been
guilty of this harm. Hence, the development of these technologies necessarily involves unethical experimentation on future children, who cannot
possibly give their consent to it.

One could reply to this by saying that there are plenty of risks to a naturally   **937**
developing fetus — it may fail to implant in the uterus, spontaneously abort,
or develop a congenital defect; and the risk to a fetus in a "test tube" is not
significantly greater. The rejoinder is that this is an illegitimate justification,
even if your statement about the relative risks is true, because the fetus
would not have been exposed to any risks at all had you not meddled in the
first place; the fetus simply would not have existed to begin with. A rough
way of paraphrasing this argument is that if you run over a person with your
car and break his back, you cannot justify your action by pointing out that
people run over by automobiles quite frequently get broken backs.

Despite this reminder of the responsibility assumed by the genetic engi-   **938**
neer, it seems strange to be so concerned about the lack of consent of the
child-to-be. Did any of us give our consent to be born? The world is full of
risks, both in utero and outside it; nobody asked our opinion before exposing us to them. Assuming that the techniques for genetic engineering (such
as in vitro fertilization) had been perfected through the appropriate experiments, and assuming we could imagine the child-to-be speaking on its own
behalf in advance, wouldn't we have reason to think that the child-to-be
would rather undergo the slight remaining risks rather than never to exist at
all? (Which is, we might point out, not the same thing as saying the child-
to-be has a "right to be born.")

**939** If Ramsey's argument sounds unconvincing, it may be due to a basic disagreement about ethical theory. We have been relying for the most part on a consequentialist approach to ethics, while Ramsey is committed to a deontological approach (see Appendix I). Ramsey is not able to condemn an action because it will result in harmful consequences; he must judge an action ethical or not because of its own nature. Hence, he judges this type of genetic engineering immoral because it is the nature of the act to be potentially harmful and to be performed without the consent of the individual that may be harmed. By this theory of ethics, the actual degree of ↓ harm, or its probability of occurring, is beside the point.

**940** A consequentialist, then, will probably reject Ramsey's argument as it stands because of its absolute character. Still, Ramsey's argument would serve to remind us that the individuals who will be born as a result of any genetic engineering technique need to be considered. If we think only about the good that will result for otherwise childless parents, or the good to society as a whole through the prevention of genetic disease, we will be leaving out an important ethical consideration. And, if we are willing to accept some risks, we certainly have the duty to make those risks as low as possible, since the consequences will be borne not by us but by others.

Case 59 illustrates one sort of dilemma that may place the interests of the child-to-be in conflict with the immediate reproductive desires of the par-↓ ents.

### CASE 59

**941** As a family physician in the year 1994, you are counseling a couple who have been married 3 years and wish to start a family. In the genetic screening test that is required by the government in order to get a license to have children, it was found that both Mr. and Mrs. L. carry one recessive gene for a disease that leads to severe mental retardation and death by age 10. This means that any child the Ls conceive is at a 25 percent risk to develop the disease. The Ls could bypass this risk by choosing to conceive through artificial insemination by a sperm donor, but they are opposed to this course and desire a child of "their own."

You know that for some 10 years a technique of sperm immunoselection has been in use at some centers. An antibody can be made that binds itself to sperm that carry the recessive gene; a complicated process then separates the bound sperm from the "clean" sperm, which in turn are then used to inseminate the wife.

The hitch is that children conceived from sperm treated by immunoselection have shown increased risk for developing leukemias and other childhood cancers; for some reason the cancers involved have proved rather resistant to therapy. Epidemiologists have estimated that immunoselected sperm entail a 4 percent risk of these cancers, whereas for other children the risk is less than 1 percent.

If you saw your role simply as a parent advocate for the present, you would unhesitatingly advise sperm immunoselection — the insemination would involve sperm from Mr. L., not some unknown male donor, and the risk of cancer seems small and far in the future. But, as the family doctor, you will be assuming responsibility for the child as well. **941** cont.

Do you advise

1. That the Ls accept the "natural" 25 percent risk of severe retardation, instead of the "artificial" risk of the sperm immunoselection?
2. That the Ls choose sperm immunoselection as the best solution to their present predicament, despite the future risks to the child?
3. That the Ls put aside their emotional reaction and accept artificial insemination by donor? ↓

---

Our reaction to the "unnatural" argument illustrates a good reason to reject the first option in Case 59. We could imagine someone supporting the second option as follows: "The 4 percent risk of cancer is still very low — after all, that's a 96 percent chance of not getting it. And the parents' concern over donor insemination is not just an emotional reaction affecting themselves. If they are uncomfortable with this process, marital conflicts could result, which could affect the quality of life of the growing child. Therefore, concern for the well-being of the child could justify using immunoselection." **942** ↓

Or the third option could be supported as follows: "As health professionals we have a duty not to do harm to a being, given that we have decided that that being ought to be conceived and born. Exposing sperm to immunoselection seems to entail a small but real risk of harm to the child that will result. On the other hand, we do not seem to have any duty to bring about the conception of any individual (if we did, all birth control might be unethical), or to bring about the conception of an individual with particular sorts of genes. All these considerations favor donor insemination. If this process happens to cause emotional problems for the family, those problems at least can be treated with counseling; the cancer, on the other hand, cannot be treated." **943** ↓

**944**    Notice that both these lines of argument fulfill the requirement we mentioned just prior to Case 59 — they make some attempt to include the child, not just the parents, as a morally important entity whose interests ought to be respected. There is no really clear-cut reason to prefer one argument over the other. This may well represent one of those "gray zone" cases, similar to decisions made on behalf of newborns and young children, where the decision is best left to the parents; and where, so long as the parents are well-informed and well-intentioned, there seems to be little ground for the health professional to dispute their choice. (In addition, only the parents are likely to know just how disruptive donor insemination is going to be for them.)

↓    REVIEW GRAY ZONE ↑ 405–409

**945**    What do we do, then, with the Ramsey rejoinder, that we cannot use sperm immunoselection because it would amount to putting a child-to-be at risk in a way to which it could never consent? This might make sense if applied to, say, a 12-week-old fetus when we were debating giving some drug to the mother that might harm <u>that</u> fetus. But, assuming we are not prepared in Case 59 to accept fertilization with the 25 percent risk of mental retardation, the harm to the child-to-be associated with immunoselection is a necessary condition for <u>that</u> child to be coming into existence at all — to fail to accept the risk is to opt for <u>some other</u> child, with a different genetic makeup, to be conceived through donor insemination. Since it is not even clear here <u>who</u> is unable to give consent, acceptance of this line of argument would seem to lead to some never-never land of unrealized alternatives.

    On the other hand, to choose the 25 percent risk of severe disease over the 4 percent risk of cancer because of some such concern over the hypothetical consent of the fetus would simply seem misguided.

**946**    We have now looked in some detail at the unethical means argument. Of the arguments remaining, the "bad values" argument is the most problematic. Certainly one could object to almost anything on the grounds that it reflects bad values, but this would not count as ethical decision making. One would have to specify (1) a reason for thinking that the value has negative consequences, and (2) a significant link between the bad value and the action that one is investigating. Therefore, the argument is hard to pin down firmly — many people disagree on whether certain values are, in the final analysis, good or bad, and it is often hard to trace a definite connection between one sort of action and the promulgation of values in society.

**CASE 60**

It's 1994 again, and you are on a committee of the Food and Drug Adminis-    **947**
tration (FDA) to screen new drugs and approve them for use. Fortunately,
by a recent congressional action, the FDA has been charged with looking at
new drugs from a resource-allocation viewpoint as well as the safety angle,
so that you can reject a safe drug if you judge that society could better
devote its resources to other areas.

The two pills now up for discussion have curious properties. They started
out as pills for nausea during pregnancy and were tested and approved for
use in pregnant women. Subsequently a strange feature was noticed by
chance. Of mothers who had taken pill A, 98.3 percent of the offspring
showed up with blue eyes, while in the case of pill B, 97.9 percent of the
children had brown eyes — all with no apparent alteration of the genotype.

While the mechanism is unknown, the specific chemicals responsible for
the eye color control have been isolated, and the drug company has applied for permission to release the pills for the express purpose of altering
eye color in unborn children. The chemicals have been tested further and
again no significant side effects have been noted.

The company acknowledges that certain chemicals, such as diethyl-
stilbestrol, have been found to produce deleterious effects in the offspring
when ingested during pregnancy and to show the effects when the child
reaches adolescence or later. Since this set of pills has not been tested long
enough to observe this, these long-range side effects cannot be completely
ruled out.

In its resource-impact statement, the company contends that the cost of
the pills will be quite inexpensive, and the resource allocation for this purpose will be negligible from the viewpoint of the entire industry. Therefore,
even though choosing the eye color of one's baby is not a pressing social
need, releasing the pills for general use seems justified.

Are you going to vote for or against the licensing of these pills?          ↓

---

Case 60 may well be one of those cases to which you find yourself initially   **948**
opposed without knowing why. Is the mere strangeness of the proposal
biasing your judgment? Or is there a defensible reason underlying any sus-
picions you may have? The case was hedged so as to make the resource
allocation and the ignorance aguments largely inapplicable; by the utilitarian argument, the benefits, however small, seem to outweigh the costs. It is
hard to imagine any basic rights that would be violated by the providing of
these pills. Thus, if there is an objection, it might well fall under the bad
values category. But what values are at stake here?                          ↓

**949**   Moralists are quick — usually too quick — to oppose some policy on the grounds that it would undermine marriage and the family as social institutions. We might ask: Just what sort of social policy would, in fact, undermine the institution of the family? To answer this, we might take a little while to look at the crucial functions of the family as a social institution. While the family serves many economic, educational, and other functions, let us look only at the types of relationships that exist within the family unit.

**950**   In general we have instrumental relationships with most of the people we encounter. That is, we value other people for what they can do for us and for the roles they perform. If someone else comes along who can fulfill the role of (say) supermarket cashier as well as the cashier who was there last week, we will value the new person equally, if we even notice the difference. We do have personal relationships with a small group of friends, in which we value them for who they are rather than what they do. If they were to lose their jobs, or no longer be able to play a good game of tennis, we would (we hope) still be friends. However, friends are chosen and not given, and it is common social practice to give up old friends and make new ones as one moves and changes one's interests.

**951**   The family, then, is unique in that it involves personal, noninstrumental relationships that are permanent and are not chosen by the parties. (Divorce, of course, undermines this permanence, but still family relationships, in general, are more permanent than friendships.) The family can function as a sort of psychological refuge — we can be accepted and valued just because we are somebody's father or somebody's daughter; we do not have to constantly perform and prove ourselves the way we often do in the outside world. Family relationships are mutually supportive — our relatives' readiness to accept us as persons is reinforced by our willingness to accept them, and vice versa.

**952**   However, there are strong feelings and motives that always exist in families and that constantly threaten to undermine this network of personal relationships, which is why so many families typify not peaceful bliss but rather an uneasy truce. Being close to other family members and knowing their peculiar vulnerabilities is always a temptation to try to use them to further our own selfish ends — resorting to instrumental relationships instead of personal ones. If the other family member replies in kind, the network of mutual reinforcement is broken. Children are particularly vulnerable to being used instrumentally because they can seldom, at the time, do anything to retaliate; they will tend to react lovingly to their parents and to try to please them, no matter how selfishly they may be used.

But children grow up to be adults and are then likely to treat other people as they have been taught by the examples within their own family. It follows from this that we all have a stake in how families function and in the degree to which children are raised well and are taught positive ways of interacting. We would like children to be raised to treat others as persons wherever possible, and if the children themselves are treated as objects to be used to further the interests of their parents, it is hard to see how they will learn this crucial lesson. ↓

**953**

Clearly social practices can influence the family behavior in this regard. In extreme cases it is obvious that society can undermine the possibility of intrafamilial personal relationships — imagine a society in which parents are permitted to sell their children as slaves; or Orwell's *1984* world in which children are encouraged to spy on and to report their parents. We can imagine that many other social practices, including many with laudable intentions and perhaps many other good consequences, also have a negative if more subtle impact on family life. This latter category may include those social practices that encourage parents to view their children not as separate and unique human beings to be accepted and admired for their own qualities, but rather as malleable things to be twisted to conform to their parents' ideas and their parents' needs. And this (finally!) brings us back to the blue eyes pill. ↓

**954**

To the extent that a genetic-engineering technique is offered to parents to allow them to pick and choose their children, the use of that technique encourages the replacement of personal and permanent relationships with instrumental and impermanent relationships (impermanent because of the implied threat that the children will lose their parents' love if they don't conform). In this way, increased use of genetic engineering can undermine the psychological function of the family. This may develop without conscious policy planning. Amniocentesis for chromosomal determination was originally intended to detect severe diseases such as Down's syndrome, but women soon learned it could also allow them to find out the sex of the fetus and to have an abortion if the baby were of the undesired sex. Now, women are openly demanding amniocentesis for this reason, and many physicians are reluctantly acceding to these requests. ↓

**955**

Recall Case 35 and the hypothetical IQ pill to make school children smarter. Suppose this pill could be given during pregnancy to enhance the intelligence of the unborn child. Would we have the same objections to using it as we would with the blue eyes pill? (Note once again that these hypothetical pills alter phenotype and not genotype and so are not genetic engineering in the strict sense, but the ethical issues are not dissimilar.)

**956**

We might look back on the ethical obligations of parents toward their children — to provide children with primary goods and to work toward

**956 cont.** eventual autonomy. Intelligence is a primary good in that it will be useful to the child, no matter what goals the child later decides to pursue. Having a certain eye color or having a full set of Little League baseball equipment is a secondary good — it is good for the child <u>only if</u> the child has decided to pursue certain particular goals. And if the parents, consciously or not, try to impose those goals on the child despite the child's own inclinations and natural talents, then the parents are violating their second duty to foster the child's developing sense of autonomy. We would conclude then that a harmless means to increase intelligence would not fall under the same category as our blue eyes pill (even though it might lead to a separate set of

↓ problems).

REVIEW PARENTAL OBLIGATION ↑ 383–387

**957** In summary, we can see how the bad values argument might be applied to problems of genetic engineering. It is actually the flip side of the utilitarian argument and, in final analysis, becomes a part of the latter. That is, in deciding whether the positive consequences of a proposed genetic engineering outweigh the negative consequences, we must be sure that we include under the negative consequences the possible long-range effects on social values and social behaviors. As we emphasized in Chapter 2, a consequentialist decision-making process will have to take these longer-range, more abstract consequences into account and not be overly swayed by short-range, concrete benefits.

As a practical matter, at present, our inability to predict both the short-range and the long-range risks of genetic engineering is likely to make a full assessment difficult, and so the ignorance argument may remain the best

↓ reason to be very cautious in our use of such technology.

**958** Up to this point we have been dealing with negative eugenics or with genetically neutral activities. But many of the genetic-engineering proposals for the future would fall into the category of positive eugenics — this would have been true in Case 60 had the pills changed the genes for eye color instead of merely affecting the fetus. By the "future abuse" argument, we would tend to be suspicious of any proposal to breed "superior" individuals, even more so than with proposals merely to avoid genetic diseases. But there are also additional considerations to make us wonder about positive-

↓ eugenics programs.

To start on the practical side, can we breed humans for positive traits, such **959** as good looks or high intelligence? You can do this with animals, and human beings are animals. There is, however, a problem in that most of the complex traits we might like to breed for are determined by the mutual interaction between heredity and environment, with the role played by each component unclear. Where environmental factors are important, manipulating the heredity alone may produce no change, or it may produce a worse specimen. Even when we can produce the direction of change desired by manipulating heredity, it is impossible, where there is an interaction of a number of genes, to predict the rate of change; the improvement may be too slow to be practical. ↓

And even if we forget about the environment, we must remember that **960** genes do not act in isolation from each other, but rather interact in complex ways. Each gene produces its own biochemical product, and the products do not only interact with each other, they also interact with other genes. Unless genes are turned "on" or "off" through these biochemical interactions, they remain simply inert pieces of a DNA molecule, incapable of having any effect on the traits of the individual. And we are a long way from understanding these gene interactions well enough to be able to design specific changes in complex, higher organisms. ↓

Assuming you can get over these practical difficulties, what are the ends **961** toward which the positive eugenicist should aim? Since negative eugenics aims at the elimination of genetic disease, it seems logical and laudable that the positive-minded counterpart should aim for genetic health. While we promised to talk about definitions of health and disease in Chapter 17, this creature called "genetic health" has enough peculiar features to justify considering it separately. ↓

It is revealing to watch how one geneticist, Lappé (1973), tries to elucidate **962** the concept of genetic health. He points out a number of problems along the way. First of all, there is the problem that as far as recessive genes are concerned, the phenotype does not reflect the genotype. A person can be normal in a phenotypic and medical sense and yet carry a gene that, if matched up with another like it, would produce a lethal disease. Since this gene can be passed along to children and can be expressed in the phenotype if the wrong mating occurs and two genes come together, it might make sense to say that anyone who carries such a gene is genetically unhealthy. ↓

The only problem with that reasoning is that we are all genetically un- **963** healthy. According to calculation, we all carry up to 10 recessive genes that, if matched up with another to form the homozygous condition, would produce a lethal disease. Does it make sense to have a definition of health that fits no one? ↓

**964** A further problem exists with the differences between the homozygous (two identical genes) and the heterozygous (one each of two varieties of genes for the same trait) states for certain traits. A good example is sickle-cell anemia, which appears with the homozygous state (ss). The ss individual will, without treatment, have a shortened life span, so this seems definitely to be an evolutionary disadvantage — so much so that it was a mystery as to why the gene was relatively common in the African population, since natural selection should have been working to eliminate it. It was then found that the heterozygous individuals (Ss) were more resistant to malaria than the normal (SS) individuals. If you were Ss and married an Ss in the jungle, 25 percent of your children would be ss and would be expected to die early, but 50 percent would be Ss, would have no anemia, and would be more resistant to malaria. Therefore, the net effect of the s gene was beneficial. (Nature practices statistical morality even if we don't.)

**965** In conclusion, the s gene is genetically unhealthy, in terms of fitness to the environment, only in the ss state; given a malarial environment, it is very healthy in the Ss state. How do you arrange your concept of genetic health to account for this? (It has been suggested more recently that the Tay-Sachs gene, in its heterozygous form, tends to protect against tuberculosis, which would certainly have been of benefit to Jews in Eastern Europe.)

Also, suppose you call the Ss person genetically healthy because he is resistant to malaria. Now he comes to the United States where there is no malaria, but he can still have children with sickle-cell anemia. Did he change from healthy to unhealthy in the middle of the Atlantic?

**966** As a thorough geneticist, Lappé lists all of these problems, but fails to draw the obvious conclusion — namely, that there is no such thing as genetic health. Health should be a property of a biological system (we won't say organism, because we might want to talk about, say, a healthy cell or healthy tissue). Any biological system is the result of a complex mutual interaction between its genetic program and its environment. If one of these elements by itself is messed up, the system will suffer, so we can have genetic disease. But one of these elements by itself cannot ensure the overall balance and harmony of the system — so we cannot have genetic health (or environmental health either, for that matter). By analogy, since a person will not do well if his kidneys aren't working, we can have renal diseases; but it seems silly to talk about renal health.

Therefore, we see that in addition to the practical problems of genetic ma-    **967**
nipulation, positive eugenics runs into problems in defining its goals. The
possible goals for a positive eugenics effort are: (1) a state of genetic health,
which we just saw is probably a misguided notion and impossible to specify; (2) some utopian view of the future of mankind, which is likely to
reflect the personal value biases of the planners and to be inconsistent with
the values of others, who also deserve a say in the matter; or (3) some
master-race program to serve the selfish ends of some political or ideological faction, which we would immediately condemn. We would conclude
that efforts toward genetic engineering, where acceptable at all, should
best be directed to the prevention of agreed-upon genetic disease, or to
genetically neutral efforts such as in vitro fertilization.    ↓

It is around the idea of positive eugenics and its possible abuses that much    **968**
of the negative reaction to genetic engineering has gathered. (Opposition
to other genetic technologies such as in vitro fertilization is commonly
prompted by domino theory fears that these technologies will inevitably
lead to positive-eugenics applications.) Because of the emotionalism surrounding the more extreme abuses that might be imagined, a certain irrationality may sometimes creep into debates about present-day genetic
engineering.    ↓

A case in point is recombinant-DNA research, in which genes from one cell    **969**
are introduced into another cell, which may be from a totally different species. Advantages in the near future, apart from the research potential, include the possibility of manufacturing large quantities of insulin and other
hormones by inserting the appropriate human genes into bacteria that can
then be grown in the laboratory. Fears, however, arose about new mutant
microorganisms, perhaps resistant to all known antibiotics, being inadvertently created and then escaping into the environment.    ↓

In 1974, a group of scientists headed by Berg (1974) called for a moratorium    **970**
on such research — the first time scientists had called for a voluntary halt to
a line of promising experimentation because of perceived risks. Two years
later, after much study, most scientists involved in DNA research felt that
adequate safeguards had been devised, and that the risk of real harm was
much less than had first been thought. With the approval of some government guidelines to govern laboratory procedures, these scientists urged
that the recombinant-DNA research be resumed.    ↓

**971**　In the meantime, however, other scientists had joined with various citizens' groups in opposing recombinant-DNA projects and in staging local protests outside of sites chosen to set up recombinant-DNA laboratories. These groups continued to protest such research even after the scientists who initiated the moratorium were satisfied that the early questions had been answered. In fact, the protestors seemed to be using the uncertainty argument, saying that the scientists could not <u>guarantee</u> against some future accident and that research should be stopped on that basis. Since we have already exposed the fallacy of this argument, we might suspect that these protests were motivated less by the true facts of recombinant-DNA technology and more by an emotional reaction to the increasing technology that governs our lives, and the increasing unforeseen risks of that technology.

Emotional reaction, however, is no substitute for more reasoned ethical decision making. *The more valid types of arguments we have been discussing in this chapter (after weeding out the inadequate arguments) point the way to a more rational discussion of the use and misuse of genetic engineering.*

↓

**972**　*We can summarize the more valid arguments as follows:*

1. *A utilitarian or consequentialist form of argument, weighing risks against benefits, seems most applicable; arguments based on various presumed rights seem weaker.*
2. *A consequentialist argument is most likely to give us valid answers when it includes the following elements:*
   a. *A concern for the interests of the unborn children, and not just of the parents or of society at large.*
   b. *A healthy respect for the degree of ignorance of the possible side effects of genetic-engineering technology.*
   c. *An awareness of the way in which genetic-engineering practices may alter social values and important interpersonal relationships.*

**973**　↓ CH. 16

# The Social Responsibility 16
## of the Health Professions

## CASE 61

You are a third-year medical student doing your clerkship in a community 973 hospital in Michigan. Your patient is a 68-year-old woman who is suffering from multiple illnesses; your careful history-taking leads you to the conclusion that several years of inadequate nutrition forms a major component of her problem. She lives alone in a rather run-down house, tends to be depressed, and has no appetite or incentive to eat adequate meals. You are ready to discharge her and feel that she can remain in pretty good shape for several more years at least if she could improve her diet. However, if she goes back to her old habits, you can expect to see her back in the hospital within 6 months.

You are aware that in the community there is a hospital-run program called "Meals on Wheels" that delivers one nutritious, hot meal per day to invalids or convalescents; you feel that this program is exactly what your patient needs.

In discussing this with the hospital social worker, you discover that while your patient has both Blue Cross and Medicare coverage, neither will pay the nominal $1 per day fee for the meals program. Instead, your patient would have to pay out-of-pocket, and you know that her personal finances are very tight and that she would probably not agree to pay this extra expense. "Why pay them when I am perfectly capable of fixing my own meals?" you imagine her saying, even though you know that left to her own devices she will go home and eat toast and coffee day in and day out.

The social worker makes a cynical comment that apparently Medicare and Blue Cross would rather have the patient admitted to the hospital again to run up another $6000 hospital bill rather than pay $7 a week to keep her well. This is part of the whole problem of medical-care insurance being slanted toward crisis, in-hospital care instead of prevention, she adds.

What do you do now? ↓

**974**   Case 61 can serve as a starting point to discuss the social responsibility of the health professions. Our ethical decision-making method in Chapter 2 involves taking into account all the major consequences of our actions, and this includes social, not just personal, consequences. We have also considered the social implications of many ethical issues in previous chapters — macroallocation of medical resources, legal and social implications of one's moral stand on abortion, problems in mass screening and other public health policies, and the social values implicit in proposals for genetic engineering. In this chapter we shall look at a few issues that are almost wholly social in scope and that affect health professionals.

**975**   What do we mean by social issues in health care? And what is different about these issues? A few general comments may help.

First, consider your alternatives in Case 61, assuming you have decided to do something. You could pay the daily $1 fee yourself without telling the patient, as an act of charity. You could contact the local director of Blue Cross and object to their current policies. You could propose a resolution to make exceptions for poverty cases at the next meeting of the county medical society. You could picket the state capitol carrying a sign. You could write letters to the editors of local newspapers. But all these acts fall outside of the usually accepted limits of the strictly professional duties of doctors. You would be acting less as an individual and more as a member of a constituency, and accordingly, your accountability for what you do or fail to do is less than in most of the previous cases, where you had much more power to influence the outcome directly.

**976**   Second, along with that lessening of individual accountability, we get less guidance from standard ethical theories. Our method tells us to consider social consequences, but it doesn't tell us much about how to weigh them or how to resolve any resulting value conflicts. Our focus on the values of individual autonomy and dignity also gives little help in broader social questions. It is certainly one feature of being human to value individual autonomy and dignity. But another important feature seems to be that we achieve our full human potential only as members of a society and a culture (if we can even imagine ourselves existing totally apart from society and culture). Ethical theory has not grappled with this second feature of personhood anywhere nearly as successfully as it has dealt with the first. (It certainly won't do to say that the rights and interests of individuals should be sacrificed to the greater social good, whatever that is; but if not that, then what?)

Third, we need to have a lot of practical, factual knowledge to deal with **977**
such issues successfully. For one thing, knowing the social consequences of
a proposed rule or action entails a sophisticated knowledge of economics,
sociology, and political science — and often this knowledge is not available
even to the experts, let alone the health professional who has no special
training in these fields. For another thing, actually changing policy demands
not just ethical insight but also practical, political know-how. If you don't
know when to work within the health-care system and when to go outside
it; when to negotiate privately and when to take your case to the media;
when to take legal action and when to turn instead to public persuasion
and education; you are simply going to be unsuccessful in effecting change,
however ethically correct your basic principles may be. ↓

Fourth, we might want to consider different sorts of social responsibility **978**
that might be attributed to health professionals, as Jonsen and Jameton
(1977) have suggested. In Case 61, any social responsibility assumed by the
physician or student arises directly from the care of an individual patient —
in trying to give the best possible care to this particular 68-year-old woman,
you have run into a brick wall, and any furtherance of your goal of optimal
care requires social action. We might want to contrast such responsibilities
with, say, a call to U.S. physicians to organize food shipments to various
third-world countries where malnutrition is rampant. This latter case serves
laudable social goals, and the individuals who will benefit may in fact be
much more needy than the 68-year-old woman. But they are not the physicians' patients, and so the sense of responsibility toward them is different
than it is in Case 61. (This distinction seems to make some difference; we
might argue about how much difference.) ↓

Fifth, because of the four points we have just raised, a very appealing re- **979**
sponse to Case 61 is to mutter into your beer and do nothing. Indeed, many
physicians may resent the idea that anything other than doing nothing is
ethically suspect. Friedlies (1979), replying to an editorial on holistic medicine, wrote, "Where in the name of everything holy does it say that a physician is to be more than a healer of sickness? . . . Why in the world are we
expected to be all things to all people and to take care of all of everyone's
problems?" This bemoaning may reflect merely the desire to stick one's
head in the sand; but it could also arise from an honest awareness that the
individual health professional has very little time, and perhaps even less
training, to take on complex social issues. ↓

**980**  However, there are a couple of replies that make the do-nothing response considerably less appealing as a moral stance. The first of these is a historical realization that organized medicine has traditionally held itself aloof from many pressing social issues and has attempted to assure its own privileged status even at the expense of other social groups and social institutions. Medicine has also acquired a rather sad reputation of opposing many of the major social changes that have played a part in shaping the present health-care situation. Given this rather reactionary and isolationist past, it is not too far off the mark to charge that organized medicine is itself to blame for many of the current inequities, and that physicians have a positive duty
↓  to try to correct the past failures of social conscience.

**981**  Also, even if we accept the awareness that the individual health practitioner has very little time and very little power to effect social change, we could still hold that a heavy responsibility exists to order one's actions <u>as if</u> one were in a position of greater control, because the <u>symbolic</u> value of small actions often has a much greater impact than the actions themselves. Jonsen and Jameton, arguing for this symbolic responsibility, cite the case of one physician who elected to focus attention on the widespread malnutrition among his poor patients by writing prescriptions for food and asking that Medicaid reimburse the charges. Of course, none of his patients actually got anything to eat that way, but a useful public debate ensued and indirectly helped to better the plight of his patients.

Viewed this way, doing nothing also becomes a symbolic action in a negative way — symbolizing the willingness of health professionals to stand by
↓  with hands folded in the face of social injustice.

**982**  Finally, the socially responsible behavior of health professionals is hindered by the biased viewpoint often adopted by those professionals — in particular, the tendency to see their own professional activities and goals as being of immense social importance and the work of other professions and other social institutions as being of much less worth. It's not hard to see how such biases arise when we consider the typical characteristics of people who seek the aid of health professionals:

1. They are typically experiencing a crisis that justifies their abandoning most other social duties in order to seek the help of the professional.
2. They are typically preoccupied with their health and are willing (temporarily) to give up many other goods in exchange for restoration of health.
3. They typically project unreasonable expectations upon the health professionals, such as expecting miracle cures.

If this is one's daily contact with the rest of the human race, it's easy to see how one could get an inflated sense of one's own importance and an unrealistic view of the relationship of the health-care professions to other social
↓  institutions.

Everything we've said so far can serve as a set of preliminary warnings as we    **983**
proceed to take up some social issues in health care. The list of current
issues we might take up is an imposing one — for starters consider the following:

Legal implications of the right to health care
Present health "crisis" in U.S. — real or imaginary?
History of medical societies and their roles as government lobbies
Alternative forms of financing medical care — e.g., health maintenance
    organizations, foundations of medical care
Alternative forms of delivering care — solo vs. group practice
Institutions involved in care — hospital, clinic, home care
Organized medicine as professional society and as trade union
Relationship of medical profession to the drug industry
Physicians in positions of limited options, with threat to doctor–patient
    relationship: prison doctors, military doctors
National health insurance and "socialized medicine"
Medical-care systems in other countries — communist and Western Euro-
    pean nations
Diseases of poverty, and problems of access into care system
Diseases of affluence — environmental pollution, sociocultural factors of
    obesity and overconsumption
Social responsibility of medical-education system
Means of selecting and training medical students, as ways of solving or
    perpetuating sociopolitical-economic problems                           ↓

Obviously it is beyond the scope of this book to deal with all these issues in    **984**
any depth. By way of introduction and to touch on the highlights, we will
in the remainder of this chapter look at three main issue areas: the right to
health care, government regulation of medicine, and conflicts between responsibility to individual patients and other social or personal responsibilities.                                                                          ↓

## The Right to Health Care

In discussing such issues as national health insurance, financing of health-    **985**
professions education, allocation of scarce resources to medical care, and
government regulation of physicians' activities, we frequently encounter
appeals to "the right to health care." To some, this right is a mere political
slogan with no real content; to others, it is a self-evident truth, which needs
no arguments to support it. Philosophers and ethicists have spent a lot of
effort trying to define this right, but have not come up with any firm, generally accepted conclusions.

A well-developed theory of a right to health care would have to include:
(1) what the right actually entails; (2) how this right should be limited or

**985**
**cont.** modified in light of other rights and social values that appear to, or actually do, conflict with it; and (3) how this theoretical framework is to be applied to actual policy questions to yield practical guidance. As we shall see, this is
↓ a tall order.

**986** Historically, McCullough (1979) traces the notion of a right to health care to the French Revolution and to a code of medical ethics developed in Edinburgh in the late 1700s by John Gregory. Chapman and Talmadge (1972) reveal that the idea has a long history in U.S. politics. (It may surprise some to learn that for a brief period around the First World War, the American Medical Association was an enthusiastic advocate of national health insurance.)

The recent increase in attention to this issue may be related to several factors — an increasing distrust of institutions, including medicine; the increasing power of health care to make real differences in mortality and morbidity; and the increasing recognition of the problem of scarce re-
↓ sources, as we discussed in Chapter 12.

**987** Having armed ourselves with our analysis of the concept of rights from Chapter 2, we can look at some implications of the right to health care.

One problem that arises immediately is whether we are really talking about the right to health care or the right to health. It might seem at first that it is absurd to talk about a positive right to health. (We could more easily justify a negative right to health — the right to be free from unhealthy environmental contamination, for example.) If health is a natural good for which (in large part) we cannot be responsible and for which we have limited powers to provide, we ought not enshrine it as a right. On this view, there is no way our institutions could make everyone <u>healthy</u>; but they could at least provide everyone with some health <u>care</u> — thus the health
↓ care, not the health, should be considered as a right.
REVIEW RIGHTS ↑ 72–78

**988** On the other hand, the right to health care leads to problems of its own unless it is tied to the individual's actual health. Does an individual have a right to health care that is actually ineffectual for promoting health (e.g., should Laetrile be provided for cancer patients at public expense)? Does a hypochondriac have a right to surgery for an imagined disease? Unless we look at the individual's actual health outcome, we would seem to have no way of knowing when the right to health care had been adequately
↓ fulfilled.

Even if we could specify just what we mean by the right to health care, we   **989**
would have to develop rules for judging particular social schemes for providing care to see how well alternative schemes fulfill that right. Veatch
(1979) cites two cases of what he considers to be clearly unjust schemes for
providing health care: (1) a society that has abundant resources and that
provides many services in housing, education, and so on, but that makes no
provision for health care for its citizens; and (2) a society that provides
reimbursement for hair transplants but not for childhood infectious disease.                                                                          ↓

The hair transplant example seems difficult to argue with — primarily be-   **990**
cause it represents such a peculiar inversion of values that one suspects that
the policy resulted from the selfish interests of a group of powerful, bald
politicians.
    The other example is not so clear. Engelhardt (1979) invites us to consider
a society that decides to devote the resources that would otherwise provide
health care to providing fine wines, beautiful gardens, and other esthetic
pleasures for everyone. Presumably this society would judge the greater
amenities of life, while it lasted, to be worth the risk of ill health and premature death. If this society were otherwise just, it does not seem obvious
that it should be regarded as unjust merely because it has made this odd
choice with respect to health care. And if that is the case, then even the
clear-cut examples of applying the right to health care are problematic — let
alone the tough examples, like the right to very expensive treatments such
as an artificial heart, and the right to abortions.                          ↓

Two proposals for applying the right to health care to particular social   **991**
schemes have been given wide attention — construing the right as the right
to equal access to health care, and construing it as the right to a decent
minimum of health care. The equal access view has been supported by
Outka (1974), Veatch (1979), and Childress (1979); the decent minimum
view has been argued by Fried (1976) and by Beauchamp and Faden (1979). ↓

Naturally, equal access to health care should not mean that everyone will   **992**
get the same care regardless of need. The fact that a person who has end-
stage kidney failure gets treatment with a kidney machine does not mean
that people with normal kidneys ought to go on the machine also. Veatch
therefore phrases his principle: Everyone should have access to the health
care necessary to provide for a level of health equal to the health of others,
insofar as that is possible.                                                 ↓

**993** A big problem with the equality principle is that it may not allow judgment of the overall social policy. If everyone in a society is unhealthy because of certain social policies, this principle would demand only that a person have the right to be brought up to that unhealthy standard. The principle would not allow us to condemn the entire social scheme as a violation of everyone's right to health care.

Also, a few people with chronic illnesses and congenital handicaps will never, despite indefinite expenditure of resources, come up to the level of health that is the norm for our society (barring the development of major new technologies). Can these people claim a never-ending share of the health care, even to the bankruptcy of the total health-care system? If not, where should the line be drawn? (This objection may apply equally to the decent minimum principle.)

**994** Problems also arise with the decent minimum principle. (This principle gets most of its support from the theory of social justice of John Rawls; Green (1976) shows how Rawls' theory can be applied to health care.) First, it is not clear that people can agree on what would constitute a decent minimum, and how that should be changed with advances in medical technology or with changes in the total amount of society's resources.

**995** Second, so long as a decent minimum of medical care were available to all, this principle would not find fault with providing an extremely high standard of care for an elite few (assuming they could pay for it). Some would say that this is as it should be; but others would argue that such blatant inequalities are precisely what have sparked widespread dissatisfaction with our present system − especially with the way minority groups fare under it.

**996** In addition to choosing the appropriate principle for distributing medical care, we must fulfill, for the right to health care, all the requirements we noted in Chapter 2 for full specification of a right. The following case illustrates some wrinkles.

---

## CASE 62

**997** It's no fun being a hospital administrator in the year 1990, you say to yourself, looking at the two angry individuals who have just barged into your office.

Mr. Puffer is just about to be discharged following radiation therapy for his lung cancer, and is bewailing his hospital bill. He wants to know why his national health insurance policy covers such a small percentage of the cost, when it was supposed to cover it all. Mr. Spender is writhing in pain; a cursory exam by the emergency room doctor reveals that he has acute appendicitis and will probably die without surgery − but he is being denied treatment because he doesn't have a health insurance policy and doesn't have the cash to pay. 997 cont.

You patiently explain the current national health policy. Everyone now gets a guaranteed annual income of $20,000; and for the reasonable sum of $1500 they can buy a comprehensive health insurance policy covering all routine medical care and hospital costs. However, if they choose to spend the $1500 on something else, they must either pay cash for all health services or do without. "You were guaranteed sufficient income to buy insurance," you tell Mr. Spender; "It was your own choice not to buy it."

But there is a catch — "routine" care does not cover care for illness arising directly from one's own unhealthy habits, such as smoking, overeating, or drinking. Mr. Puffer's lung cancer was linked directly to his three-pack-a-day smoking habit. "We've known for years that cigarettes cause cancer," you remind Mr. Puffer, "so you can't expect the rest of us to pay if you choose to continue smoking."

Both the gentlemen reject your explanations and holler loudly, "You're violating our right to health care."

Is this in fact a violation of rights? What would be the most just way of handling such cases? ↓

---

We saw in Chapter 2 that the mere nonfulfillment of a right does not mean that the right has been <u>violated</u>, and therefore that the action was morally unacceptable. We saw that rights could also be <u>waived</u> or <u>overridden</u>. We may now add a third feature — rights may also in some cases be <u>forfeited</u>. A person who attacks you has forfeited his right to life, and if you kill him in self-defense, you have not violated any right of his. **998** ↓

Mr. Spender's predicament raises the question of whether the right to health care is the sort of right one may waive. A strict libertarian would agree with the health insurance scheme depicted in Case 62, arguing that it would be unacceptably paternalistic either to force Mr. Spender to buy the insurance, or to stick the rest of society with the tab if he doesn't. His premature death would be the result of his own free choice and thus would not be ethically unfortunate. On the other hand, one could argue that because poor health is such an unpredictable occurrence, some degree of paternalism is demanded, as otherwise prudent people might be tempted to forego the insurance but would later regret their choice. By this argument, the right to health care should not be waivable by voluntary action. **999** ↓

**1000**  Mr. Puffer, by contrast, is considered by the principles of the insurance plan to have forfeited his right to health care (or to a portion of it at public expense), by virtue of having voluntarily engaged in behavior known to increase his risk of disease. Do we want the right to health to be forfeited in this way? Arguments to the contrary point to the dubious sense in which habitual behaviors like smoking are truly "voluntary" and to the unacceptable police state that might be required to tell who has engaged in unhealthy habits and who hasn't.

Clearly, any complete defense of the right to health care will have to
↓ specify the conditions under which it can be waived and forfeited.

**1001**  Finally, we have to consider a direct assault on the right to health care from the libertarian standpoint — the argument that no such right could exist because it would violate the physician's right to decide when, how, and for what price he will treat any patient. Sade (1971) argues that, derivatively from the right to life itself, there exists a right to earn one's livelihood and to spend one's earnings without interference. Thus a physician has the right to total control over his work and his earnings; a social scheme that forced him to deliver medical care when he didn't want to, or at a lower fee, would
↓ be violating his rights and robbing him of his livelihood.

**1002**  Several responses to Sade are appropriate (in addition to the observation that, given how physicians' salaries compare with other people's, Sade's views are unlikely to arouse much public sympathy for doctors). First, his extreme libertarian view is at odds both with the practices of our own society and with many other theories of social justice. Regulations and restrictions that interfere with how one earns one's livelihood are the norm, not the exception, in our complex society; and many, if not most, such restrictions are ethically justifiable — consider pure food and drug laws and prohi-
↓ bitions of the sale of dangerous substances to young children.

**1003**  Second, Ruddick (1979) observes that the purported right to earn one's livelihood argues for, not against, a right to health care. After all, ill health prevents one from earning a livelihood; so if the right to a livelihood is (as Sade claims) as important as the right to life itself, there would seem to be strong
↓ grounds for a right to health care.

A third point has to do with Sade's motives rather than his argument per se. **1004** Sade claims, in the final analysis, that his upholding of physicians' rights has nothing to do with selfish interests. Rather, his concern as a physician is "the absolute priority of the welfare of his patients," and this would be jeopardized by the heavyhanded government interference a right to health care would mandate. We will see that sociologic evidence is against this argument, but it is also worth noting that Sade sees no conflict between claiming that patient welfare is his primary goal and denying patients any substantial rights in the medical care system. Individual autonomy, by this approach, is seen to be a good thing for the doctor but not for the patient — a return to the priestly model we encountered in Chapter 2.                                ↓
   REVIEW PRIESTLY MODEL ↑ 127

Out of all this muddle, has anything been learned about the so-called right **1005** to health care? Without reaching any final answers, we can at least make some useful generalizations. First, the difficulty in specifying what such a right means might suggest one of two conclusions. The right to health care may in fact be shorthand for a cluster of distinct but closely related rights, some positive and some negative, and these will have to be sorted out explicitly. Alternatively, *it may be more useful to ask, "How would health care be provided for in a society with such-and-such values and resources, if the greatest degree of social justice prevailed?"* instead of *"Is there a right to health care?"* This is not to say that theories of social justice do not give rise to their own problems; it is to say only that reference to rights in this area may produce further obscurity rather than greater clarity.                    ↓

Second, and supporting the first point, *it should be clear that any right to* **1006** *health care we may decide on is not discovered, but rather is created by us in the furtherance of certain social values and conceptions of justice.* If there are any natural rights, which have an independent existence apart from our knowledge of them, the right to health care is certainly not one. It is clearly a tool of our devising to order our society in a certain way for certain purposes.                                                              ↓

Case 63 has implications for the right to health care and also leads us into **1007** the next issue we will discuss — government regulation of medicine. Returning to Sade's argument, we might reject the position that there is no right to health care because we can permit <u>no</u> interference with the wage-earning freedom of physicians; but we are left then with the important question of <u>how much</u> interference we are willing to allow. To put it another way, <u>recognizing</u> a right to health care means (as we just saw) reordering the distribution of social goods in order to better serve a set of needs that are now being ignored; but how far are we willing to alter the social matrix to meet those needs when other basic needs and rights come into conflict?                                                                   ↓

## CASE 63

**1008**   The debate in the Political Action Committee of the American Society of Medical Students (ASMS) grows increasingly heated. At issue is the stand the ASMS will officially take on the bill, recently voted out of the Senate Health Subcommittee, to require 2 years mandatory public service after completion of medical training for all newly graduating U.S. physicians.

Those opposing the bill claim to be in favor of better health care for the underserved population and admit that medicine's past record is not impressive. But they adamantly oppose a measure that would address these problems only by nearly total denial of the personal freedom of the young physician; and they further question the quality of the health services that would be delivered by "conscript labor." In the future, they lament, the best students may choose not to go into medicine just to avoid this heavy-handed regulation. Surely financial incentives and other means can be found to encourage physicians to give more health care to the needy.

There is another group, however, that urges the ASMS to come out in favor of the bill. Financial incentives and other measures just haven't worked, and right now the public approval of physicians is at its lowest ebb in decades. The only way to turn around these unpleasant trends is to support this new measure boldly — not as an acceptance of loss of freedom, but as an acceptance of public responsibility. If the medical profession acts now to get behind the measure, this argument goes, there may be some leeway to increase the wages that will be paid for the compulsory service and also to increase financial aid to medical students (to reverse the current trend of only the children of the rich being able to afford medical school). If physicians oppose this measure, the proponents add ominously, perhaps even worse restrictions lurk down the road.

↓ How do you vote?

---

### Government Regulation of Medicine

**1009**   Presently, no one is seriously considering a law such as that envisioned in Case 63 — although some would see little difference between a law and the present situation in which medical school tuitions are being raised to levels beyond most students' ability to pay, and wherein the only financial aid available requires "pay-back" in the form of mandatory service. In many other ways, the United States government, stimulated by the idea of the right to health care and other major national interests, is imposing an increasing degree of regulation upon a profession that has been historically notable for an amazing degree of autonomy. The results are being hotly debated, as a quick look at the editorial columns of almost any current ↓ medical journal will show.

Major issues in government regulation include:     **1010**

1. Movement toward a national health insurance policy, which could either be a voluntary option or a compulsory replacement of private insurance.
2. Regulations to contain the increasing cost of medical care by prohibiting new hospital construction, acquisition of expensive machinery, etc. unless proven need exists.
3. Attempts to force further self-policing by physicians to ensure the quality of medical care and to develop uniform standards of quality.
4. Attacks on so-called monopolistic practices in medicine, such as sanctions against advertising by physicians and the imposition of standard fee scales.
5. Regulation of the drug industry to assure safety, which, according to critics, keeps new and useful drugs off the market.     ↓

A glance at this list might suggest that we are mistaken in including the     **1011** issue of government regulation in this book in the first place. We seem to have generated a list of economic and political issues, not ethical dilemmas. For example, it might appear that there is nothing ethically sacrosanct about physicians not advertising. If there is anything wrong with allowing physicians to advertise, it would have to do with the deleterious economic and political consequences that might result. Further, the main support for the idea of allowing advertising comes from the hope that more free enterprise would bring down the cost of medical care; but some economists argue persuasively that health care simply does not work by the same rules of competition as other segments of the economy, and hence allowing advertising would not have the hoped-for result. This factual argument against advertising seems to be more persuasive than one based on ethics.     ↓

However, this dismissal of the value of ethical decision making in resolving     **1012** these issues may be premature. The issues of government regulation have to do with what Jonsen and Jameton (1977) term the form of health care, which they designate as one broad area of the health professional's social responsibility. This responsibility may be justified on the grounds that the form of health-care organizations will influence the behaviors and the values of the health professionals, and these changes may have a positive or a negative impact on the care the patient from an ethical standpoint.     ↓

**1013** Suppose, for example, that the government were to carry to extremes the quest for standardization of quality-of-care criteria (possibly also motivated by predictions that we could save money by making health care more uniform). This could result in very rigid formulas for the sort of care that would be allowed for any individual's sickness. But this form of health care conflicts in a basic way with the contractual model of the doctor–patient relationship, which becomes less meaningful as fewer options are offered to the patient. If only one sort of care is offered, we have reverted to the priestly model, only with the government agency rather than the doctor occupying the priestly role. If we can indeed argue that the contractual model is ethically more sound, it follows that the ethical health professional should oppose this rigid standardization.

↓ REVIEW MODELS ↑ 127–131

**1014** On the other hand, suppose that a new way of financing medical care were proposed that had potential for increasing the decision-making role of the patient and for aiding patient education so that more informed decisions would result. For the same reasons that we would oppose the rigid standardization policy, we would, from an ethical standpoint, approve of this new plan (assuming that it did not have some other deleterious conse-

↓ quences).

**1015** Our basic ethical method ought also to suggest that regulations be looked at with suspicion. If we have reserved a very basic place in our value framework for individual autonomy, we should not rush to embrace external controls on our behavior. It would seem better, as a means of promoting desired social change, to first try various sorts of persuasion, education, and

↓ voluntary incentives.

**1016** But against this observation must be placed the realization that regulation and even overregulation is more the norm than the exception in our complex society. Physicians, responding to the biased viewpoint we mentioned earlier, have often reacted as if their activities were of such high importance to society that no interference was tolerable, and that they themselves knew better than anyone else how medicine ought to be practiced and financed. While for a long time medicine, compared to other social institutions, was largely free of government regulation, physicians have tended to see the rather belated extension of regulatory activities to medicine as an example of medicine being unfairly singled out. In the generally angry response to proposed government regulations, it is hard to separate the genuine concern for patients' interests from the self-serving defense of the tradi-

↓ tional physicians' privileges.

If we sweep away the biases and the self-serving rhetoric, we might be left     **1017**
with an argument against government regulation something like this:

We rely on individual physicians for technically competent and humane
care of patients, and we rely on the entire medical profession for further
scientific advances and new medical technology for the future. On the individual level, autonomy is necessary to allow individualized choice and
the personal relationship of doctor with patient. On the professional level,
autonomy is necessary to protect medical knowledge from restrictions imposed by the scientifically incompetent. Therefore, both for the profession
as a whole and for the individual professional, regulations by outside agencies diminishes the ability of the profession to carry out its assigned tasks.  ↓

You will notice that this argument relies in part on an empirical assertion —     **1018**
the actual, practical consequences of government regulation. We could
test this assertion by looking at medical systems that already operate under
a high degree of government regulation — not a difficult problem, since the
United States is virtually the only developed country in the world that has
not adopted some form of socialized medicine. Defenders of the traditional fee-for-service method of financing medicine point to such social-
ization as the first major step in stripping away professional autonomy.
Therefore, it would be useful to study the actual practices of the medical
profession in other societies (so long as we restrict the comparisons to general issues; the differences in the social environments among different
countries are likely to make any detailed, point-by-point comparison invalid).                                                                        ↓

Friedson (1970), a medical sociologist, devotes much attention to the study     **1019**
of how medicine fares under different social systems. At heart, Friedson is a
strong supporter of professional autonomy, claiming that autonomy is precisely what is essential to make medicine a "profession" in the strict sense
of the word. Were it not for professional autonomy, medicine would find it
hard to develop a firm and expanding body of knowledge; it would be
blown this way and that by changing social demands and whims — more
like clothing fashions.                                                        ↓

But Friedson is also careful to distinguish various aspects of the medical     **1020**
enterprise: the accumulation and interpretation of medical knowledge, the
economic and social conditions under which the knowledge is to be applied, and the goals and consequences of the application.                      ↓

**1021** Friedson's review of many studies of socialized medicine, in which the governments and not the physicians dictate the economic and social conditions for medical practice, leads him to conclude that this sort of government regulation does not in fact lead to lessened professional autonomy in the "core" area — that is, the accumulation and interpretation of medical knowledge. The tendency in many socialized nations is for the medical profession to guard jealously this core autonomy, even while accepting government regulation of how medical care is to be financed.

**1022** In the third area, the goals and consequences of the application of medical knowledge, there is simply no question of the need for government regulation. The use of medical technology affects the entire populace, not just physicians; and it would be simply intolerable if physicians were to choose to apply their knowledge in ways contrary to the public interest, just as it would be intolerable for industrial engineers to decide unilaterally to discharge toxic wastes into the public water supply.

**1023** Of the three aspects of the medical enterprise, Friedson concludes from his sociologic perspective that the argument about the absolute need for autonomy applies properly only to the core aspect. (An example of a loss of this core autonomy would be, say, if the government decided that diagnosis of sickle-cell anemia was unfairly discriminatory against blacks, and ordered all references to sickle-cell anemia removed from medical textbooks. The very outrageousness of this example suggests that we are in little danger of this sort of loss of autonomy, although it did befall the science of genetics in Stalinist Russia.)

**1024** If Friedson is correct, then, government regulation of the economic and social organization of medicine, and of the application of medical knowledge, does not in and of itself destroy professional autonomy and the ability of the physician to give appropriate care to his patients. Of course, the specific regulations might be so noxious or burdensome as to make proper patient care impossible. Therefore, we cannot argue against government regulation just because it is regulation. We are obligated to assess the impact of specific proposed regulations in light of the practical economic, social, and ethical consequences.

**1025** In assessing the impact of proposed regulations, any general appeal to medical ethics in the abstract, or to traditional oaths or codes of ethics, will not aid in understanding the issues and is likely to be viewed as self-serving rhetoric. Furthermore, pious expressions of concern for the patients' welfare are not likely to win points — the public has too much reason to think that doctors get excited about patients' welfare only when their pocketbooks are affected.

A reasoned response to proposed regulation from an ethical standpoint,

then, demands appeals to particular ethical issues such as the ones we ana-    **1025**
lyzed in the first several chapters of this book: the doctor–patient relation-    cont.
ship, patient autonomy, confidentiality, informed consent, quality of life,
and so on. In addition to the more general formula of weighing the consequences of the proposed regulation against our scale of values, these generally applicable ethical issues provide a checklist to assess the likely ethical
impact of the regulations.    ↓

As we noted, Jonsen and Jameton (1977) state that the issues of government    **1026**
regulation have to do with the health professional's social responsibility for
the form of health care. They also cite another area of responsibility — for
the uses of medical or health care skills. In the next section we shall look at
situations where the use (or nonuse) of skills seems to involve the health
professional in a conflict between competing responsibilities.    ↓

---

## CASE 64

The nurses at the inner-city, 700-bed County Hospital have been accus-    **1027**
tomed to low wages for a long time. What has incited them to a fury are
newly announced economic cutbacks by the local government. Nursing
coverage has been cut back on all wards, making one nurse responsible for
more patients at one time. In addition, many housekeeping and other support personnel have been laid off. Now nurses must clean up spills and take
specimens to the lab as well as perform their usual patient-care duties.

You attend a meeting called by the nurses' organization. Many of the
nurses are ready to go out on strike. They want to demand restoration of
adequate staff coverage as the condition for returning to work, and they
argue that the public will support them, especially since they are not asking
for more money for themselves. They propose to maintain nursing coverage
of the emergency room and the intensive care units. Patients on the other
wards will have to be cared for by the supervisors, interns, and residents or
be transferred to other hospitals.

Many nurses, however, are opposed to the strike. They point out that the
county really has no choice, faced with escalating costs and a diminishing
tax base. Even if sympathetic to their plight, the county supervisors may be
helpless to change things. More basically, they say that their duty as nurses
is to give the best possible care to patients, and the second-rate care they
now have to give is better than refusing to give care at all.

Do you support the strike of your fellow nurses or urge alternative measures?    ↓

## Conflicts of Responsibility

**1028** Case 64 depicts a situation becoming increasingly common in United States health systems, as more and more health workers see themselves more as union members aligned against management in an adversarial relationship rather than as professionals allied in a common cause. Strikes by nurses and house-staff physicians have taken place in many cities, mostly under conditions similar to those described in Case 64. As Badgley and Wolfe (1968) describe, physicians in Saskatchewan went out on strike in 1962 to protest the government's new publicly financed health plan. A 1972 survey of U.S. physicians revealed that a majority said they would strike, given sufficient provocation.

**1029** If Sade is correct in the extreme view that the right to earn a living without interference should be the most basic consideration governing the behavior of health professionals, there can be no objection to such strikes, no matter how flimsy the provocation. But Sade could not then claim, as he does, that the health professional does what he does out of concern for the welfare of the patients. Health professionals are just that and not health workers, because they have assumed an obligation (implicit in our contractual model) to put the interests of the patient ahead of their own monetary gain to some extent. This point is made in an epigram quoted by Kaplan (1972): "The professional man, it has been said, does not work in order to be paid; he is paid in order that he may work."

**1030** Does that mean, then, that we can never justify a strike by health professionals on ethical grounds? There might be grounds to make this sweeping claim. From the way we have characterized the contractual model, the unilateral pulling out of the relationship by the caregiver would seem to be a violation of the health professional's basic ethical obligation (as well as possibly a commission of the legal tort of abandonment). And yet, there might be cases in which the health professional–patient relationship was already so severely jeopardized that a strike would add no further injury. Suppose the County Hospital in Case 64 decided to further economize by selling off their entire stock of medicines, syringes, bedpans, and everything; and then ordered the nurses to appear for work and carry out their duties. We could easily argue that whether the nurses showed up for work the next day would really be immaterial insofar as patient care would be concerned. (With patient care no longer at issue, the nurses, due to the symbolic responsibility mentioned before, could have a positive ethical duty not to show up.)

In Case 64 we have a middle position, in between striking purely for mone- **1031**
tary gain and striking because any sort of decent care is impossible. Clearly
the nurses have a responsibility to the patients now in the hospital, and the
strike would amount to a violation of that responsibility. But is there a
larger community responsibility to protest the inadequate conditions? Or,
if one does not strike and hence forces the existing patients to go on with
substandard care, could one be said to be violating a responsibility to those
patients, too? ↓

There are many situations in which one can promote social change by caus- **1032**
ing harm to a small number of people. (Consider those who expose illegal
or improper medical practices by deceitfully posing as patients or by stealing confidential patient records.) From a consequentialist standpoint, the
greater social good may seem to justify such actions. But an ethical analysis
in terms of duties and responsibilities would challenge this conclusion. By
this analysis, there are many alternative ways to achieve social change, and
one individual has only limited power to do so. On the other hand, the
individual often has considerable power to harm one other person or a
small group of people. We would conclude from this that the duty to avoid
harming other individuals should be given stronger weight than the duty to
help bring about positive social change. (Our emphasis on individual dignity in our value scale would tend to go along with this analysis.) ↓

This argument may lead us to conclude that the nurses in Case 64 ought not **1033**
strike. This conclusion is further supported if, as a strictly practical point,
the strike is unlikely to succeed. But note once again that there might be
more extreme cases in which this line of argument would justify a strike. ↓

A threatened strike is only one example of how a health professional may **1034**
be involved in a conflict of ethical responsibilities. A very common sort of
conflict exists when the health professional is bound to an employer whose
interests may not coincide with the interests of the individual patient. This
situation exists for health professionals working in "total institutions" such
as the military or the prison system and to a lesser extent for professionals
employed by industry and by insurance companies.

But conflicts of responsibility can arise in much more mundane settings,
and at one time or another affect all health professionals. ↓

---

## CASE 65

You are just completing your family practice residency at the University of **1035**
Virginia and are about to set up a solo private practice in the small town of
Piney River. Knowing the dangers of setting up a practice without careful

**1035**
**cont.** financial and managerial planning, you are giving the matter careful thought.

One of the things that attracts you to Piney River is the need for a physician in that area. Many of the rural folk drive the 40-odd miles to the University for their care, and still others do without medical attention entirely. You suspect that the town could eventually provide a comfortable practice for two physicians, and that you will probably be very busy on your own once you become settled.

On the other hand, you are committed to giving personal attention to your patients, and to try to spend a little time with them rather than rushing them through your office. The patients in Piney River might appreciate "assembly-line care" more than no care at all, but that would not fit with your own image of the ideal family physician. You are also committed to spending time with your family, and you know that the demands of solo practice often conflict with personal and family life to a significant degree.

One way you have of controlling these factors is to limit the number of patients you will accept into your practice and to limit the number of patients you will see in a day. Seeing fewer patients a day will allow you time for the style of medicine you prefer. It will also limit your practice by, in effect, creating a waiting list for nonemergency visits. But it will probably leave many of the citizens of Piney River without consistent medical attention.

↓ What approach do you take in designing your practice?

---

**1036** Case 65 presents a microallocation problem similar to some of those that we discussed in Chapter 12. Here, the scarce commodity is not money, artificial hearts, or cadaver kidneys, but the individual physician's time. Clearly this new family doctor would like to serve all the needy of Piney River, spend enough time to get to know each patient, devote attention to his family, and also get a good night's sleep every night; but there aren't enough hours in the day to accomplish that, so the conflicting responsibilities need to be rank-ordered in some way.

**1037** Don't the arguments we just raised about strikes dictate against limiting this physician's practice? Isn't it just as bad to withhold health care from the citizens of Piney River as it is to withhold it from the patients at County Hospital in Case 64?

However, on closer investigation the two cases are quite distinct. In the language of the contractual model, a strike involves cutting and running from a contract already in force. Case 65 involves limiting the number of contracts the physician will enter into, and also setting some of the terms of his end of the contract (i.e., that it may be harder to get in to see him, but when the patient does have an appointment, he will get the doctor's full and devoted attention).

In Chapter 12 we mentioned Fried's (1974) concept of a right to personal    **1038**
care, which required that a course of treatment, once begun, should be
continued to the end (thus the problem with strikes). Another feature that
Fried cites is that personal care, if it is to be tied to the dignity of the individual patient, is at some point indivisible and incapable of wider distribution. That is, in the normal work day, our Piney River doctor may choose to
see 30 patients for 15 minutes each, or perhaps 45 patients for 10 minutes
each. But if he tried to see 450 patients for 1 minute each, or 900 patients for
30 seconds each, we would not be inclined to praise him for distributing
the benefits of his care over a wider group; we would say that he has
stopped giving care altogether. Thus, at some point, seeing more patients
stops becoming giving more health care. (This is also the case, of course, if
seeing more patients means that the patients see a doctor who is tired, irri-
table, or who lacks the time to keep up with current medical knowledge.)    ↓

As we noted, the conflict faced by this family doctor is different from the    **1039**
case of deciding whether to strike. We characterized the strike dilemma as
that of weighing the harm to a few against the possible benefit to many. But
the family doctor has to weigh the various benefits he might bestow, so
long as he stays within the limits of personal care — benefits to his patients,
to his family, and to himself. Therefore, the principle that served as some
guide in the strike case — that possible benefits to many do not outweigh
harm done to a few — will not help this family doctor make his choice.    ↓
   CONSEQUENTIALIST? * 1041

In the end, it would seem that the choice this physician makes will have to    **1040**
be highly individualized. Some physicians can work very long hours and
still have time and energy left for family and personal pursuits; others need
much more rest and relaxation and need to guard their time more carefully.
Some families proceed nicely even with the husband or wife absent much
of the time; others need a great deal of attention and shared time. It seems
unlikely we could develop any general rules to assist this physician, other
than to make sure that his assessment of the needs of his town, his family,
and himself are realistic.    ↓**1042**

---

* We mentioned above that the greater duty to avoid harm, as opposed to    **1041**
the duty to provide benefits, flows more smoothly from a duty-based rather
than a consequentialist ethic (see Appendix I). But we can give a consequentialist justification for it as well. We are aware of the follies committed
by many past reformers and revolutionaries, in which they tended to overestimate the real benefits likely in the future and to underestimate the actual degree of harm they were inflicting. If this is a psychological fact about
how the zeal to reform is likely to bias our judgment, then good consequences would follow from a rule that made us pay more attention to the
harms.    ↑**1040**

**1042** We have now looked at three general issues arising from the social responsibility of health professionals — the right to health care, government regulation, and conflicts of responsibility. Recalling the list of issues we presented near the beginning of the chapter, however, you will see that we have just barely scratched the surface of this complex topic. For more detailed discussion of some of the specific issues, you will want to consult the ↓ references for this chapter.

**1043** We will conclude this chapter with one final case and will leave the discussion of the case to you. This case rounds off the chapter because it represents an example of one of the sorts of conflict of responsibility we mentioned — the dilemma of doctors (in particular, psychiatrists) serving in the military. This case also leads us into a discussion highlighted in the next chapter — how are judgments made in deciding on the presence of health and disease? In particular, what role do value judgments play in such deci- ↓ sions?

---

### CASE 66

**1044** The following news item regarding an event during the Vietnam War appeared in an Air Force military surgeons' newsletter of December, 1966.

Fear of Flying: A 26-year-old SSgt AC 47 gunner with 7 months active duty in RVN (Republic of Vietnam), presented with frank admission of fear of flying. He had flown over 100 missions, and loss of several aircraft and loss of several crews who were well known to the patient, precipitated his visit. He stated he would give up flight pay, promotion, medals, etc., just to stop flying. Psychiatric consultation to USAF Hospital, Cam Ranh Bay, resulted in 36 days hospitalization with use of psychotherapy and tranquilizers. Diagnosis was Gross Stress Reaction, manifest by anxiety, tenseness, a fear of death expressed in the form of rationalizations, and inability to function. His problem was "worked through" and insight to his problem was gained to the extent that he was returned to full flying duty in less than 6 weeks. This is a fine tribute to the psychiatrists at Cam Ranh Bay.

1. Were the Air Force psychiatrists serving the best interests of the patient? What was the nature of their contract?
2. What do you think of the diagnosis reached in this case? Do you think that a "disease" was indeed present? If the sergeant displayed diseased behavior, what would have constituted "normal" behavior under the circumstances?
3. Are anxiety, tenseness, fear of death, and inability to function symptoms of disease whenever they appear, or only in some circumstances? What sorts of value judgments play a role in determining these circumstances?
4. If you were the psychiatrist at Cam Ranh Bay in charge of this case, what would you have done?

(Case brought to our attention courtesy of Robert G. Newman, M.D., and H. Tristram Engelhardt, Jr., M.D., Ph.D.)

**1045** ↓ CH. 17

# Defining Health and Disease 17

In this chapter we will look at the concepts of health and disease, and we **1045** will see how a clear understanding of these concepts might aid our understanding of medical practice. The issue we will be most concerned with is the role that values play in the concepts of health and disease. Back in Chapter 2, we pointed out that all medical decisions have ethical components — that is, that they include value judgments along with factual, empirical data. We concluded that value judgments were an inseparable part of the practice of medicine. But this still leaves open the possibility that values play no important role in the science of medicine — that when medical scientists say that an individual is healthy or diseased, they are merely describing facts and no value judgments are present. Now in this chapter we will present a more radical thesis — that the very concepts of "health" and "disease" include value judgments on a fundamental level and no value-free science of medicine is possible. ↓

REVIEW FACTS VS. VALUES ↑ 19–26

Before we turn to arguments in support of this thesis, we need to discuss **1046** some important introductory points. To begin, we might consider one criticism leveled at modern medicine — that we are too busy worrying about disease when our primary concern should be preserving health. From this, one might conclude that we need to look at the concept of health first, and then consider the concept of disease as a secondary case. In doing so, we might avoid the pitfalls of getting very interested in diseases and then defining health in a purely negative way as the absence of disease. ↓

Certainly we ought to stress health maintenance and preventive medicine **1047** much more than we have tended to do in the past. The only question is: Does focusing our concern on the concept of health rather than disease give us any practical assistance in this project? Unfortunately, as some of the following discussion may illustrate, it turns out that analysis of the concept of disease has been much more fruitful. (Maybe this is because health professionals perhaps ought to be more concerned with health but actually are much more preoccupied with disease.) However, this does not mean we have to give up on health altogether, and we will see later how the systems perspective may help to accommodate both health and disease. ↓

**1048**  As a second point, we may distinguish between another pair of concepts — "disease" and "illness." This distinction seems to have started among anthropologists studying sickness in different cultures, but it has many useful features. Disease refers to the description or explanation applied to the patient's experience, while illness refers to that experience itself. For example, a person might develop fever, muscle aches, nausea, and diarrhea (illness) and then think to himself, "I must have caught that flu bug that's going around the office" (disease). In such common cases the ill person may himself apply the disease description; in more serious cases he will turn to the doctor.

**1049**  As we develop sophisticated theories of disease, there is not always a nice correspondence between disease and illness. For instance, our research has led us to consider hypertension a serious disease when untreated, leading as it does to increased risk of heart attack and stroke. But people with undiagnosed high blood pressure generally feel fine and have no symptoms. It seems that they have a disease but no illness. On the other hand, many people have a variety of symptoms for which they repeatedly visit doctors, but thorough investigation fails to detect any disease of the sort that is written about in medical textbooks. Doctors, if kind, may call these patients "hypochondriacs" or "psychosomatic complainers"; if unkind, they are likely to dismiss these patients as "crocks." These patients are certainly suffering illness by our definition, but according to the theories of these doctors they have no disease. (Is this a reflection on the patients, or on the theories of disease used by these doctors?)

**1050**  Clearly it may be stressful to the doctor–patient relationship if the patient's illness and the doctor's ideas of disease do not correspond. But it can also be stressful if the theories and assumptions about the disease that is present differs for doctor and patient. Kleinman (1978) discusses how "explanatory models" may be divergent, especially among people of different cultures.

**1051**  Consider, for example, a Puerto Rican patient who subscribes to the "hot–cold" theory of disease, a well-established aspect of the Hispanic folk culture. According to this theory, diseases and remedies are categorized as either hot or cold: a hot remedy will cure a cold disease while a cold remedy will make a cold disease worse. The common cold is considered one of the cold diseases. Thus, the physician who gives this Puerto Rican patient the useful advice to drink a lot of fruit juices for a cold is likely to be ignored and held in lower esteem by the patient, who regards fruit juices as a cold remedy. Here the explanatory models employed by the doctor and the patient to explain the same disease differ markedly.

But we do not have to look to these extreme cases to see how the doctor— **1052** patient relationship is affected by divergent explanatory models. Consider the middle-class American doctor treating the middle-class American patient for weight loss and fatigue. The doctor does a careful evaluation and concludes that the patient is suffering from depression brought about by some marital problems, which the patient tends to deny. But the patient refuses to believe that his suffering could have an emotional basis (or be "all in his head," as he might put it). His own explanatory model holds that he must have a hidden cancer that the doctor can't find (which makes him all the more depressed, to boot). If this patient is not to embark on a doctor-shopping tour, which may result in many unneeded x-rays, lab tests, and surgery, some sort of negotiation will have to take place between doctor and patient to allow them to bring their explanatory models into better harmony. ↓

Seeing how explanatory models of disease differ has important practical **1053** applications, as these two cases show. But it also helps us in our understanding of the concept of disease. When we see how concepts and explanations of disease differ between cultures and even within the same culture in different historical periods, we see how variable specific concepts of disease can be. But people of all cultures and all periods must be talking basically about the same thing — disease. We can, then, look for the underlying concept of disease that is shared to some extent by these varying specific concepts of disease. (We also get to be a bit more humble about our own highly touted theories of medicine; perhaps 100 years from now our theories will look as silly as the hot-cold theory does to us today.) ↓

We can now turn back to the question that we started with — how values **1054** are fundamentally bound up with the concept of disease. *Basically, we will argue that the terms healthy and diseased are used by medical scientists to describe phenomena that occur in the world; but that specifically, these phenomena are so called because they are desirable (healthy) or undesirable (diseased). Without the value judgments about what states are desirable and undesirable, we have no concepts of health or disease.* ↓

Imagine a scientist excitedly running out of his lab to announce the discov- **1055** ery of a new disease. We ask him to tell us more. He describes the disease in detail, and then goes on to say that it's the sort of state that makes no difference to the individual whether he has it or not. We ask about how one would treat this disease; and the scientist replies that he isn't concerned at all with treatment — since it makes no difference to the individual whether or not he has this disease, it would make no difference whether or not he were treated, either. ↓

**1056** We would probably greet this scientist's announcement with some skepticism. Our skepticism would <u>not</u> be directed at the facts that the scientist claims to have discovered; we might agree with all of them. Rather, we would say that the state of affairs he has described is not a disease at all; or at best, he is using the word disease in a very peculiar way. This is to say that the idea of being undesirable, unwanted, to be changed if one could, and so on is a fundamental feature of the concept of disease.

**1057** This is an illustration of the point, not an argument in its favor. What arguments could we use to convince someone who thought that the concept of disease can be characterized in a value-free way?

We might have a good deal of sympathy with such a position. After all, we were taught back in grade school that science is value-free, and that science began to make progress precisely when people saw that it was possible to leave their value judgments outside the laboratory. As examples of the ways values could interfere with scientific progress, we learned about the persecution of Galileo for teaching an astronomy that was at odds with Church doctrine, and about the Scopes "monkey trial" where religious zealots tried to stifle Darwinian theory. Some might think, then, that to admit values back into concepts basic to medicine would be to turn the clock back to before the Renaissance.

**1058** Hopefully, we will show that admitting values back into medical science will not prove to be all that bad, but first we have to make the argument that they should be admitted.

One form our argument might take is to line up all the different concepts of disease that have been used in the past or present. If we can show that each has value components, we may convince the opponents that values are fundamental to the more general concept of disease.

**1059** A historical survey is a good place to start in listing the various concepts of disease. Medical historians have aided us here by dividing most of the disease concepts into two broad categories — ontologic and physiologic approaches to disease.

**1060** The <u>ontologic</u> approach considers <u>disease as a distinct entity</u>. Disease entities are seen as having some sort of independent existence (just what sort is often a debated issue). A healthy individual becomes sick when he has one of these disease entities visited upon him, after which he becomes a sort of amalgam of individual-plus-disease. Diagnosis becomes a process of deciding which of a known set of disease entities is present in this case, and treatment is the process of removal of the disease entity.

The importance of the ontologic concept spans the history of Western medicine. Very early disease theories, in which sickness was seen as being caused by demon or spirit possession, is an extreme form of ontologism. The success of Linnaeus' system of classification according to genus and species in botany in the 1600s prompted physicians like Sydenham to try similar classifications of diseases. The ontologic approach achieved its present height with the rise of the germ theory of disease and the development of antibiotics.    1061

↓

The second major approach, the <u>physiologic</u> approach, considers <u>disease as deviation from the norm</u>. The disease is not an entity that exists apart from the sick individual; it is merely a state of affairs that exists when one or more physiologic functions of the individual deviate from their normal or proper activity. Diagnosis, then, consists of identifying the offending physiologic function, and treatment would be directed at getting it back to within normal limits.    1062

Often, in a physiologic disease schema, diseases come in pairs. Looking at physiologic function X, we often find that individuals can have either an excess or a deficit of X, so we can have both hyper-X and hypo-X disease. ↓

For many centuries, the physiologic approach held sway in Western medicine in the form of the theory of the four humors of the body (blood, phlegm, black bile, and yellow bile), which was in turn derived from the Greek theory of the four elements of nature (earth, air, fire, and water). Disease was felt to arise from too much or too little of any of the humors, or its presence outside of its proper location within the body. Health, then, was a sort of harmony in which all the humors were in equilibrium. Similar theories are found in traditional Arabic, Indian, and Chinese medicine. (In fact, the Hispanic hot-cold theory of disease probably arose from the humoral theory, showing how yesterday's scientific theories can become today's folk theories.)    1063

↓

We should note that it is often difficult to make a hard-and-fast distinction between the ontologic and the physiologic views, and that both play a role in modern medicine. If, for instance, we say that a normal person may become diseased through hyperfunction of the thyroid gland, we are sticking closely to the physiologic approach. When we start to notice that certain symptoms are characteristic of this disease, and to apply the diagnosis of hyperthyroidism when this symptom complex is present, the ontologic approach is starting to creep in. And if we refer to "the case of hyperthyroidism in Room 306," we have pretty much sold out to the ontologic approach (even to the extent of leaving out the patient).    1064

↓

**1065**  At any rate, the reason for bringing up the different approaches is to see if we can detect value judgments in their operation.

Clearly, in applying the ontologic approach, a considerable degree of selectivity is going on. We look at the various observables that are present in patients, and when certain collections of observables are present, we say that a disease entity exists. For example, if we see a patient with the set of observables including joint pain, uric acid crystals present in the joint fluid, and so on, we declare the presence of the disease "gout." But there are an infinite number of potential observables, and hence an infinite number of such collections. What possible reason could we have for picking out a rather limited number of them to be called diseases and ignoring the rest? The real reason seems to be that certain collections are correlated with <u>un-desirable</u> states of affairs. We consider it <u>important</u> to detect those collections because, where possible, we want to change or to prevent the undesirable state of affairs. And these key value words signal the fundamental
↓ role of values in this approach to disease.

**1066**  There is a similar selectivity going on in the physiologic approach. Once again, there is a much larger number of physiologic functions we could conceivably observe and measure than there are identified disease states. We could rather easily measure the rate at which people's toenails grow, determine an average range, and then set up nationwide screening programs to detect hypo- and hyper-toenail growth rates. We do not in fact do this (nor would Blue Cross reimburse for such screening!), not because rate of toenail growth is objectively different from level of thyroid function or other physiologic variables, but because change in rate of toenail growth has not been linked in any useful way to states that we consider undesirable. (On the other hand, if we discovered that a change in the rate of toenail growth is a reliable, early sign of cancer, then such a string of screening
↓ clinics might make a lot of sense.)

**1067**  We also see selectivity in the physiologic approach when deviation in only one direction is considered to represent disease. Looking at our patient's laboratory test, we may get very concerned about an abnormally high bilirubin level in the blood, which may signal liver disease or certain types of anemia; we do not get at all excited about abnormally low bilirubin levels, which are not connected with any known undesirable states. Similarly, we regard people who have IQ values a certain number of points <u>below</u> the mean as having the handicap (if not the "disease") of mental retardation; but we do not apply any such label to those who have IQs that number of points <u>above</u> the mean, since higher IQ is regarded as a desirable rather
↓ than an undesirable trait.

These examples do more than illustrate how values are fundamentally in-    **1068**
volved in disease ascriptions. They also show how easy it is to miss the
value component — simply because most of the value judgments are ones
on which almost everyone would agree. No matter what historical period
or what culture one comes from, one would readily agree that gout, hyperthyroidism, jaundice, and so on are all bad states of affairs. Because
agreement among many different observers is one criterion we use to test
the truth of empirical data, we might be misled by this widespread agreement on disease ascriptions into assuming that disease ascriptions were
purely empirical observations. But this would be to miss the fact that we are
talking fundamentally about goodness and badness, and hence about
values.                                                                      ↓

This point becomes more obvious when we look past the cases in which    **1069**
widespread agreement holds. There are many states considered diseases by
one culture, or in one historical period, but not by others; and investigation
usually reveals that the difference lies much of the time in value orientation. We already mentioned that low IQ in our culture is designated as a
disease or handicap; in a simple agrarian culture it would probably go unnoticed unless it were very severe. Some rain-forest tribes suffer from what
we would call skin diseases, but which they consider the normal state of
affairs; it is the ones without the splotchy skin, which we would call
healthy, that the tribespeople consider abnormal and refuse to allow to
marry the "normals." In our own past history, Engelhardt (1974) has called
attention to the nineteenth century disease of masturbation, which was
thought to lead to epilepsy and insanity and was often treated surgically;
and the pre-Civil War South disease of draepetomania, an "abnormal" condition of slaves in which they suffered from an "irrational" desire to run
away. And finally, in our present society, we see the arguments over
whether alcoholism and homosexuality should be regarded as diseases or
as morally deviant behavior.                                                 ↓

Examples like alcoholism and homosexuality point out the connection be-    **1070**
tween disease and deviance. As sociologists put it, deviant behavior elicits
generally negative value judgments and usually results in some sort of social ostracism. Deviance can be the result of one's own free actions, as in
morally deviant behavior; or it can result from biologic phenomena beyond
one's direct control, as with disease or with skin color in a racist society.
What separates disease as a subcategory of deviance from, say, having a
minority skin color, is that the disease is seen as temporary, not as part of
one's permanent nature. (Clearly, cases of congenital disease or chronic
disease strain this model.)                                                  ↓

**1071**   For this reason all cultures have evolved a "sick role" as the socially acceptable behavior for one who is sick. The sick individual is excused from his usual work and family responsibilities and is expected to present himself to that culture's approved "healer" and to follow that healer's advice. By this set of social expectations, one may not be directly responsible for getting sick, although one may be indirectly responsible if one failed to wear galoshes when going out in the rain, failed to offer the proper prayers to the spirits, and so on. However, one is expected at least to take responsibility for trying to get well. Indeed, if the sufferer fails to act out his proper part of the sick role, the social group may revise the original ascription of disease, and decide that the person is really a malingerer trying to evade legitimate duties.

**1072**   When we argue about whether alcoholism and homosexuality are diseases, then, we are arguing <u>only in part</u> about the "facts." Certainly new knowledge about the psychodynamics of alcohol addiction, about how early in life one's sexual preferences are established, and whether homosexuals have too much or too little sex hormones, and so on plays a role in our decisions about how much free choice is involved in these conditions. In addition to the factual issues, there are the value issues of the degree of "badness" represented by these conditions — many who declared homosexuality bad 15 years ago are now prepared to say that it is neutral from a value standpoint — and the political issues about which institutions in society ought to be responsible for their regulation. To say that such conditions are diseases, then, is to make the political decision that the health-care establishment, and not the police, the clergy, or the individuals themselves, ought to have the appropriate authority to handle the deviant behavior.

**1073**   Let's stop a minute and see where we are. Our argument has shown two things: (1) the two most generally acceptable approaches to disease, the ontologic and the physiologic, both fundamentally make use of value judgments, and (2) so long as we include problems such as alcoholism and homosexuality under the category of disease, and not just broken bones and heart attacks, the value elements cannot be ignored.

But we are still trying to convince the skeptic who wants to endorse the idea of a value-free medical science. What will the skeptic say in reply?

Our skeptic might say, first, that if we have shown the value content of    **1074**
traditional disease approaches, we have not shown the <u>impossibility</u> of a
value-free medicine; we have just shown the weaknesses of those approaches. It is our job to come up with a new disease conceptualization
that will eliminate the offensive value elements.    ↓

Further, the skeptic would argue, why shouldn't there be such a value-free    **1075**
conception of disease? Aren't the sciences of physics and chemistry, and
biology by extension from them, value-free? Isn't "E equals mc²" a simple,
empirical description of the world and not a hidden value judgment? And if
a scientist uses that formula to build a bomb, can't we separate our value
judgments about how the knowledge is <u>applied</u> from the value-free character of the <u>knowledge itself</u>? Just as physicists may be dragged into the political arena because of their power to manipulate matter, doctors may end
up playing a political role when disease states, such as alcoholism, become
profound social problems. But (the skeptic concludes) the value content of
medical <u>practice</u> shouldn't confuse us by making us think that values ought
to be involved in medical <u>science</u>. The debate over homosexuality, for instance, merely shows us that we need better objective criteria before we
can decide whether it is a disease.    ↓

There is a lot at stake in getting an answer to this dispute. If the skeptic is    **1076**
right, we had better drop all this carrying-on about values, get back to the
laboratory, and find some "objective criteria" to tell us whether homosexuality (or whatever else troubles us) is a disease or not. On the other hand, if
our account so far in this chapter is correct, then those so-called objective
criteria <u>simply don't exist</u>. Certainly we want to go on doing research and
finding out more about homosexuality, but we don't want to fall into the
trap of thinking that this research, by itself, will finally decide the disease
question.    ↓

Where, then, can we look for a flaw in the skeptic's argument? First, we    **1077**
might note that the skeptic is relying heavily on the assumption that physics
and chemistry are value-free sciences. If we could show that value judgments occur fundamentally in physics and chemistry, in ways similar to
what we have seen in the various approaches to disease, then the skeptic's
argument loses most of its punch. For, if the natural sciences themselves are
value-laden, then medicine, as an applied science, ought to be even more
value-laden.    ↓

**1078**   The argument about values in science would take us very far beyond the field of medical ethics (Engelhardt [1976] provides a quick summary of some recent work in this field). All we can mention here is that philosophers studying science have largely given up the idea that scientific inquiry is value-free. Some of the arguments relate to the problems of selectivity we mentioned in the context of the ontologic and the physiologic approaches to disease — out of all the potential observables, scientists choose to look at some and not others; and their choices are based in part on preconceptions about what will be useful and worth knowing. Other arguments relate to the very basic assumptions of science, such as the uniformity of nature — assumptions that must be <u>accepted</u> as true in order to
↓ do science at all, but that no scientific discovery can ever <u>prove</u> to be true.

**1079**   But we can illustrate in a small way the fundamental role of values in a scientific view of human beings, which will dictate by implication a role of values in defining health and disease. We can do so by moving beyond traditional concepts of health and disease to a "unified systems theory" of health and disease, similar to the view described by Engel (1977) as the "biopsychosocial model" of medicine. This model has the virtue of integrating the biologic sciences with human behavior and the social sciences, allowing us to look at mental health and social concepts, such as the sick role, along with physical disease. It also makes use of new advances in science, such as information theory and systems theory. It is also a model that some have looked to to provide a really value-free concept of disease — so that if we find a basic role for values here, we will have hammered another
↓ nail into the coffin of the value-free hypothesis.

**1080**   To start, we have to be clear on some terms, including system, information, and hierarchy. The essence of this concept is the nature of man as a biologic system. A "system" is an organized set of subcomponents; it is made up of a number of subsystems, and each subsystem could be considered a system with its own subsystems, and so on down the line. These systems, as we rank them in order of complexity, form a "hierarchy." In biology, we are familiar with the idea of a hierarchical system with the individual at the highest level. At the next lowest level are the organ systems, and each of them in turn has the organs as their subsystems. Each organ has a variety of tissues as its subcomponents. We can carry this down through cells to mol-
↓ ecules or atoms.

We can imagine a collection of organs, tissues, cells, and so on, all lying in a heap on the floor of an anatomy laboratory. What distinguishes a biologic system from this heap of the different subcomponents? We already mentioned the orderly nature of a system, but of what does this order consist? The order is maintained by information flow within the system, and between the system and its environment ("information" here is being defined in a very broad sense, as something that has the potential to change the activities of a component of the system). Very commonly the information flow pattern takes the form of "feedback loops," in which component A influences component B, and the new state of B in turn acts upon A, so that it is possible to maintain a balance. In this way a system can maintain its orderly structure — if one subsystem starts to get out of line, the other subsystems act on it to set things right. If your cardiovascular system starts to pump blood too fast, it activates neural and hormonal feedback mechanisms, which work to restore the normal state. Thus, each subsystem has the freedom to do what it chooses within certain limits, but once it crosses those limits, feedback loops are activated to return it to its proper place. **1081** ↓

What we have just described is no more than the physiologic concept of homeostasis. However, we want to go beyond the levels of the hierarchy that are usually considered in purely physiologic terms. Why stop with the individual organism? First we might want to include some allowances for behavior. We can say that simple motor behavior is at a lower hierarchical level than behavior that requires the use of language; and that sophisticated problem-solving behavior is at a still higher level, and so on. So we might want to subdivide the individual or "person" into these different levels of behavior and experience. Further, we note that persons are not content to remain isolated, but form themselves as the subcomponents of still higher-level systems such as families, communities, nations, and so on. If we are going to have a really comprehensive view of human beings, it would seem that our systems view would have to include all these hierarchical levels. **1082** ↓

Clearly, the exact nature of the information flow is going to be different at different levels of the hierarchy. Atoms in a molecule keep each other in line by means of electrostatic attractions and repulsions; family members keep each other in line mainly by language behavior; and cultures keep their individual members in line mainly by transmitting values. However, if we are willing to regard all of these examples as information flow (and information theory provides a basis to do this), then the basic characteristics, such as the nature of the feedback loop, should be applicable to each level of the hierarchy. **1083** ↓

**1084** Figure 4 summarizes what we have just described; it shows the levels of the hierarchy and describes some of the types of information flow that occur between two adjacent hierarchical levels. There are also information-flow circuits between levels more widely spaced, as when the nation feeds back directly to the person, say, to order him to produce his income tax. Also do not forget that each level of the hierarchy has information circuits to connect it with the environment. Since it takes energy to move all this information around, it is characteristic of biologic systems that they must take in ↓ energy from the environment to maintain themselves.

**1085** Now, take a look at the picture just drawn of this biologic system we call "man." It is maintaining itself as an orderly array of subcomponents. It is taking energy in from the environment, and it is interacting with the environment in other ways to maintain the fitness we mentioned earlier. Each of its subcomponents at all the different levels is "doing its own thing" within the limits allowed, while the various feedback circuits are standing ready to be activated once those limits are crossed and the subcomponent embarks on a course that could threaten the stability of the whole system. It would be reasonable to identify this state of overall equilibrium as what we ↓ mean by a healthy system.

**1086** However, this idyllic state of affairs does not always prevail. Every once in a while a subcomponent oversteps its bounds (often as a response to some disruption originating in the environment, which the usual feedback loops were unable to prevent). Or in some cases, the limits imposed by the feedback circuits might become too rigid, so as not to allow the subcomponent any breathing room and thus hampering its function. In either way, the particular level of the hierarchy has its equilibrium disrupted, and we could say ↓ that a disease has occurred.

**1087** But as a rule, the disease does not stop at one level, since all the levels are interconnected by the information circuits. Therefore, a disruption at one level is bound to be transmitted to levels above and below, although the degree of disruption may decrease in the process (unless the disruption is major). In theory, we can say that a disruption at one level ought to lead to a disruption at all levels, even though as a practical matter the effects at distant levels are negligible. For instance, if we want to call diabetes a disruption at the biochemical level, we can observe that it leads to pathologic changes at the cellular level at various places in the body, and that when these accumulate the end result can be disruption of the functions of various organs, such as the kidney or the eye. But it is safe to assume that the structure of the atoms in that individual's body are untouched for all practical purposes. Likewise, the disease changes the individual's behavior and may disrupt his family and possibly even his local community, but the country in which he lives probably goes about its business pretty much ↓ oblivious to the plight of this one individual.

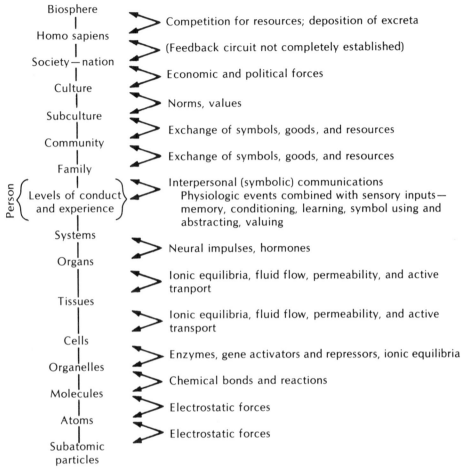

**Figure 4.** *Systems approach to the nature of human beings, showing levels of the hierarchy on the left and the nature of the information flow between different levels on the right.*

What happens to the system after a disease occurs and its disruptions have **1088** been transmitted up and down the hierarchy? There are two possibilities. First, if enough of the components of the system, in the key places, are still reasonably intact, they can call into play new circuits of information flow (often circuits held in reserve for just this purpose) to remedy the disruption of the other components, or at least to sequester them so that they cannot disrupt the system further. If some subcomponents "die," they can be replaced by growth processes; and eventually the system restores itself to its equilibrium state. However, to accomplish this, it has required a greater supply of energy than it would have needed simply to maintain itself in a healthy state. Also, while this process of correction was going on, the system was less able to respond to any other insults that the environment might have thrown at it, and so was at risk for catching a more serious disease. ↓

**1089**  The other possibility is that the disruption was too large, or that it spread up and down the hierarchy too rapidly, for the system's defenses to be mobilized. In that case we could have the final stage of disruption, which is death; but as we just noted, death itself can occur at one or more hierarchical levels. Cells in our bodies are dying all the time without noticeable effect; occasionally we can even have an organ die and survive as an individual. Going farther up the hierarchy, occasionally a nation will collapse after the death of a political leader, but most often the effects of an individual's death do not go much beyond the family. And, in the other direction, we know that an individual might be dead while many of his cells
↓  and tissues go on living for some time afterward.

**1090**  Because most of the information circuits in the system are in the form of feedback loops — bidirectional instead of unidirectional — we can conclude that the disruptions associated with disease can move down the hierarchical levels as well as up. The differences between different disease entities (as described by the ontologic view) may be related to such factors as where the initial disruption arises, which hierarchical levels are most affected, and so on. It should also be noted that often what we take to be signs of disease may be the efforts of the system to restore order — fever is a
↓  common example.

**1091**  For further illustration, Figures 5 and 6 explain two disease processes in systems terms. In Figure 5, a case of genetic disease resulting in physical and mental retardation is shown; the initial disruption is presumed to be radiation from the environment that produces a mutation in the reproductive cells of one parent, and the resulting spread of disruption is up the hierarchical levels. In Figure 6, a case is shown of so-called psychosomatic disease resulting from emotional stress on an individual — here, an airplane engineer thrown out of work by budget cuts. The initial disruption is at the
↓  national level, and the spread of disruption is downward.

**1092**  Since the idea of therapy is closely tied up with the idea of disease, how does therapy fit into this model? We would have to say that therapy is a disruption from the environment that is intended to counteract the disease-disruption and aid the system in returning to a state of equilibrium. If diseases and therapies are both disruptions from the environment, what is the difference between them? None — other than the value judgment
↓  placed on the final results, or the predicted final results, of the disruption.

**1093**  Now, the disadvantages of this systems concept of health and disease are obvious. Not only are the practical applications hard to imagine; but in addition we seem to have been deliberately obscure by redefining a number of familiar concepts in unfamiliar terms. On the other side of the ledger,
↓  what are some of the advantages of this system?

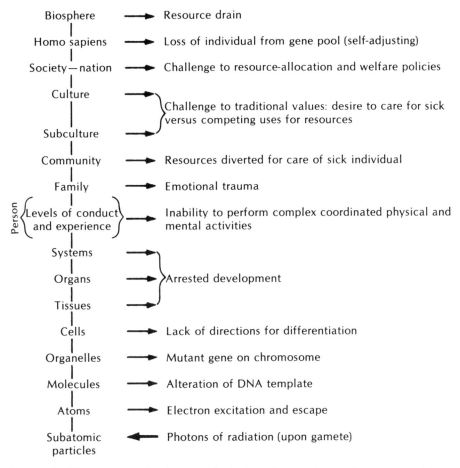

**Figure 5.** *Disease example. Severe physical and mental retardation caused by radiation-induced mutation in the gamete: example of spread of disruption upwards through the hierarchy.*

*Key:* ← = *Initial perturbation;* → = *Resulting disruption*

First, it does represent an increase in unification. It takes into account the physiologic view of disease, since the physiologic processes of homeostasis and deviation from normal limits are already being explained in terms of feedback loops. By showing the possibilities of differences between diseases in terms of what kind of disruption may cause them, on what levels their primary manifestations are located, and so on, the systems view indicates that there is utility in adopting at least some of the classifications of the ontologic view, even if we want to deny the theoretical validity of the "separate entity" concept. Furthermore, since the various levels are all interconnected, we expect that diseases involving organ and tissue disruptions also have associated disruptions on the behavioral levels; so the behavioral concept of disease is explained as a view that focuses on one particular aspect of the total picture. 1094

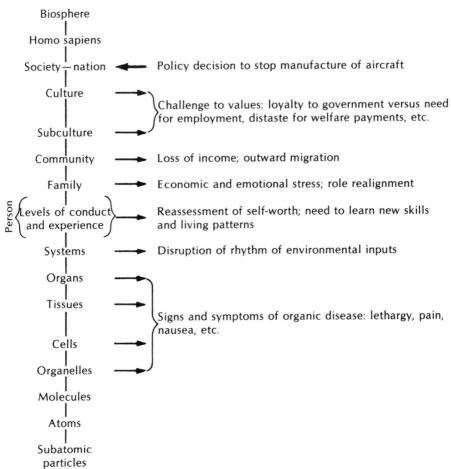

**Figure 6.** *Disease example. Stress-related psychosomatic illness in an unemployed aerospace engineer: example of spread of disruption downward through the hierarchy.*

*Key:* ← = *Initial perturbation;* → = *Resulting disruption*

**1095**    This leads us into the second advantage, that of eliminating the sharp distinction between organic and mental diseases, which has been plaguing medical thought recently, and which has been adhered to despite accumulating evidence that it is dysfunctional. If disruptions can move equally well up and down the hierarchical levels, as was illustrated in Figures 5 and 6, there is no reason why psychosocial disruptions cannot cause tissue or biochemical manifestations, and vice versa. Under the old concepts, medicine has tended to act surprised when it was discovered that such interconnections existed — for example, when it was discovered that persons with certain personality traits were more likely to develop certain types of organic disease, such as ulcer, or that a procedure such as kidney dialysis could lead to severe psychiatric problems. Applying the systems model, we should be surprised if these interconnections <u>did not</u> exist.

In abolishing this sharp distinction between types of disease, we also abol- **1096**
ish the sharp distinction between the biologic and the behavioral and social
sciences. We drew an analogy between things like social values and hormones — they are both part of the system's information circuitry, but they
occur at different levels. We know that it is easier to measure and quantify
hormones than values, but it seems erroneous to extend that and say that a
science that tries to observe information flow at one level of the hierarchy
is less scientific in any way than a science that addresses itself to another
level.                                                                        ↓

A third advantage is particularly useful in ethical discussions, which, as we **1097**
saw, often come to grief by looking only at the anticipated results and not
at possible undesirable side effects. If we start with the idea that all levels
are interconnected, we are not only reminded that side effects are bound to
occur; we also have a handy check list as to where to look for them. All we
have to do is follow each of the feedback loops — we have to look at other
levels, at other subsystems in the same level, and at the environment. Of
course, there are actually an (almost) infinite number of these feedback circuits, which explains why we can never exhaustively explore all the possible consequences before making a decision.                                    ↓

Here a caveat is appropriate: remember how the ontologic view comes to **1098**
grief when the disease entities are viewed as real things and not as concepts. Similarly, the levels of the hierarchy should be seen as ways of guiding us in our search for interrelations among real-world phenomena, not as
real-world phenomena in themselves, although they agree well with some
of our intuitive views. Thus Engelhardt agrees in saying that disease-
concepts must be seen as complex relations among many different factors,
but he avoids any specific hierarchical or other model of these factors.      ↓

This search for side effects is especially important when applied to therapy. **1099**
Again, the medical field tends to act surprised, even when it should know
better, when a drug turns out to have a side effect.                          ↓

As a matter of fact, from the systems perspective, it is little short of a mira- **1100**
cle that there are any therapies at all whose benefits outweigh all the possible side effects. This alone serves to remind us that modest attempts to aid
the natural restorative reactions of the system are often to be preferred to
heroic intervention. This also reminds us that longer-range changes in the
system, which make it more adaptable and better able to cope with
stresses, are to be preferred to one-shot interventions after the disease has
occurred. Thus, while antibiotics have to be regarded as one of the greatest
medical advances of this century, their effect on the infant mortality statistics in the United States was only a fraction of the effects of chlorinating
city water supplies and pasteurizing milk.                                    ↓

**1101**    A fourth advantage comes from the fact that disruption at one level leads to disruptions at many other levels, and the level of primary manifestation (if there is one) is not necessarily the level of the initial insult. Likewise, while ideally we might want to direct therapy at the "primary cause" of a disease, this primary cause may not exist if the disease was caused by a constellation of factors. (For example, psychiatric depression is probably a complex response to psychological stress, genetic predisposition, and biochemical state of the brain, among other factors.) Even where there is an identifiable primary cause, it may be better from a practical standpoint to direct the therapy-disruption at a different level.

**1102**    If these are kept in mind, we can avoid the simplistic notions that hamper much of medical understanding, such as those of confusing the level of intervention with the level of disease. From the fact that the complex constellation of interactions which we call depression can be treated with certain drugs, we cannot deduce that therefore depression is simply a disease of the biochemical level and nothing more. Similarly, if an illness gets better because of the "placebo effect" (which is intervention on the language-behavior level), we cannot conclude that the person was not "really" sick and that it was "all in his mind." (The symptoms of incurable cancer have been shown to respond to placebos.)

**1103**    Hopefully we have now shown why this systems approach to health and disease has many useful features and why it is being used more frequently by physicians seeking a more comprehensive understanding of their task. But we must still return to our old friend the skeptic and ask whether this systems model aids us in arguing against a value-free conception of disease.

**1104**    We might start by pointing out that values are involved in the systems hierarchy as one sort of information flow. But the skeptic doesn't mind this — indeed, this is one reason why some have seen in systems theory a vindication of the hypothesis of a value-free science. For if the systems model merely <u>describes</u> values as they function in the real world and refrains from making value judgments <u>about</u> the values, then the model itself can be value-free. That is, it is possible to imagine a value-free science of values.

**1105**    Instead, we have to realize that the systems model itself represents a value-laden approach to reality. As we mentioned briefly, systems organization and hierarchical levels are not merely descriptions of reality, but are rather complex interpretations of reality. Our empirical observations of the world force us to conclude that some entities are simple and some are complex, and that simple entities occasionally join together to make up more complex ones. But our observations do not force us to recognize these particular hierarchical levels and not others, or to draw the boundaries between the system and the "outside" environment where we do. And nothing in our observations forces us to look at some phenomena at one level and not

at others — for instance, to prefer to look at DNA molecules when we are    **1105**
looking into the basis of genetics, and to look at family communication    cont.
patterns when we are worried why Johnnie is afraid to go to school.    ↓

Churchman (1968) has emphasized that there is always a certain arbitrary    **1106**
element to a systems approach. We give up the idea of having one true way
to look at a natural phenomenon, and instead gain several alternative ways
to look at it (in our case, corresponding to the different levels of the hierarchy in our model). Like the proverbial blind men and the elephant, we
can never get the true picture by looking at only one level (as in saying, "a
human being is nothing but a collection of cells," or "a human being is
nothing but a single cog in the great machine of society"). As we put together what we learn by looking from our different points of view, we start
to approach a "true" overall picture. But we never quite arrive there — first,
because there are very likely some important points of view that we left out
of our model, and second, because we can never look at the phenomenon
from all points of view simultaneously.    ↓

What, then, are we to do, if the true overall picture will always be just be-    **1107**
yond our reach? Again, we will have to be selective. We will have to choose
to look from one viewpoint or from a few viewpoints. And how we choose
will depend on our values and goals: what we want to accomplish and what
we consider to be important. Particularly, in medicine, we will choose the
points on the hierarchy to make our observations and our interventions in a
very pragmatic way. Knowledge of the complexity of the human system is
all well and good, but what we really want to do is make sick people better,
and we will select our observations and our interventions with this goal
firmly in mind. We will obey the law expressed by Willie Sutton of questionable memory who, when asked why he robbed banks, replied, "That's
where the money is."    ↓

We will assume at this point that our friend the skeptic has finally fallen    **1108**
silent, and is prepared to grant that the concepts of health and disease are
fundamentally bound up with value judgments. Before leaving this chapter,
we will look briefly at three related matters: practical and ethical implications of our conclusion; possible problems with the concept of disease in
the future; and finally, some specific conclusions we can make about the
doctor–patient relationship.    ↓

**1109** First, we can look at practical implications of the concepts of health and disease. As we have hinted in the discussion of alcoholism and homosexuality, we tend to treat people whom we consider diseased in a way very different from the way we treat other sorts of social deviants. In these sorts of problematic cases, calling the individual diseased is likely to arouse a degree of sympathy and support that is not offered to other deviants. But there is also a risk of dehumanization in all this, as to say that the individual is diseased is also to say that he is not responsible for his own actions.
↓ Clearly such judgments have important ethical consequences.

**1110** Recall Case 66 and the airman suffering from the "disease" of fear of flying. The dehumanizing element is very prominent in that case, where the behavior called sick was really what we would consider a rational assessment of risks and a realistic emotional reaction to a horrendous situation. By contrast, the "cured" behavior consisted of a denial of this rationale and a willingness to go out cheerfully and be killed. Throughout the entire process, the airman was regarded as a child incapable of knowing his own best interests. But the military psychiatrists might reply, reasonably enough, that they were doing the airman a favor by treating him that way — since the most likely alternative way of responding to his behavior, within the mili-
↓ tary reality, was a charge of willful disobedience and court-martial.

**1111** Controversial instances of "disease" like homosexuality and fear of flying represent the most extreme cases. However, even in the more commonplace examples, the physician's basic concept of disease may have subtle but important effects on his practice of the profession. For instance, Fabrega (1972) contends that the prevalence of the ontologic approach in medical thinking reinforces episodic care of acute illnesses and steers medical attention away from preventive medicine and more comprehensive types of care. Recall that the ontologic view has a tendency to see the individual as completely normal when the disease "entity" is not present. By this view, there is little support for looking for factors in the individual that would predispose toward later disease, or for preventing disease by inter-
↓ vening in some way before disease is actually present.

**1112** The unified systems model, we argued, avoids many of the flaws and oversimplifications present in traditional disease models and also has some practical implications of its own. For one thing, if health is viewed as a property of the entire hierarchy of systems, it becomes clear that many of the disruptions that lead to ill health — on the family, community, and national levels, for example — fall outside of the realm of health professionals as we now train them. This means that preserving health demands more than physicians and other health professionals can do by themselves. As we have seen in discussing the allocation of resources, we can sometimes do more to promote health by allocating available funds to nonmedical programs. Blum (1976) has outlined a national approach to health policy that is
↓ based on the unified systems model we have used here.

Second, we need to be aware of how a current change in our ideas about    **1113**
disease may have important future consequences. Recall Case 62 and the
dilemma of Mr. Puffer, the smoker with lung cancer who was being made
to pay for his own hospital care because he was "responsible" for his own
disease. In our outline of the concept of disease, we laid stress on the lack
of responsibility (at least of direct responsibility) on the part of the sick
individual. It seems that this lack of responsibility is a crucial element in
eliciting the helping and caring responses from the friends and family of the
sick person and in securing the services of the healer.    ↓

Currently medical research is hard at work discovering new ways in which    **1114**
our deliberate choices, our life styles if you will, contribute to disease. In
addition to alcohol and cigarettes, overeating, lack of exercise, and improper sleep and rest patterns are all being indicted as promoters of disease. Also, we are increasingly aware of industrial hazards, such as chemical
carcinogens. In some sense, people who "choose" to continue working in
high-risk industries may be said to be contributing to their own diseases.    ↓

This trend has had very valuable results. Health professionals and lay peo-    **1115**
ple alike are using this new knowledge to modify life styles in more healthy
directions, and medical research has gained important clues into disease
causation. Changes in human behavior are no longer the special province
of the mental health professional, but are now seen as an important part of
general medicine.    ↓

At the same time, we might wonder about a more subtle change in our    **1116**
basic concept of disease. The idea that an individual can be responsible for
his or her own disease is a radical break with the concept of disease as it
seems to exist presently. Will we come to have a two-class system of health
services — care for those who appear truly not to be responsible for their ill
health, and disgusted, demeaning tolerance for the overeaters, underexer-
cisers, and smokers? If the case of Mr. Puffer strikes a responsive chord, this
possibility may not be too far-fetched.    ↓

The issue of the relationship between disease and personal responsibility,    **1117**
then, will be an important issue, and new medical discoveries in the future
will have to be assessed with this issue in mind. Right now we can imagine
three ways of trying to take personal responsibility for life-style illnesses
into account without altering our basic concept of disease.    ↓

**1118**  One response is to turn around and deny personal responsibility all over again. We see alcohol and heroin addictions as states in which the individual has diminished responsibility; similarly we could view smoking and overeating as addictions for which the individual loses control and is unable to help himself. Thus, we preserve the concept that the sick individual is not responsible for his own illness.

The addiction model is a useful one in planning practical strategies, such as campaigns to get smokers to quit, but as a philosophical position it seems to do too much. It dehumanizes the smoker or overeater to a degree that doesn't seem warranted by the evidence. After all, we all know of people who have <u>chosen</u> to quit smoking or stop overeating. And almost everyone occasionally pursues bad habits that they know they shouldn't, without feeling powerless or not in control of their lives. It seems a gross
↓ oversimplification to deny personal responsibility in such cases.

**1119**  The observation that all of us have some bad habits leads to a second response, which is to say that people are indeed responsible for the diseases that are brought on by their unhealthy behavior, but that all of us engage in some sort of unhealthy behavior, so no one has clean enough hands to blame anyone else. Since this engaging in unhealthy habits is the common lot of humanity, we may as well be humane about it and not deny care to anyone on that basis. We should treat others as we would like to be treated ourselves.

This solution sounds nice but is based on some questionable assumptions. There may be those who do not engage in any unhealthy habits at all. And of the remainder, there is clearly a large difference among individuals
↓ in the amount of unhealthy behavior engaged in.

**1120**  The third response is the most complex but probably the most satisfactory. It is to engage in a much more detailed analysis of "responsibility" in these sorts of cases to discover different degrees, different sorts, or different levels of responsibility.

For example, what do we mean when we say a cigarette smoker is responsible for the lung cancer he developed? We do not mean that he intended to get cancer, in the same way a person putting a loaded gun to his head and pulling the trigger intends to die. He knew perhaps that smoking increased his risk of cancer; but he may have reasoned that he would be one of the lucky ones who smoke and don't get cancer; or he may have judged the pleasures of smoking to be worth the risk. (Driving an automobile is very risky too, but we do not hold that one intends to have an accident or is responsible for one if it happens, just by the act of driving.) We might conclude that the smoker is clearly responsible for his smoking but not responsible in any meaningful way for the cancer. By this analysis, our current concept of disease would be preserved, while we would still be able to hold individuals personally responsible for their voluntarily as-
↓ sumed habits.

Finally, what have we learned in this analysis of the concepts of health and    **1121**
disease that will help us understand the doctor–patient relationship? When
we placed that relationship at the basis of our approach to medical ethics
and outlined the contractual model as the most appealing model for the
relationship, we had no fundamental view of the ethical responsibility of
the health professional. What is the fundamental ethical duty of the health
professional?

A traditional answer, at least insofar as doctors are concerned, is that the    **1122**
physician is supposed to cure disease. This view of the medical duty has
been criticized as leading to overly technological, episodic, and often inhumane health care. Certainly these criticisms are valid if one's concept of
disease does not go beyond the ontologic view: if the physician is concerned more with the disease entity than with the sick person. Our unified
systems model helps to mitigate this criticism. If the doctor is to understand
and treat the disease, he must be aware of all levels of the disruption —
familial and emotional as well as biologic.

But, as we saw in Chapter 6, many of the most difficult ethical dilemmas
arise when cure is not possible, or where continued treatment would promote greater suffering. In these difficult situations, a duty to cure disease
hardly seems to come close in defining the doctor's basic ethical responsibility.

Another answer that seems good to modern ears is that the duty of the    **1123**
health professional is promotion of health. But, in this chapter, we have run
into some problems with this notion. First we saw that the concept of
health, as compared to the concept of disease, was more difficult to pin
down — and the more vague a concept, the harder it is to apply it as a basic
ethical duty. Once again, turning to the euthanasia and quality-of-life cases
in Chapter 6, it is not clear how a duty to promote health would help the
doctor understand his ethical obligations any better. Also, we saw that the
duty to promote health, by our systems model, must be shared with many
other professionals and social institutions.

But the more basic objection to both **these** answers is that they risk forget-    **1124**
ting about the patient — after all, that was why we looked at the relationship between doctor and patient in the first place. If our thinking back in
Chapter 4 was valid, then whatever the basic ethical duty of the health professional is, it must be owed to the patient and not defined solely in relation to some abstraction like "disease" or "health."

**1125** Fried, in developing the concept of the right to personal care that we have mentioned several times, uses an interesting phrase — that the physician ought to be the "servant . . . of the life plans of his patients." We might expand this idea a little: *The fundamental ethical duty of the health professional is to be a servant to the life plan of the patient, within the capabilities of medical technology, and within the framework of broader social obligations.*

↓

**1126** This formulation becomes clearer when considered one element at a time. A "servant" is supposed to be subservient to the values of the master that he serves (but notice that the master here is the life plan, not the patient). But the servant is not a slave; he has his own values and responsibilities, his own standards for what counts as work well done. The servant expects to be paid for his services and can terminate the relationship if asked to render some service that conflicts with his own ethical values. He also has the freedom to choose who to serve.

↓

**1127** The service here is owed to the "life plan" of the patient. It is not owed to the desire or request of the patient (as would be the case in the engineering model). That is, a person's values, desires, and interests are seen as being most reflective of that individual's personhood and autonomy when they form a part of a reasonable and coherent set of goals and purposes, which guide the individual both in the present and into the future. This cluster of values and purposes, which are more basic than temporary desires or attractions and which account in large part for the uniqueness of the individual, is what Fried calls the life plan.

↓

**1128** Serving a person's life plan is a tricky business. In general, a person knows his own life plan best, and so doing what the person requests is the best way to fulfill the duty. But occasionally, when irrational or emotionally overwrought, the individual may express desires that are contrary to his basic life plan; or he may be unconscious and unable to express any desires at all. The servant in such cases may have to make his own informed judgment about what would best further the life plan. He may, then, be justified in acting paternalistically.

↓

**1129** But the life plan he serves must be the life plan of the patient, that life plan autonomously chosen, and not some idealized or culturally approved life plan selected by the health professional or by society. The life plan may in fact be one that the health professional disapproves of and would not choose for himself (so long as he does not find the life plan positively immoral). This feature eliminates the priestly model as a possible description of the fundamental ethical duty.

↓

The next restriction on the service is "within the capacities of medical tech-    **1130**
nology." It may be part of the patient's life plan to gain promotions in his
office or learn to play several musical instruments, but the health
professional's service stops short of these so long as medical technology
includes no special skills to serve these ends. This restriction is a pragmatic
one, as there is no firm, theoretical formula to determine whether some
skill ought to be included under the title of "medical." And clearly this
body of skills will change over time, leading to differing expectations on the
part of the patient.                                                             ↓

EXPECTATIONS REALISTIC? * 1133

Finally, we add the restriction, "within the framework of broader social ob-    **1131**
ligations," to remind us of our discussions in Chapter 16. Health professional and patient approach each other as individual persons, but they are
also members of society, and do not shed their social responsibilities at the
door of the doctor–patient relationship. We have discussed at length how
social responsibilities may conflict with the particular modes of serving the
patient's life plan and how some of those conflicts may be negotiated.        ↓

In saying that the basic duty of the health professional is to be a servant to    **1132**
the life plan of the patient, within the capabilities of medical technology
and within the framework of broader social obligations, we are really restat-
ing in more detail the contractual model of the doctor–patient relationship
from Chapter 4. *And the notion of "contract" reminds us that we are
describing a mutual endeavor. The basic duty of the health professional is
not to do battle with disease or champion health, but to enter into this
mutually negotiated, ongoing, personal relationship with the patient.*         ↓**1134**

---

* We live at a time when unrealistic expectations are often being projected    **1133**
onto the medical profession. Won't this description of basic ethical duty
foster more of this — by suggesting that whatever one's life plan, medicine
will be available to help fulfill it? We would have to modify our general
statement by noting that many diseases and injuries simply make the original life plan impossible, as when a rising young athlete has to undergo amputation of a limb. The medical duty then switches to helping the patient
adjust emotionally to his loss and to begin to formulate a revised life plan
to meet the realities of his true prognosis.                                   ↑**1131**

**1134**   In looking at the concepts of health and disease, we have now come full circle, returning to the doctor–patient relationship and other matters from the earliest chapters of this book. *It should not surprise us that values (as they are embodied in the patient's life plan) ought to get so much attention in defining the health professional's basic duty, for we have now seen that whether some state of affairs can properly be called a disease depends in part on whether it will form an obstacle to the life plans of the average person (and hence will be regarded as a dysvalue). The fundamental role of values in the concepts of health and disease reinforce our earlier statement about medicine as a fundamentally ethical enterprise.*

But we have not yet explored the question of the basis of the values that we have been alluding to throughout this book. Our final chapter will take up this issue.

**1135** ↓ CH. 18

# The Foundations 18
## of Values

We have now looked at the full spectrum of ethical issues in medicine and **1135** at some of the fundamental concepts of medicine and the doctor–patient relationship. But we still have some unfinished business before we can close. Back in Chapter 2, we described a consequentialist ethical decision-making method that requires one to apply one's own system of values in order to test the consequences of possible ethical actions. We also added a further stipulation that the values of individual dignity and autonomy were to be considered fundamental in an ethical value system; this stipulation would prevent anyone holding a Nazi-type value system from imposing his values on others, on the grounds that "one person's ethical opinion is just as good as another's." And, in the following chapters, we saw how the decision-making method and the value placed on autonomy and dignity could help us to work through various ethical dilemmas in health care. ↓

But all this still leaves us with some work to do. We have not really said **1136** much about what values are and what role they play in determining behavior. We have not shown how to justify adherence to one particular value when, as often happens, values come into conflict. And finally, if individual dignity and autonomy is to play such a basic role in our value framework, we need to do a better job of understanding just what the individual person is and consists of and of justifying why the individual should occupy this important role (e.g., why not make the good of society our basic value?). ↓

We need to understand clearly that we are now getting into questions that **1137** are very basic to the whole field of ethics. Philosophers since Plato have argued about these issues, and as yet no unanimity has emerged on these basic questions. It would be preposterous to think that we could resolve these issues in any final fashion in one chapter of a book of this size. But if we do not at least make the attempt at reaching a preliminary understanding, we would have to admit that all of our ethical conclusions so far have no firm foundations to support them, and most people find this an unsatisfactory and therefore unacceptable position. ↓

We might start by trying to flesh out a bit our concept of "values." A useful **1138** metaphor or model to describe the role of values is the idea of cultural evolution. Going back to the systems hierarchy we described in Chapter 17, we could envision classical Darwinian, biologic evolution as applying to the levels of the hierarchy below the individual level. The same general concepts (such as random variation and natural selection), when applied to higher levels of the hierarchy, give rise to cultural evolution. ↓

REVIEW SYSTEMS HIERARCHY ↑ 1079–1103

**1139**   Where do our values come from? Basically, we get our values from our indoctrination into the culture into which we are born, usually at an early age and continuing through our schooling and social interactions. Cultures, in turn, get their values as a part of the process of cultural evolution, analogous to Darwinian biologic evolution. Values arise in response to the society's needs, often related to changes in the environment, which the society must cope with. Then, by a process of selection, those values that have survival value for the culture are maintained and strengthened by being associated with social institutions, while useless values are dropped ↓ along the way.

**1140**   There are a couple of reasons why we might want to improve upon this process. By analogy with Darwinian evolution, it would appear that a culture with nonadaptive values will die out and be replaced by new, better fitted cultures. But if we are a member of the condemned culture, we cannot be expected simply to sit back and let this happen; we will want to make modifications in our values to head off this fate. In effect, the only alternative to letting evolution take its course is for us to take our evolution ↓ into our own hands.

**1141**   The other reason for avoiding a laissez-faire approach to values comes about because of the present rapid rate of change in our society due to the exponential increase in technology. Today we can change the environment as much in one decade as would have taken thousands of years in the prehistoric times when man was evolving as a biologic creature. Man is still evolving biologically, but biology alone cannot keep pace any more. Up until a few centuries ago, the chance that values would become obsolete due to sudden changes was less than the chance that useful values might be lost due to failure to transmit them from one generation to the next. Therefore, it made good sense from the cultural-evolution standpoint to "rigidify" good values in self-perpetuating social institutions, such as the church, which could transmit them to succeeding generations with a minimum ↓ of distortion.

**1142**   The result is that now, when maintaining static values is no longer necessarily in our best interests, we are prevented from making progress by these same institutions that resist change; social institutions, by their design, are made to transmit values and not to reexamine them. This problem is not just one of social policy. All of us have gone through the same cultural indoctrination, and all of us have come to identify emotionally with our social values and institutions, so we are all hard-pressed to reject these values and institutions, even when our reason tells us that failure to do so may have dire consequences. The job of personal reform is as hard or harder ↓ than the job of social reform.

Now, if both social institutions and individuals go to that much trouble to   **1143**
hang onto values, values must be rather important. We are used to thinking
of values as rather abstract sorts of things, soft and mushy. But the systems-
hierarchy model characterized values as one sort of information flow in the
hierarchy of systems. As the science of information theory has been telling
us for the last 30 years, information is anything but abstract and static; indeed, what makes information what it is is precisely its power to change
things. Figure 7 provides a model of how values participate in various sorts
of change. (Figure 7 could be looked at as a sort of "blowup" of one set of
information circuits within the whole hierarchy of systems.)   ↓

Figure 7 shows what we already noted, that values come into being through   **1144**
an interaction between our view of the world and concerns or anxieties,
which are often precipitated by changes in the environment. These values
then go on to become embodied in social institutions and are transmitted
by symbols. These institutions and symbols then go on, as we are indoctri-
nated into the ways of our culture, to determine our behavior at many
levels — from simple biologic-sustenance behavior all the way up to abstract and symbolic thought.   ↓

The sum of the resulting behaviors could be termed our "life style." Our life   **1145**
style, of course, must take place within the physical–biologic world, and
because of the feedback loops between the person and the environment,
our life style will have an environmental impact — as the ecology movement has taken pains to show us in recent years. The impact may change
the environment to the extent that the environment no longer fits in with
our existing world-view. This creates an anxiety and the cycle starts over
again.   ↓

What we just described can be, in cybernetic terms, either a positive or   **1146**
negative feedback system. If it is a negative feedback system, the life style
will change the environment in a way that reverses the original environmental challenge. For example, suppose the original challenge that creates
anxiety is the observation that our environment is littered with tin cans. If
we then change our life style so that we recycle all cans instead of throwing
them away, this is negative feedback and the problem is corrected. But
there is no guarantee that this will be the case; our new life style may make
the matter worse instead of better. This is positive feedback or the proverbial vicious circle, which is an inherently self-destructive situation.   ↓

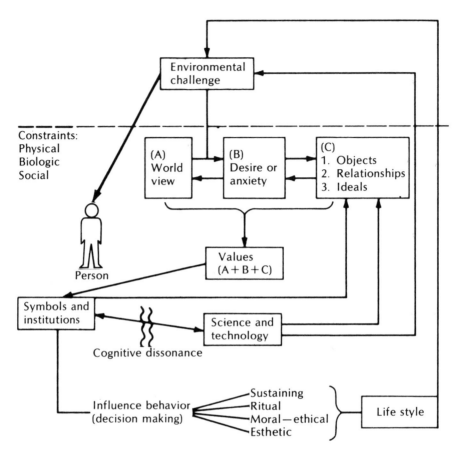

**Figure 7.** *Feedback circuits of information flow connecting science and values within the realm of human activity. Arrows beneath the horizontal broken line represent information circuits within the human hierarchy; arrows crossing broken line represent flow between human beings and external environment.*

To make the circuit a little more complicated, Figure 7 shows science and technology as a separate social institution. It has interrelations with other social institutions, and we have already seen that these interrelations have significant potential for "cognitive dissonance." That is, the messages we get from science about the nature of the world may conflict with the messages we are getting from other social institutions. This can lead (following the arrows backwards) directly to an alteration in our values. **1147**

↓

Through its direct applications, technology also acts directly on the environment to produce change. This sets up the opportunity for some additional instances of positive and negative feedback. Technology A can counteract technology B's effects, such as the use of catalytic converters to control auto emissions. When a technology produces undesirable environmental changes, we can change our life style, possibly in such a way as to require less of the commodity produced by the technology. Or, where some aspect of our life style other than technology is responsible for a change, technology can be called into play to correct the situation. But in all these circuits, note that values are important intermediate steps in the process. **1148**

↓

Figure 7 teaches us a negative lesson also: If our values lead to technological behavior that leads to a changed environment in which our prosperity or survival is threatened, we could also have a failure of the "feedback" circuits. And if we fail to see what is happening and refuse to alter our values, the negative changes in the environment will continue to mount up. By the time we are finally forced to see what is happening, it may be too late to make any corrections that would stave off disaster. **1149**

↓

Currently some areas of scientific research and technology assessment and forecasting are sending us some definite danger signals about the deleterious side effects of modern technology — signals that our social and political institutions are proving reluctant to accept. The most obvious threats looming on the horizon are the outbreak of a major thermonuclear war; increasing pollution of the earth's physical environment; out-of-control population growth with an inability of existing resources to keep up with demand; and the rapid exhaustion of currently usable energy sources before new sources can be developed. It may be going too far to say that any of these would lead to man's biologic extinction as a species; but it is likely that any of these developments would gravely endanger our present idea of the human culture. **1150**

↓

**1151** Still, this sort of argument could get us into trouble. We are saying that values are bad and should be rejected if they lead to technological changes which in turn lead to negative environmental consequences. But how do we know if an environmental consequence is good or bad, if not by referring to our values? And this would put us in the position of saying that the way we know whether our values are good or bad is because of our values. And this would seem to be a circular argument. Clearly, we are going to have to take up the question of how values can be supported and justified ↓ in a noncircular way.

CIRCULAR THINKING? * 1154

**1152** We can look at three general sorts of justification to support ethical values and general ethical principles. The first is the sort we have just been talking about, and which we found to be circular and hence unsatisfactory. We can call this "common-sense justification" because it is the sort of man-on-the-street ethical reasoning that people tend to adopt when they have not bothered to analyze issues carefully. This mode of justification is dia-↓ grammed in Figure 8.

**1153** People who think more deeply about ethical matters generally reject the common-sense justification and adopt a position that we could call "deductive justification." This resembles the deductive arguments in logic. A fundamental value, or rule, is presumed to be given; then more specific rules and decisions about particular cases follow deductively from the fun-**1155** ↓ damental rule or value.

---

**1154** * When we look at specific values, and not values in general, the apparent circularity of Figure 7 is not necessarily detrimental. For example, suppose we are motivated to cut health-care costs and, with this in mind, introduce some new medical technology. But then we do some research that shows that this new technology actually has as a consequence the increase of health-care costs. Certainly we would change our behavior on this score, and we would have learned some useful information.

But suppose someone challenged us to say why cutting costs is a worth-while value to pursue. We might then say that the value of cutting costs might lead to new technologies; and these new technologies (if effective) would have the consequence of cutting costs; and the new environment of reduced costs would be a change for the better. But this is circular reasoning in the bad sense — it says that cutting costs is good because cutting costs is good. And that is the sort of reasoning that we must avoid in ethical **1152** ↑ thinking.

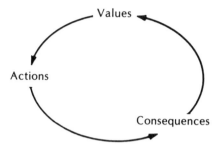

**Figure 8.** *Common-sense model of ethical justification.*

An example of this sort of reasoning would be: Accept truth as a fundamen-  **1155**
tal value. One deduces next a general rule, "Always tell the truth." Then,
faced with the question of whether to tell Mrs. Jones that she has cancer,
one can proceed by deductive logic: One should always tell the truth; telling Mrs. Jones about the cancer is a case of telling the truth; therefore I
should tell Mrs. Jones that she has cancer. This process is diagrammed in
Figure 9.                                                                                        ↓

But so far we have sidestepped the real issue, which is how the fundamen-  **1156**
tal value or rule is itself justified. Here there are different schemes for doing
this, depending on what school of ethical theory one follows (see Appendix I). Frequently one adopts a religious justification, saying that the fundamental values or rules are those revealed by God; but this type of argument
leads to its own problems in turn (see Appendix II). Other ethical philosophers try to ground their fundamental values in a theory of natural law, or
in a purely logical analysis of ethics or of the language in which ethics is
expressed.                                                                                       ↓

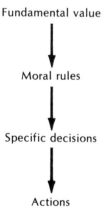

Fundamental value

Moral rules

Specific decisions

Actions

**Figure 9.** *Deductive model of ethical justification.*

**1157**   All of these theories about what supports the fundamental values are open to criticism, which often takes the form of an infinite regress — if you say that A is supported by B, I will turn around and ask what supports B, and so on to infinity. But those who accept deductive justification often reply that, regardless of the difficulties, we have to assume that there <u>is</u> firm support <u>somewhere</u>. After all, they might add, how could we have ethics if one such firm, absolute fixed point did not exist? We are presented with a dichotomy — either we have a firm foundation, however hard it might be to grasp this concept, or all our ethics are totally relative, founded on shifting sands, and we have indeed fallen into the pit of "one person's opinion is just as good as anyone else's." And if the idea of having an absolute, fixed point seems to leave out any chance for growth, change, or flexibility, that is simply the
↓ price we must pay in order to have a secure foundation for our ethics.

**1158**   We may, then, accept the challenge: Can we find some other means of justifying values that avoids the dangers of circularity and infinite regress, while leaving room for flexibility and change in our ethical thinking? One answer can be found in the model of "equilibrium justification." The best recent statement of equilibrium theory appears in the work of social philos-
↓ opher John Rawls (1971).

**1159**   The equilibrium model accepts the idea that to avoid circular thinking, we must somewhere have a fixed point. But it turns deductive justification on its head by looking for this fixed point not in our most general values, but in our judgments about specific actions. Consider these specific judgments: "Slavery is wrong." "It is wrong to murder your grandmother in order to inherit her monogrammed set of china." We hold these to be as nearly true as anything we know. If someone told us that these judgments are not correct, we might well ask what judgments <u>could</u> possibly be correct. (We would ask this even though we might know of some culture or society that did not share those judgments.) And we would be very likely to reject any theory of ethics if the theory purported to support slavery or murder for
↓ gain.

**1160**   Now we can see a way to justify general ethical principles and our overall value system. We can compare any proposed general principle to our set of basic judgments about specific actions. We can modify the principle in various ways until it "fits" with those basic judgments. When that happens, we have a sort of equilibrium state between our basic judgments and general principles (without having logically deduced either one from the
↓ other).

But we need not stop there. In addition to our most basic judgments, we **1161** have a lot of less basic judgments, where we think we know what is right but are not as certain as we were with the most basic judgments. And then we have problematic judgments, where we are not very sure what is right (as happened in many of the cases in this book). We can also try to extend our equilibrium so that it encompasses these other judgments as well. In doing so, we need not restrict ourselves to modifying the general principle; we might also make modifications in the specific judgments, since these are not our most basic judgments and hence more open to revision. And, when we finally get overall equilibrium, we have no guarantee that it will be permanent. Some new case may come up that requires new judgments and that in turn may require modification of other judgments or of our general principles.                                                                 ↓

It's hard to see how the equilibrium process would be carried out unless we **1162** look at an example. Consider a case of a newborn with severe meningomyelocele who will be physically handicapped and mentally retarded and whose parents request that life-prolonging surgery not be performed. Suppose that our judgment is that it is acceptable for the parents to make this decision. (This would clearly be a more problematic judgment and not one of the most basic judgments.)                                                     ↓

We might next look for a general principle, or value, on which to base this **1163** particular judgment. We might first try the principle, "The family is in the best place to decide the fate of an incompetent family member." Or, expressed as a value, we might call this the "value of family privacy." So far we see a good fit between our specific judgment and our general principle.     ↓

But now consider the case of a newborn who will never be retarded or **1164** handicapped at all and who needs a very minor operation to survive, but whose family refuses the surgery on the grounds that they would rather buy a motor boat with the money they would otherwise spend on food and clothing for this new child. Our judgment is that it would be wrong to allow this family to make this choice. And this is now a more basic judgment, similar to our being opposed to murder for gain — we feel we are unlikely to be mistaken about it.                                                              ↓

**1165** But we now see that our general principle does not fit with this more basic considered judgment. We can try to remedy the matter by modifying the principle: "The family is in the best place to decide the fate of an incompetent member, so long as the family is concerned with the best interests of that member." Or, in the form of a value statement, we might say that in our value system the value of protecting the interests of the incompetent takes precedence over the value of family privacy when the two conflict. With this revision of the general principle, we have a good fit among the principle, our basic judgment, and the more problematic judgment; so we have accomplished a sort of mini-equilibrium. A diagram of this procedure
↓ appears in Figure 10.

**1166** We should note that this equilibrium-justification model is different from the decision-making method discussed in Chapter 2. The decision-making method is on the "level of moral rules" according to Aiken's scheme of four levels; we will actually use this in practice. But our equilibrium-justification model falls in between the "level of ethical principles" and the "postethical level." It is important as a general scheme to see what we might be thinking of when we speak about justification. Therefore, its value does not depend on how easy it would be to use it in practice. (In fact, getting a full-scale
↓ equilibrium state would seem to be very difficult.)

**1167** How does the equilibrium justification stack up against deductive justification? To the extent that it allows for change and revision, the equilibrium model is not absolute. But neither is it relativistic in the bad sense — as we saw, it would reject any ethical principle that runs counter to our most basic judgments.

We might view the system of deductive justification as a building that gets its support from one single, very strong pillar, which in turn rests on a foundation of bedrock. By contrast, the equilibrium justification resembles a building that has no single, firm foundation and gets its strength instead from the interconnections between many mutually supporting members. It is like the ingenious models of bridges built out of toothpicks; any one toothpick is easily snapped, but the whole structure, made up of hundreds of toothpicks each supporting the others, is quite strong. If you somehow remove the bedrock foundation of the deductive building (e.g., by disagreeing with the revealed religion from which the values arise), the whole support fails. On the other hand, if you snap a few of the toothpicks in the
↓ equilibrium structure, the strength of the whole is lessened only a little.

**1168** In a small way, the approach we have taken in this book might incline us toward the equilibrium-justification model. By the deductive model, discussion of specific cases can never change the fundamental values and general principles; all case study can do is to serve as an educational tool illustrating the correct application of the principles. But, by the equilibrium model, our judgments about specific cases can modify principles and
↓ values.

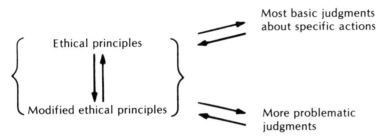

**Figure 10.** *Equilibrium model of ethical justification.*

There is another line of thought that lends support to the equilibrium-   **1169**
justification model and that has to do with some newer concepts of science. Back in Chapter 2, of course, we were very careful to distinguish between empirical and ethical statements, so as not to confuse science with
ethics; and those differences remain valid, since our method of ethical decision making is very different from methods of scientific inquiry. But, in
this chapter, we are more interested in similarities between science and
ethics, and, in particular, in what ethics can learn from science. (With this
in mind we were willing to stretch a point just now and refer to our basic
ethical judgments as being "true," even though we said before that truth or
falsity applies to empirical and not ethical statements.)   ↓
REVIEW ETHICAL VS. EMPIRICAL ↑ 19–26

The view of science that most of us were taught in grade school has a cer-   **1170**
tain straight-line quality similar to our deductive model of ethical justification (Figure 11). By this view, the scientist, surveying the facts, develops a
new scientific hypothesis. He deduces from this hypothesis the outcome of
a particular experiment. He then performs the experiment and the hypothesis is confirmed if the new facts produced by it match the predicted
outcome. On this view, hypotheses may be accepted or rejected, but the
facts are unassailable, and form the bedrock on which scientific knowledge
is based.   ↓

However, as we saw in the last chapter, this simple view of science has   **1171**
come under strong criticism. Without going into philosophy of science, we
may note that this hypothetico-deductive model of science is being replaced with new models, some of which have features similar to our equilibrium model of ethical justification.   ↓
REVIEW CRITICISM ↑ 1077–1078

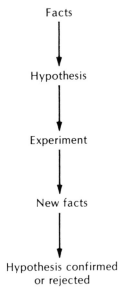

Facts

Hypothesis

Experiment

New facts

Hypothesis confirmed
or rejected

**Figure 11.** *Deductive model of scientific justification.*

**1172** By an equilibrium model (Figure 12), the goal of scientific inquiry is not to deduce theories from unassailable facts, but rather to get the best fit between a system of interconnected theories and basic laws and the established data. In achieving this fit, the theories may be modified and secondary theories introduced; and also some data that are not so well established may be rejected or reinterpreted. (As we saw in Chapter 17, there is a lot of selection going into which data scientists choose to gather; and also much of the data in modern science come by means of sophisticated instruments and so are subject to the theories of how those instruments work. Hence, much scientific data is "contaminated" with theories.) The strength of the scientific knowledge, then, rests on the good fit between theories and facts and not on the primacy of one or the other. If this model is acceptable, then there is a good deal of similarity between the justification of scientific theories and the justification of basic ethical ↓ values.

**1173** The great power of science in generating new and useful knowledge has naturally led thinkers to try to apply scientific methodology to ethics. The crudest efforts have been to deduce ethical principles from scientific facts. But all such attempts run afoul of the basic difference we noted between ethical and empirical statements, so that one sort of statement cannot be logically deduced from the other. All systems of ethics supposedly derived from science, such as the social Darwinism that was used to justify capitalist exploitation early in this century, turn out on examination to have value ↓ judgments smuggled in under the guise of facts.

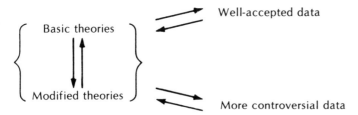

**Figure 12.** *Equilibrium model of scientific justification.*

Our equilibrium models have shown that logical deduction is not the only    **1174**
useful way that different sorts of statements can be connected. If we can
talk about good or bad fit between basic ethical judgments and general
principles, or between scientific laws and theories and bodies of data, we
can at least explore the notion of a fit between science and ethics. We have
already said many times that scientific knowledge is necessary to determine
the consequences of actions, in order to apply a consequentialist mode of
ethical decision making. Now we must see whether there is a more basic
level of fit.    ↓

One approach to linking science and ethics comes from the "bioethics"    **1175**
developed by a biologic scientist, V. R. Potter (1971). Potter has noted many
of the points we have already made in this chapter — the importance of
accurate scientific predictions in a consequentialist ethic; the need to
change values if they are shown to lead to negative changes in our environment; and appreciation of the danger signals about negative consequences
of science and technology.    ↓

But another feature of Potter's bioethics is the emphasis on scientific    **1176**
theories and discoveries about human nature. *If our values are to be "hu-*
*man" values, they ought to be consistent with the best scientific knowl-*
*edge about human beings, their potential, their activities, and their needs.*
*It would be wrong, as we saw, to try to deduce human values from any set*
*of scientific observations. But, at the same time, it would be silly to adopt or*
*to propose some values that fly in the face of human nature as science sees*
*it* (e.g., to base an ethical system on a theory of either total selfishness or
total altruism).    ↓

**1177** Potter also proposes a respect for value pluralism as a basic part of bioethics. We adopted a similar stance based on our respect for persons and individual autonomy. Potter is motivated more by an awareness of the analogies between Darwinian and cultural evolution. Just as a greater variation among members of a species provides the best insurance against future changes in the environment, greater variation among values will help cultures survive in the face of rapid technological change, so long as those values that lead to the most adaptive behaviors are allowed to rise to the ↓ top.

**1178** Potter's bioethics cannot claim to be a comprehensive and well-thought-out ethical theory. But it can stand as a valid criticism of traditional theories of ethics, including those discussed in Appendix I. It helps, in getting a handle on some proposed ethical theory, to ask: What fundamental theory ↓ about human nature does this ethical system seem to take for granted?

**1179** One of the most influential ethical theories in Western philosophy has been that of Immanuel Kant. Looking for what he called the "foundations of the metaphysics of morals," Kant started out by trying to imagine a community of rational beings and asked what sort of moral system might be developed to regulate behavior in such a community. He felt that in order to be a pure theory of morals, the moral system would have to come <u>only</u> from the fact that the members of the community were rational beings and not from any other facts about their desires, interests, or circumstances. For Kant, a rule could be truly a moral rule only if any rational being would view the rule as binding on his own behavior, simply because he was a ra- ↓ tional being.

**1180** Another highly influential ethical theory is the utilitarianism developed by Jeremy Bentham and John Stuart Mill. The utilitarian system is based on the observation that people can feel pleasure or pain, and that they view pleasure as good and pain as bad. Generally it is argued that more complex values can also be broken down into some combination or amalgamation of pleasure and pain. Then, in order to know what is ethical, one must decide which action creates the greatest net gain in pleasure over pain (and of course, in order to decide, one must look at the consequences of actions, ↓ not at some a priori set of rules).

The point we want to make here is that each of these two ethical theories **1181** seems to focus on a very narrow feature of what we have been calling "human nature." Kantian deontologic ethics looks at a human being's capacity for rationality and isolates that as the most important human trait for an ethical viewpoint. (It is interesting that Joseph Fletcher, the "situation ethicist," who is about as far as possible from being a follower of Kant, also is willing to isolate rationality as the single most important human characteristic — see his "indicators of humanhood" in Appendix VIII.) By contrast, the utilitarian looks at the human capacity to feel pleasure or pain — that is, at humanity as sentient existence — and isolates this feature of human nature as the ethical base.

↓

Recall that we saw, when looking at abortion, that an ethical theory does **1182** more than prescribe moral rules; it also defines, even if implicitly, a moral community among whom its rules apply. Isolating different features of human nature on which to base an ethical theory leads to very different boundaries for the moral community. Kant acknowledged that angels (assuming they exist) would be part of his moral community of rational beings, despite the fact that they are immortal and presumably have few of the desires and interests that motivate human beings. On the other hand, a consistent utilitarian would seem to be obliged to count as members of his moral community all sentient beings — since many animals are just as capable as we are of feeling pleasure and pain, there is no logical justification for excluding them when we come to add up the net result of the consequences of our actions.

↓

It seems to make a big difference which features of human nature one picks **1183** when laying the groundwork for an ethical theory. So it is disturbing that some of our most hallowed ethical traditions seem to be based on such very narrow views of human nature. Surely we can feel pleasure or pain; and surely we have the capacity for rational thought. (Of these two characteristics alone, the latter would seem more important — hence our emphasis throughout this book on individual dignity and autonomy, which grow out of our status as free, rational agents.) But on reflection we would probably say that we are made up of much more than any one of these characteristics.

↓

**1184**   What, then, would count as a more comprehensive view of human nature on which to base an ethical theory? And in what way could we use the tools of science to help define and clarify this view?

*In the last chapter we looked at a view of the person as part of a hierarchy of natural systems. This systems approach regards the person in part as a complex biologic system made up of organs, cells, and molecules — a result of a continuing interaction between heredity and environment, which is governed by the laws of physics and chemistry. The person is also a part of higher-level social and cultural systems and is in large part a product of cultural influences and social interactions. And, finally, the person is a person — a unique level of the hierarchy of systems, an entity in his own right, not ↓ just a mass of smaller subcomponents or a small cog in some larger system.*

**1185**   Ideally, an ethical theory would be grounded in a view of human nature that included the entire sweep of the systems approach. This would embrace theories of human nature from the biologic, the behavioral, and the social sciences.

The systems hierarchy reveals that just being "scientific" is no guarantee of being comprehensive. We have recently been treated to a series of books and articles about human nature from zoologists and other scientists, many of them based on new discoveries about the evolution of prehistoric man, which single out certain traits like aggression or territoriality as the key to being human. Some have then tried to derive ethical and social imperatives from these speculations. But scientific analyses of this sort are no better than the older philosophical analyses, since they isolate only a few facets of human nature and ignore the much broader scope of the hierarchy of sys-↓ tems.

**1186**   If there is a feature of human nature missing from most ethical theories, it is the social and cultural element. This may be a reaction to past excesses, such as the distorted Hegelian philosophy that was used to justify fascism, which tended to view the state as everything and the individual as nothing. Certainly no sound, ethical theory can support total devotion to a social group while renouncing all individual values and interests, or can approve of acts when committed by the state that would be condemned as atrocious if committed by individuals. But by the same token it is silly to pretend that morality is simply a matter of regulating the interactions of individuals who come into contact and then go their own way like billiard balls ↓ on a table.

Take, for example, so basic a tool of morality as language. It takes language to frame moral rules — indeed, it takes language to think rationally. But words and sentences are simply meaningless sounds, and alphabets are merely meaningless scribblings, unless they are a part of a more-or-less stable and enduring culture. (Without some generally accepted cultural expectations about when a word is used in the right way, words mean whatever we want them to mean — which is to say they don't mean anything.) ↓   **1187**

Persons, then, are not isolated atoms, but are by their very nature participants in culture and society, although cultures and societies can take many different forms. It would seem that an ethical theory that focuses primarily on the individual level would have serious deficiencies, especially when trying to come to grips with social problems. In our discussions, we have noted the problems of traditional ethical theories in dealing with complex social issues, such as the macroallocation of scarce resources.   ↓   **1188**

So far we have looked at ways that science can tell us more about the nature of persons and therefore more about ethics. But since an equilibrium is based on fit, it has to work both ways — that is, we have to learn about the nature of persons also as a result of our ethical analyses. We have seen two examples of this sort of reasoning in previous chapters.   ↓   **1189**

In Chapter 6, we argued that some members of the species homo sapiens might not be persons in the ethical sense (e.g., those in irreversible vegetative states). By looking at what it means to have rights and interests, we concluded that such individuals could not be said really to be moral agents and hence were not persons. (Of course, in following this line of argument, we were swayed by the assumption that individuals in this sort of coma experience no thoughts or memories, and this assumption is grounded in modern neuroscience. The key to this argument about personhood is not scientific fact, but a philosophical analysis of what it means to be a moral agent.)   ↓   **1190**
REVIEW PERSONHOOD ↑ 280–290

Then, in Chapter 10, we looked at the troublesome issue of abortion. We determined that this argument is the sort that will never be settled purely by discovery of new scientific facts (say, about the brain function of the fetus). Instead, we will have to make an ethical judgment about how fetuses ought to be treated. If we decide that fetuses have rights and ought to be protected, we will in effect be deciding that fetuses have some status as moral agents within our moral community; if we decide that fetuses can be killed at whim, we will be excluding them from our moral community. In either case, we will be making an important decision about what it means to be a moral agent, what it means to be a person.   ↓   **1191**
REVIEW FETUS ↑ 615–620

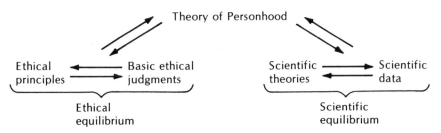

**Figure 13.** *Overall equilibrium model embracing both ethical and scientific systems, linked by a theory of personhood.*

**1192**  *Perhaps we can now, at long last, catch a glimpse of what it would mean to have an ethical value system that is justified according to the equilibrium model. The key to the justification is to have a comprehensive and cohesive theory of personhood. On the one hand, this theory will fit with the set of scientific theories and facts about human beings at all levels of the hierarchy of systems. On the other hand, it will fit with our ethical principles and values and our considered judgments about specific actions. This overall model of equilibrium is shown in Figure 13.*

**1193**  Of course, in this book, we have not laid out in any detail an ethical value system that fits this description. Nor have we developed in any explicit way a full-scale theory of personhood. Both of these may in fact be life-long tasks that an ethical and reflective individual may choose to undertake, and not the sort of thing one can find laid out ready-made in cookbook fashion. But Figure 13 at least shows us the dimensions of the problem and how we might go about testing our theories and conclusions.

**1194**  We have started our line of inquiry with that branch of ethics that deals specifically with decisions in medicine and health care, and we have now come to questions that underlie and even go beyond the entire structure of ethics. But we are still dealing with issues of central importance to medicine, for, as we saw in the last chapter, a proper understanding of the doctor–patient relationship (by extension of the contractual model) forces us to see the physician as the servant of the life plan of the patient, and this patient is a person. Only by understanding personhood — especially what it means to have a life plan, which is to have autonomously chosen goals and values — can the physician understand the nature of his most basic professional obligation. And it is, finally, on such an understanding that ethical decisions in medicine will be based.

# Appendix I
## Alternative Ethical Methods

The ethical decision-making method outlined in Figure 1, which we will be using as a basis for further discussion, is not the only legitimate ethical method. Philosophers have proposed a number of ethical theories, and no single theory has succeeded in emerging as a knockdown favorite. In this appendix we will list some of the more popular theories that have arisen in Anglo-American philosophical thought. (See Chapter 18 for further discussion of these theories and what counts as justification for one's ethical values.)

Different ethical theories often agree on specific decisions. (Both utilitarian and deontologic ethicists will readily agree that murder and robbery are immoral.) The differences between various ethical theories emerge primarily in the more problematic cases and often have to do with where the real "bite" in ethical reasoning is seen to come. One general division is between teleological (ends-based) and deontological (duty-based) ethical reasoning. To the teleologist, what gives ethical principles their bite is that they serve to maximize some good — that is, their ends or results. For the teleologist, what is, in the long run, the "right" thing to do is based on what is the "good" thing to do. Teleologists may then differ among themselves on what should be the ultimate scale of goodness. But, having once decided what is good, the teleologist should theoretically have no trouble deciding what is right.

To the deontologist, however, merely serving the good is not an adequate foundation for ethics — after all, serving some narrow conception of one's own good is usually the basis for most unethical activities. The deontologist argues that the only way ethical principles can have any real bite is if they are based on some rules or principles that are known to be right independent of whether they serve good ends. That is, for the deontologist, the right principle is independent of the good result, although he will, of course, want to promote the good result whenever he can do so without violating one of his moral rules. Deontologists will then disagree among themselves on what constitutes those principles that can be known to be right. Some deontologists rely on religious values for this. Others, especially followers of Immanuel Kant, hold that some principles are universally valid because any rational party would agree to accept those rules (i.e., universalizing the opposite of the rule would involve one in some sort of logical self-contradiction, such as trying to square a circle). Regardless of the rationale, principles such as honesty, avoiding harm to others, justice, and autonomy are commonly cited as the basis for deontologic ethical methods.

Figure 14 shows how a deontologist might go about making an ethical

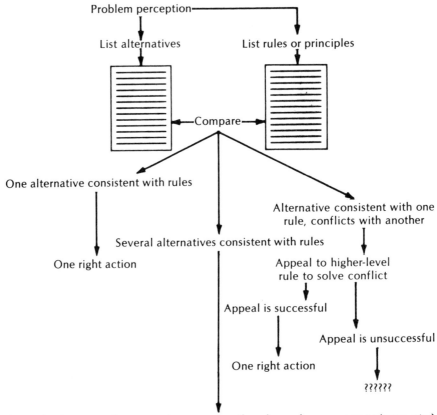

Several right actions (one may choose among them by preference, convenience, etc.)

**Figure 14.** *Deontological ethical method.*

decision. He first lists the alternative courses of action and compares these to his list of rules or principles. If his comparison shows that one and only one alternative is in accordance with his rules, he is home free with a decision. If several alternatives are acceptable, he can choose among them on other grounds — for instance, he can pick his favorite conception of the good and choose that alternative that maximizes the good. If none of the alternatives fits the rules, or if an alternative fits some rules but contradicts others (e.g., if the only alternative that would avoid harm to another is one that requires dishonesty), the deontologist has a problem. He may have to develop a priority scale among his rules to see which one is more important, or he may have to appeal to some higher-level ethical principle to settle the dispute. (Note that our own decision-making method in Figure 1 could encounter the same problem. But that method has a feedback loop that allows us to modify the original rule if it turns out to have unacceptable consequences. This step is generally not open to the deontologist, who feels that his rules are right independent of their consequences.)

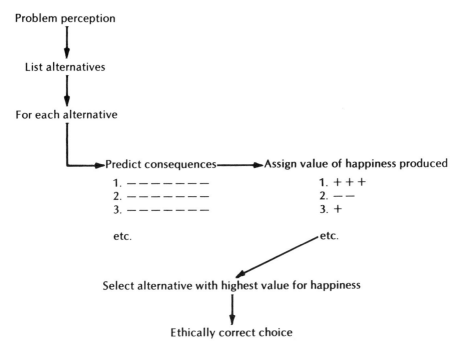

**Figure 15.** *Act-utilitarian ethical method. This method fails if: (1) one is unable to predict consequences accurately, or (2) one is unable to estimate accurate happiness values.*

Within the general category of teleologic ethical theory, the most popular method is <u>utilitarianism</u>. To the utilitarian, promoting the good means creating the greatest happiness, or the greatest net increase in pleasure over pain. The purest form of utilitarianism, "act-utilitarianism," is shown in Figure 15. The act-utilitarian lists alternative courses of action, and for each one calculates the net amount of happiness that would arise from all the consequences of the action. He then chooses the action that would produce the most happiness, or, failing that, the least unhappiness. (To apply this method properly, he is not allowed to increase his own happiness at the expense of others; he must consider one person's happiness as equal in value to another's.) This decision-making method will fall down if the act-utilitarian fails to predict consequences accurately, or, having predicted the consequences, if he is unable to decide what happiness value to assign to them.

Joseph Fletcher's "situation ethics" resembles act-utilitarianism, except that the measure of the good is not happiness but "agape," which can be translated from the Greek as "general goodwill" or "love for humanity." In one sense the label "situation ethics" is a misnomer, since an act-teleologic ethics has no corner on the "situation" market. Any ethical reasoning that is not merely silly takes the situation into account — the teleologist to predict the most likely consequences, the deontologist to decide which of his rules best apply.

Another popular variety of utilitarianism is "rule-utilitarianism." From the act-utilitarianism standpoint, rule-utilitarianism will seem to be an impure form of utilitarianism, but its defenders would respond that it merely takes into account what deontologists have always recognized — that rules are a valuable means for promoting ethical behavior, and that people seldom have the energy or the insight to approach each new situation in a totally fresh way. We could picture rule-utilitarianism as a two-level decision process. The higher-level process is the selection of the rules, which will follow a procedure very similar to Figure 1 — the difference being that the proposed rules will be compared not with some set of values, but with the amount of happiness or unhappiness the rules will produce were they to be put into general practice. Once the rules with the highest "utility value" are chosen, the lower-level process, to decide what to do in a particular case, will proceed much like Figure 14.

Questions of rights illustrate the difference between the rule-utilitarian and the act-utilitarian approaches. Most of the time, we would think, allowing free speech will lead to the greatest general happiness. But there may well be a few instances where this will not be true. The act-utilitarian, then, will oppose the concept of any universal "right to free speech," preferring instead to judge each case on its own individual utility value. But the rule-utilitarian will defend a right to free speech on the grounds that more happiness will occur in a society that acts according to such a right than in one that does not. He will argue that the act-utilitarian is more likely to make a mistake in calculating his individual utility values and hence inadvertently produce unhappiness, than an individual who follows the idea of a right to free speech as a general rule.

Since the rule-utilitarian, higher-level decision process is similar to Figure 1, the rule-utilitarian can use our feedback loop to modify his rule, if it should turn out that in some cases the original rule fails to promote the greatest happiness. This modification will often take the form of restricting the scope of the rule. For instance, "The right to free speech doesn't include the right to shout 'fire' in a crowded theater" might be how a rule-utilitarian would modify his original rule once he sees that it has unintended, negative consequences as originally stated.

We can now see that our own ethical decision-making method in Figure 1 would fall under the category of a rule-teleologic method. It determines the right by reference to the good — that is, to the set of personal values we hold. But we can also include among those values some of the principles that are found in deontologic theories, most notably the principle of personal dignity and autonomy (or what is described in Kantian ethics as "treating others as ends and never as means only").

For coherence, we will generally turn to the decision-making method of Figure 1 for the remainder of this discussion, but as we saw, no one ethical theory is so clearly superior to all others that we would be justified in using it exclusively. It may turn out that for some ethical issues (as we argue in Chapter 6, especially), concepts from deontologic theory seem to fit the problem better than an approach based solely on the consequences of actions. It might be wise to adopt a nondogmatic approach and to think of different ethical theories like different carpenter's tools; the wise carpenter tries to select the right tool for the task at hand. One way to select the best ethical tool is to think of the sort of error one is most likely to fall into when discussing that particular ethical issue. If decision makers in the past have erred primarily by adhering rigidly to rules and by failing to see the peculiarities of individual cases, a teleologic approach might counteract this tendency. But if past decision makers have tended to cause unhappiness and indignity for others because of their short-sighted pursuit of the good as they have idiosyncratically defined it, a deontologic approach might be called for.

Our approach to ethical decision making reflects a modern bias toward seeing ethics in terms of actions; questions of what constitutes virtue, good character, or the "good life" become less important and are defined in terms of the sum of a large number of individual actions. The situation was very different in the classic philosophy of Plato and Aristotle, where good character and virtue were the cornerstones of ethical theory and individual actions were merely temporary and imperfect reflections of character. The change may reflect the evolution of simpler, unified cultures in which there was little dissent over what was right, good, and virtuous, into complex, pluralistic societies in which many different values compete in the cultural marketplace. Some philosophers suggest that our current value pluralism is merely a way station, and an unsatisfactory one at that, on the way to a future value synthesis that will once again give our culture an unquestioned direction and purpose. But such matters are clearly unresolvable within the scope of this book. Representative books and articles on general ethical theory will be found in the first section of References and Suggested Readings.

# Appendix II
## Ethics and Religion

Martin Benjamin, Michigan State University

In what ways, if any, and for what reasons, if any, do matters of religion bear upon ethical decisions in medicine? I will argue that although religious beliefs and practices cannot provide the justification for our basic ethical principles, any such principles must acknowledge the importance of religious beliefs in the lives of both patients and health-care professionals.

### Religion as the Basis for Ethics

It is widely held that all ethical decisions are ultimately grounded upon, and inseparable from, some set of religious beliefs. If this is correct, people in a religiously pluralistic society will be unable to develop a systematic framework for resolving basic ethical disagreements. Ethical differences will be regarded as a function of religious differences, and ethical reasoning and discussion will be interpreted as an attempt at religious conversion.

But what does it mean to say that ethical decisions are ultimately grounded upon, and inseparable from, religious belief? For some, this statement may mean simply that our ethical principles are causally or historically rooted in one or another religious tradition. Even if this is true, however, it does not follow that the principles cannot be justified on their own terms, quite apart from the tradition from which they developed. We do not, for example, say that the validity of modern chemistry depends on the validity of Renaissance alchemy, even though the former had its origins in the latter; nor does the fact that astrology is the mother of modern astronomy imply that controversies that arise in the latter cannot be resolved without appeal to the former. Similarly, even if there is a causal or historical connection between religion and basic ethical principles, we cannot conclude that the validity of an ethical principle depends upon the validity of the religious tradition from which it emerged.

But when people claim that ethics is based on religion they may not mean that ethics is simply causally or historically grounded in religion; they may also mean that only religion can provide the ultimate justification of our most basic ethical principles. Thus it is often said that an ethical principle is correct if and only if it has been issued by God. If this is true, a secular ethical framework will have no foundation, and basic ethical differences will be beyond the reach of ordinary standards of reason and evidence.

Further consideration, however, reveals that the notion of "God," or any other purely religious authority, as the ultimate source of ethical justification runs into insuperable problems. Even if we ignore the considerable difficulties involved in determining the existence of God, how do we discover the basic ethical principles that He has set for us? There are, it seems, only two ways to become aware of them: (1) we are informed of them directly by God, or (2) we learn of them indirectly from others who claim to have been informed by God. In both cases there is ample room for doubt. First, how is one to know that the "voice" directly conveying God's principles is not that of the Devil or the result of an hallucination? And second, if God's principles are relayed through an intermediary, such as a priest or a document, how does one know that the transmission of God's views is accurate, or that it is God, and not an hallucination or the Devil, that is the source of the principles?

Suppose, for example, one hears a voice identifying itself as God that says that we are now ethically permitted to kill the retarded, or suppose that a certain religious order suddenly advocates killing the retarded and defends itself by appealing to a recent communication from God. In either case we would reject both the ethical judgment and the claim that it came from God. But why? The answer, I think, is that those who claim that ethics is grounded in religion believe that God is the source of ethics not only because He is all-knowing and all-powerful, but also (and perhaps mainly) because He is perfectly good. And a god who is perfectly good, they would maintain, would never advocate killing the retarded. Therefore pronouncements of this kind must be attributed not to God, but rather to hallucinations, madness, or the Devil.

This line of reasoning, however, actually undermines the claim that ethics depends on religion, for it assumes the independent validity of certain ethical considerations. The judgment that a perfectly good god would not permit killing the retarded assumes that we have some idea of what a perfectly good god is like and whether such a god would permit those acts. But what is the source of this knowledge? To say that such knowledge comes from God is simply to relocate the question, not to answer it, for the problem of distinguishing God's principles from those attributable to hallucinations, madness, or the Devil would now be transformed into a problem of distinguishing God's account of His perfect goodness from accounts attributable to hallucinations, madness, or the Devil. It adds nothing to our understanding to say that a certain ethical principle would not be issued by God because God is perfectly good, unless we have some source other than God Himself for learning what a perfectly good god is like. Therefore we can say that a perfectly good god would not permit the killing of the retarded only if we can appeal to certain values that shape our conception of God's goodness and that are justifiable quite apart from their having God as their source. These secular considerations, then, are more fundamental for human understanding than any God may be said to issue, for without them we could have no idea of the nature and values of a perfectly good god.

Therefore appeals to religion as the justification for our basic ethical principles are either: (1) unable to distinguish God's commandments from those of the Devil or hallucinations, or (2) assume the validity of some non-religiously grounded ethical principles that are used to identify the commandments of a perfectly good god.

This conclusion suggests that insofar as people of various religious persuasions come to some rough agreement on the nature of a perfectly good god, it is because they already agree upon some religiously neutral ethical standards. Such standards, when clearly identified and defended, may thus provide the foundations of a common framework for resolving ethical disagreements. If so, patients and health professionals of various religious persuasions, as well as agnostics and atheists, will be able to appeal to this framework in making and justifying ethical decisions. Moreover, those who are strongly committed to one or another religious tradition will, in some cases, be able to develop secular arguments to support what may presently be regarded as religiously based principles. As a result they will be able to preserve certain values and persuade others of their worth without being accused of imposing their religious beliefs on those who do not share them. For example, someone who has previously been able to defend the Golden Rule only by appeal to religious authority should welcome the efforts of Kant and contemporary philosophers like Hare and Donagan to show that versions of this rule can be supported solely by secular arguments.

## Religion as a Basic Concern of Ethics

At first glance, our conclusions about the limitations of religion as the basis for ethical principles may seem to compromise the Jewish and Christian traditions. But, as we shall see, these limitations in no way imply that people's religious beliefs, principles, and practices are irrelevant to a secularly grounded ethical framework. On the contrary, they are of central importance.

As Alan Donagan has recently emphasized, both Judaism and Christianity have traditionally distinguished between that part of their ethical frameworks that is binding upon all persons simply in virtue of their being rational (this corresponds to Kantian ethics, as described in Appendix I), and that part that depends upon divine commandments and a way of life specified by religion. The former is supposed to be known and justified simply by appeal to human reason and is therefore binding on all rational creatures, whatever their particular religious beliefs or affiliations.

> The conception of morality as a law common to all rational creatures by virtue of their rationality, although endorsed by the Stoic, Jewish, and Christian religious traditions, is not itself religious. Except with regard to divine worship, neither Stoics, Jews, nor Christians found it necessary to resort to premises about the existence and nature of God in stating the various provisions of the moral law.*

This, of course, is the way it had to be if Jews and Christians were to be able to appeal to ethical principles in their dealings with those who did not share their particular religious views.

Religions such as Judaism and Christianity go beyond these basic secular principles, however, by including them within a religiously oriented <u>way of</u>

---

* A. Donagan, *The Theory of Morality*. Chicago: The University of Chicago Press, 1977. P. 6.

life, where provisions and ideals are grounded in faith and comprise the notion of a full Jewish, Catholic, Presbyterian, Lutheran, Methodist, Jehovah's Witness, and so on way of life. They include participating in various religious observances and obeying, as the case may be, certain restrictions with regard to diet, alcohol, contraception, sterilization, and so on. In addition, such ways of life will often include high ideals of such virtues as charity, forgiveness, and self-sacrifice that, unlike proscriptions against causing harm, are not so easily justified on secular grounds. A religiously grounded way of life may thus be considered to enhance and supplement, rather than to rival, a more limited secular framework.

An acceptable secular framework must, nonetheless, recognize the importance to various people of a religious way of life. Insofar as one's religious beliefs form a part of one's identity as a person, respecting a person's exercise of these beliefs is part of respecting him or her as a person. Whenever possible, then, a secular framework that values respect for persons should allow considerable freedom of religious observance and practice. In the context of health care, this requires that health professionals respect the importance of a patient's religious beliefs when these beliefs play a major role in his or her basic values and life plan. For example, religious holidays, dietary restrictions, attitudes toward contraception, sterilization, autopsy, and so on are always of significance in determining a patient's course of treatment.

In some cases, however, one requirement of a religiously based way of life may conflict with the requirements of the basic secular framework. We may agree, for example, that when a competent adult Jehovah's Witness refuses a life-saving blood transfusion (as in Case 23), his or her freedom to act in accord with his or her religious way of life is of primary concern. But we may be inclined to respond quite differently when Jehovah's Witness parents refuse to consent to life-saving transfusions for their children. Here the religious injunctions seem to clash with the requirements of secular morality. Conflicts of this sort involve complex issues and concerns and must be given close, careful examination.

Although strictly religious beliefs and practices are not directly relevant to the justification of basic ethical principles, they are nonetheless important in determining their content and application. The most plausible secular principles will be those that are able to acknowledge and respect a wide variety of religious beliefs and practices. Where conflicts arise between religious and secular precepts, every effort should be made to accommodate the religious values at stake. In some cases, however, this will be impossible; and then, as a rule, the secular precepts will be regarded as being of overriding importance.

# Appendix III
## Patient's Bill of Rights

American Hospital Association, November, 1972

1. The patient has the right to considerate and respectful care.
2. The patient has the right to obtain from his physician complete current information concerning his diagnosis, treatment, and prognosis in terms the patient can be reasonably expected to understand. When it is not medically advisable to give such information to the patient, the information should be made available to an appropriate person in his behalf. He has the right to know by name, the physician responsible for coordinating his care.
3. The patient has the right to receive from his physician information necessary to give informed consent prior to the start of any procedure and/or treatment. Except in emergencies, such information for informed consent should include but not necessarily be limited to the specific procedure and/or treatment, the medically significant risks involved, and the probable duration of incapacitation. Where medically significant alternatives for care or treatment exist, or when the patient requests information concerning medical alternatives, the patient has the right to such information. The patient also has the right to know the name of the person responsible for the procedures and/or treatment.
4. The patient has the right to refuse treatment to the extent permitted by law, and to be informed of the medical consequences of his action.
5. The patient has the right to every consideration of his privacy concerning his own medical care program. Case discussion, consultation, examination, and treatment are confidential and should be conducted discreetly. Those not directly involved in his care must have the permission of the patient to be present.
6. The patient has the right to expect that all communications and records pertaining to his care should be treated as confidential.
7. The patient has the right to expect that within its capacity a hospital must make reasonable response to the request of a patient for services. The hospital must provide evaluation, service, and/or referral as indicated by the urgency of the case. When medically permissible a patient may be transferred to another facility only after he has received complete information and explanation concerning the needs for and alternatives to such a transfer. The institution to which the patient is to be transferred must first have accepted the patient for transfer.
8. The patient has the right to obtain information as to any relationship of his hospital to other health care and educational institutions insofar as his care is concerned. The patient has the right to obtain information as to the existence of any professional relationships among individuals, by name, who are treating him.

9. The patient has the right to be advised if the hospital proposes to engage in or perform human experimentation affecting his care or treatment. The patient has the right to refuse to participate in such research projects.
10. The patient has the right to expect reasonable continuity of care. He has the right to know in advance what appointment times and physicians are available and where. The patient has the right to expect that the hospital will provide a mechanism whereby he is informed by his physician or delegate of the physician of the patient's continuing health-care requirements following discharge.
11. The patient has the right to examine and receive an explanation of his bill regardless of source of payment.
12. The patient has the right to know what hospital rules and regulations apply to his conduct as a patient.

No catalogue of rights can guarantee for the patient the kind of treatment he has a right to expect. A hospital has many functions to perform, including the prevention and treatment of disease, the education of both health professionals and patients, and the conduct of clinical research. All these activities must be conducted with an overriding concern for the patient, and, above all, the recognition of his dignity as a human being. Success in achieving this recognition assures success in the defense of the rights of the patient.

# Appendix IV
## A Living Will*

To my family, my physician, my clergyman, my lawyer —

If the time comes when I can no longer take part in decisions for my own future, let this statement stand as the testament of my wishes:

If there is no reasonable expectation of my recovery from physical or mental disability, I, _____, request that I be allowed to die and not be kept alive by artificial means or heroic measures. Death is as much a reality as birth, growth, maturity and old age — it is the one certainty. I do not fear death as much as I fear the indignity of deterioration, dependence and hopeless pain. I ask that medication be mercifully administered to me for terminal suffering even if it hastens the moment of death.

This request is made after careful consideration. Although this document is not legally binding, you who care for me will, I hope, feel morally bound to follow its mandate. I recognize that it places a heavy burden of responsibility upon you, and it is with the intention of sharing that responsibility and of mitigating any feelings of guilt that this statement is made.

Signed _____

Date _____

Witnessed By: _____

_____

_____

* Prepared and distributed by the Concern for Dying, 250 West 57th Street, New York, N.Y. 10019. This form has also been used as a model for "death with dignity" bills introduced into state legislatures.

# Appendix V
## Christian Affirmation of Life*

To my family, friends, physician, lawyer, and clergyman:

I believe that each individual person is created by God our Father in love and that God retains a loving relationship to each person throughout human life and eternity.

I believe that Jesus Christ lived, suffered, and died for me and that his suffering, death, and resurrection prefigure and make possible the death-resurrection process which I now anticipate.

I believe that each person's worth and dignity derives from the relationship of love in Christ that God has for each individual person and not from one's usefulness or effectiveness in society.

I believe that God our Father has entrusted to me a shared dominion with him over my earthly existence so that I am bound to use ordinary means to preserve my life but I am free to refuse extraordinary means to prolong my life.

I believe that through death life is not taken away but merely changed, and though I may experience fear, suffering, and sorrow, by the grace of the Holy Spirit, I hope to accept death as a free human act which enables me to surrender this life and to be united with God for eternity.

Because of my belief:

I request that I be informed as death approaches so that I may continue to prepare for the full encounter with Christ through the help of the sacraments and the consolation and prayers of my family and friends.

I request that, if possible, I be consulted concerning the medical procedures which might be used to prolong my life as death approaches. If I can no longer take part in decisions concerning my own future and if there is no reasonable expectation of my recovery from physical and mental disability, I request that no extraordinary means be used to prolong my life.

I request, though I wish to join my suffering to the suffering of Jesus so I may be united fully with him in the act of death-resurrection, that my pain, if unbearable, be alleviated. However, no means should be used with the intention of shortening my life.

I request, because I am a sinner and in need of reconciliation and because my faith, hope, and love may not overcome all fear and doubt, that my family, friends, and the whole Christian community join me in prayer and mortification as I prepare for the great personal act of dying.

* Prepared by Rev. Kevin D. O'Rourke, O.P., as an alternative to the "Living Will" (Appendix IV), and available from the Catholic Hospital Association, 1438 South Grand Boulevard, St. Louis, MO 63104.

Finally, I request that after my death, my family, my friends, and the whole Christian community pray for me, and rejoice with me because of the mercy and love of the Trinity, with whom I hope to be united for all eternity.

Signed _____ Date _____

# Appendix VI
## Directions for My Care*

I, _____, want to participate in my own medical care as long as I am able. But I recognize that an accident or illness may someday make me unable to do so. Should this come to be the case, this document is intended to direct those who make choices on my behalf. I have prepared it while still legally competent and of sound mind. If these instructions create a conflict with the desires of my relatives, or with hospital policies or with the principles of those providing my care, I ask that my instructions prevail, unless they are contrary to existing law or would expose medical personnel or the hospital to a substantial risk of legal liability.

I wish to live a full and long life, but not at all costs. If my death is near and cannot be avoided, and if I have lost the ability to interact with others and have no reasonable chance of regaining this ability, or if my suffering is intense and irreversible, I do not want to have my life prolonged. I would then ask not to be subjected to surgery or resuscitation. Nor would I then wish to have life support from mechanical ventilators, intensive care services, or other life prolonging procedures, including the administration of antibiotics and blood products. I would wish, rather, to have care which gives comfort and support, which facilitates my interaction with others to the extent that this is possible, and which brings peace.

In order to carry out these instructions and to interpret them, I authorize _____ to accept, plan, and refuse treatment on my behalf in cooperation with attending physicians and health personnel. This person knows how I value the experience of living, and how I would weigh incompetence, suffering, and dying. Should it be impossible to reach this person, I authorize _____ to make such choices for me. I have discussed my desires concerning terminal care with them, and I trust their judgment on my behalf.

In addition, I have discussed with them the following specific instructions regarding my care:

(Please continue on back.)

Date _____ Signed _____

Witnessed by _____ and by_____

* Reprinted with permission of the author and publisher from Sissela Bok, Personal directions for care at the end of life. *New England Journal of Medicine* 295:367–69, 1976.

# Appendix VII

## "Directive to Physicians" from California Natural Death Act*

Directive made this _____ day of _____ (month, year).

I, _____, being of sound mind, willfully, and voluntarily make known my desire that my life shall not be artificially prolonged under the circumstances set forth below, do hereby declare:

1. If at any time I should have an incurable injury, disease, or illness certified to be a terminal condition by two physicians, and where the application of life-sustaining procedures would serve only to artificially prolong the moment of my death and where my physician determines that my death is imminent whether or not life-sustaining procedures are utilized, I direct that such procedures be withheld or withdrawn, and that I be permitted to die naturally.

2. In the absence of my ability to give directions regarding the use of such life-sustaining procedures, it is my intention that this directive shall be honored by my family and physician(s) as the final expression of my legal right to refuse medical or surgical treatment and accept the consequences from such refusal.

3. If I have been diagnosed as pregnant and that diagnosis is known to my physician, this directive shall have no force or effect during the course of my pregnancy.

4. I have been diagnosed and notified at least 14 days ago as having a terminal condition by _____, M.D., whose address is _____, and whose telephone number is _____. I understand that if I have not filled in the physician's name and address, it shall be presumed that I did not have a terminal condition when I made out this directive.

5. This directive shall have no force or effect five years from the date filled in above.

6. I understand the full import of this directive and I am emotionally and mentally competent to make this directive.

Signed _____

City, County, and State of Residence _____

The declarant has been personally known to me and I believe him or her to be of sound mind.

Witness _____

Witness _____

(Note: This directive is legally binding under the law only if the patient is terminally ill at the time of signing and has completed Section 4; otherwise the directive is of informational value only.)

* Contained in the California Natural Death Act, Assembly Bill No. 3060, signed into law September, 1976. The California law recognizes only those directives executed exactly in this form. Key terms such as "terminal condition" and "life-sustaining procedure" are defined elsewhere in the law.

# Appendix VIII
## Criteria for Determining Quality of Life*

"Tentative Profile of Man" by Joseph Fletcher: Fletcher, a theologian and professor of medical ethics, has proposed a set of positive human criteria specifically designed to serve as indicators of personhood in decisions regarding abortion, allowing to die, and so on. With brief explanation, his list consists of:

1. Minimal Intelligence: Below 40 on Stanford-Binet or similar IQ test is questionably a person; below 20 is not a person.
2. Self-awareness
3. Self-control: If condition cannot be rectified medically, individual without self-control is not a person.
4. A sense of time: A sense of the passage of time and of the need to allocate time.
5. A sense of futurity: A sense of time to come; looking forward and planning.
6. A sense of the past: A sense of time gone by; memory.
7. Capability to relate to others: Includes both inter-individual and diffuse social relationships.
8. Concern for others: While role this trait actually plays is debatable, its absence is indicator of psychopathology.
9. Communication: Completely isolated individual who cannot communicate, as opposed to being disinclined to communicate, is not a person.
10. Control of existence: When absent leads to state of irresponsibility (compare No. 3).
11. Curiosity: "Man is a learner and knower as well as a tool-maker and user."
12. Change and changeability: Of one's mind and conduct.
13. Balance of rationality and feeling: Person can be neither coldly rational nor given over completely to feelings.
14. Idiosyncrasy: Must have recognizable identity.
15. Neo-cortical function: All other traits hinge upon this; offers legitimacy of brain-function approach to defining death.

For purposes of clarification, Fletcher also lists five points of negative human criteria, which he deems not essential to personhood: (1) man is not non- or antiartificial (i.e., technology is a normal part of human existence); (2) man is not essentially parental and can be fully a person without reproducing; (3) man is not essentially sexual; (4) man is not a "bundle of rights";

* Adapted from the *Hastings Center Report*, Vol. 2, November 1972, with the permission of the Institute of Society, Ethics and the Life Sciences, Hastings-on-Hudson, N.Y. 10706.

and (5) man is not a worshipper ("Faith in supernatural realities . . . is a choice some human beings make and others do not.")

Fletcher acknowledged many problems with his list and proposed it as a start for discussion rather than as a final product. He noted that some items may be essential for human existence where others might merely promote optimal existence. He was unable to suggest how to rank-order the criteria. While he did state that the potential cannot be treated equivalently to the actual, he did not state how to regard precisely such "potential" persons as normal fetuses. He did not say just how many indicators, or which ones, had to be absent before the individual is no longer worthy of medical protection.

As noted in the text, in 1974 Fletcher had revised his notions to the extent that he acknowledged the primary importance of No. 15, cerebral function, and was willing to make life-and-death decisions based on that criterion alone.

### Other Personhood Criteria

Other authors have developed lists of traits that they consider essential for humanhood, but that were developed for other purposes and so are not directly applicable to medical-ethical decisions without clarification.

G. G. Simpson has listed the following activities that he considers to be the biologic basis of human nature:

1. Abstracting.
2. Communicating.
3. Tool-making.
4. Ethicizing or valuing.

These, of course, are stated in the most abstract form, and thus are of limited practical use in deciding specific cases.

T. S. Clements, in an attempt to explicate the philosophy of scientific humanism, lists a number of "personality atoms," which are part of what he calls the "good life." These include the following:

1. Desire to be loved.
2. Desire to be excited.
3. Desire to satisfy curiosity and exercise intelligence.
4. Desire for order.
5. Desire to feel healthy and unified.
6. Desire to feel meaningfully related to world and to others.
7. Desire to share experiences socially.

Again, the "good life" label suggests that these are criteria for optimal existence, rather than the minimal criteria needed for making quality-of-life decisions in a medical-ethical context.

# Appendix IX
## Declaration of Helsinki*
Recommendations Guiding Doctors in Clinical Research

### Introduction

It is the mission of the medical doctor to safeguard the health of the people. His or her knowledge and conscience are dedicated to the fulfillment of this mission.

The Declaration of Geneva of the World Medical Association binds the doctor with the words, "The health of my patient will be my first consideration," and the International Code of Medical Ethics declares that, "Any act or advice which could weaken physical or mental resistance of a human being may be used only in his interest."

The purpose of biomedical research involving human subjects must be to improve diagnostic, therapeutic and prophylactic procedures and the understanding of the aetiology and pathogenesis of disease.

In current medical practice most diagnostic, therapeutic or prophylactic procedures involve hazards. This applies *a fortiori* to biomedical research.

Medical progress is based on research which ultimately must rest in part on experimentation involving human subjects.

In the field of biomedical research a fundamental distinction must be recognized between medical research in which the aim is essentially diagnostic or therapeutic for a patient, and medical research, the essential object of which is purely scientific and without direct diagnostic or therapeutic value to the person subjected to the research.

Special caution must be exercised in the conduct of research which may affect the environment, and the welfare of animals used for research must be respected.

Because it is essential that the results of laboratory experiments be applied to human beings to further scientific knowledge and to help suffering humanity, The World Medical Association has prepared the following recommendations as a guide to every doctor in biomedical research involving human subjects. They should be kept under review in the future. It must be stressed that the standards as drafted are only a guide to physicians all over the world. Doctors are not relieved from criminal, civil and ethical responsibilities under the laws of their own countries.

### I. Basic Principles

1. Biomedical research involving human subjects must conform to generally accepted scientific principles and should be based on adequately

---

* Resolution adopted at the 18th World Medical Assembly, 1964, by the World Medical Association, of which the American Medical Association is a member, and revised at the 29th World Medical Assembly, 1975.

performed laboratory and animal experimentation and on a thorough knowledge of the scientific literature.

2. The design and performance of each experimental procedure involving human subjects should be clearly formulated in an experimental protocol which should be transmitted to a specially appointed independent committee for consideration, comment and guidance.

3. Biomedical research involving human subjects should be conducted only by scientifically qualified persons and under the supervision of a clinically competent medical person. The responsibility for the human subject must always rest with a medically qualified person and never rest on the subject of the research, even though the subject has given his or her consent.

4. Biomedical research involving human subjects cannot legitimately be carried out unless the importance of the objective is in proportion to the inherent risk to the subject.

5. Every biomedical research project involving human subjects should be preceded by careful assessment of predictable risks in comparison with foreseeable benefits to the subject or to others. Concern for the interests of the subject must always prevail over the interests of science and society.

6. The right of the research subject to safeguard his or her integrity must always be respected. Every precaution should be taken to respect the privacy of the subject and to minimize the impact of the study on the subject's physical and mental integrity and on the personality of the subject.

7. Doctors should abstain from engaging in research projects involving human subjects unless they are satisfied that the hazards involved are believed to be predictable. Doctors should cease any investigation if the hazards are found to outweigh the potential benefits.

8. In publication of the results of his or her research, the doctor is obliged to preserve the accuracy of the results. Reports of experimentation not in accordance with the principles laid down in this Declaration should not be accepted for publication.

9. In any research on human beings, each potential subject must be adequately informed of the aims, methods, anticipated benefits and potential hazards of the study and the discomfort it may entail. He or she should be informed that he or she is at liberty to abstain from participation in the study and that he or she is free to withdraw his or her consent to participation at any time. The doctor should then obtain the subject's freely given informed consent, preferably in writing.

10. When obtaining informed consent for the research project the doctor should be particularly cautious if the subject is in a dependent relationship to him or her or may consent under duress. In that case the informed consent should be obtained by a doctor who is not engaged in the investigation and who is completely independent of this official relationship.

11. In case of legal incompetence, informed consent should be obtained from the legal guardian in accordance with national legislation. Where physical or mental incapacity makes it impossible to obtain informed consent, or when the subject is a minor, permission from the responsible relative replaces that of the subject in accordance with national legislation.

12. The research protocol should always contain a statement of the ethical considerations involved and should indicate that the principles enunciated in the present declaration are complied with.

## II. Medical Research Combined with Professional Care (Clinical Research)

1. In the treatment of the sick person, the doctor must be free to use a new diagnostic and therapeutic measure, if in his or her judgment it offers hope of saving life, reestablishing health or alleviating suffering.

2. The potential benefits, hazards and discomfort of a new method should be weighed against the advantages of the best current diagnostic and therapeutic methods.

3. In any medical study, every patient — including those of a control group, if any — should be assured of the best proven diagnostic and therapeutic method.

4. The refusal of the patient to participate in a study must never interfere with the doctor-patient relationship.

5. If the doctor considers it essential not to obtain informed consent, the specific reasons for this proposal should be stated in the experimental protocol for transmission to the independent committee (1, 2).

6. The doctor can combine medical research with professional care, the objective being the acquisition of new medical knowledge, only to the extent that medical research is justified by its potential diagnostic or therapeutic value for the patient.

## III. Non-Therapeutic Biomedical Research Involving Human Subjects (Nonclinical Biomedical Research)

1. In the purely scientific application of medical research carried out on a human being, it is the duty of the doctor to remain the protector of the life and health of that person on whom biomedical research is being carried out.

2. The subjects should be volunteers — either healthy persons or patients for whom the experimental design is not related to the patient's illness.

3. The investigator or the investigating team should discontinue the research if in his/her or their judgment it may, if continued, be harmful to the individual.

4. In research on man, the interest of science and society should never take precedence over considerations related to the wellbeing of the subject.

# References and Suggested Readings

## Ethics, General

Donagan, A. *The Theory of Morality.* Chicago: The University of Chicago Press, 1977.

This philosopher argues that the moral system enshrined in the Judeo-Christian ethical tradition is supportable on rational-philosophical grounds, and not just on narrowly theological grounds.

Dworkin, G. Paternalism. In R. A. Wasserstrom (Ed.), *Morality and the Law.* Belmont, Calif.: Wadsworth, n.d.

The question of paternalism and when it is ethically justifiable runs through much of medical ethics, and Dworkin here gives a concise summary of this issue.

Fletcher, J. *Situation Ethics.* Philadelphia: Westminster, 1966.

Hailed as the "new morality" of the early 1960s, Fletcher's modified act-utilitarianism has appealed strongly to some medical thinkers and outraged others. See discussion in Appendix I.

Frankena, W. K. *Ethics* (2nd ed.). Englewood Cliffs, N.J.: Prentice-Hall, 1973.

Frankena's introductory textbook remains one of the best works of its size on ethics and provides an excellent starting point to the study of contemporary ethical theory.

Gert, B. *The Moral Rules.* New York: Harper and Row, 1970.

Gert's book is a creative recent effort to construct an ethical system based on rules rather than on consequences.

Gustafson, J. M. *Theology and Christian Ethics.* Philadelphia: United Church Press, 1974.

Gustafson is one of the more distinguished theologians contributing to the current ethical literature and has written on several medical issues as well.

Hare, R. M. *Freedom and Reason.* New York: Oxford University Press, 1965.

Hare is one of the most prominent representatives of the attempt to study the foundations of ethics by analyzing the language in which ethical statements are expressed — especially by analyzing the concept of universalizability.

Kant, I. In R. P. Wolff (Ed.), *Foundations of the Metaphysics of Morals.* New York: Bobbs-Merrill, 1969.

First published in 1785, Kant's work is the classic of deontologic ethical theory. See discussion in Appendix I.

MacIntyre, A. Why is the search for the foundations of ethics so frustrating? *Hastings Center Report* 9(August 1979): 16–22.

In this provocative article, MacIntyre argues that our inability to agree upon a foundation of morality reflects a broader cultural malaise in which we no longer have a picture of our culture and the human community in a whole, interconnected fashion.

McCormick, R. A. *Ambiguity in Moral Choice.* Milwaukee: Marquette University Press, 1973.

McCormick, a liberal Catholic theologian, has also written extensively on medical ethics.

Mill, J. S. Utilitarianism; On Liberty. In M. Cowling (Ed.), *Selected Writings of John Stuart Mill.* New York: Mentor, 1968.

These classic statements of utilitarian ethics and of the right of noninterference first appeared in 1863 and 1859, respectively. See discussion in Appendix I.

Rawls, J. *A Theory of Justice.* Cambridge, Mass.: Harvard University Press, 1971.
Rawls' large and difficult book is the most creative modern treatment of what constitutes a just society and how we can tell a just society from an unjust one.

Smart, J. J. C., and Williams, B. *Utilitarianism: For and Against.* New York: Cambridge University Press, 1973.
A good collection of essays summarizing the modern debate over the validity of utilitarianism.

Stevenson, C. L. *Facts and Values: Studies in Ethical Analysis.* New Haven, Conn.: Yale University Press, 1963.
Stevenson studies the relationship between facts and values and shows that ethical and scientific thinking are not as far apart in some ways as we suppose.

## Medical Ethics, General

Ashley, B. M., and O'Rourke, K. D. *Health Care Ethics.* St. Louis: Catholic Hospital Association, 1978.
This theologically oriented book looks at rights and responsibilities of patients, the healing profession, and difficult bioethical decisions.

Bandman, E. L., and Bandman, B. *Bioethics and Human Rights: A Reader for Health Professionals.* Boston: Little, Brown, 1978.
Coedited by a teacher of nursing and a philosopher, this anthology offers a number of readings organized according to rights — the right to life, the right to health care, the rights of the aging and the mentally ill, and so on. Each section begins with an introduction discussing that right.

Beauchamp, T. L., and Childress, J. F. *Principles of Biomedical Ethics.* New York: Oxford University Press, 1979.
This textbook, after discussing moral theory in general, looks at medical decisions as falling under four broad principles: autonomy, nonmaleficence, beneficence, and justice. As such, it could in fact be used as a general textbook of ethics, not just medical ethics. The authors strengthen their discussion of the principles by referring to a set of 29 illustrative cases.

Beauchamp, T. L., and Walters, L. (Eds.). *Contemporary Issues in Bioethics.* Encino, Calif.: Dickinson Publishing, 1978.
This anthology covers general ethical theories and specific issues in medical ethics. Articles included are by physicians, philosophers, theologians, and lawyers. (Cited below as "Beauchamp.")

Campbell, A. V. *Moral Dilemmas in Medicine.* Baltimore: Williams and Wilkins, 1972.
This short text, published first in Britain, looks at ethical issues under such headings as "the individual conscience," "the common good," "rules and situations," and so on. Each section starts with several cases illustrating the dilemmas.

Clouser, K. D. Some things medical ethics is not. *Journal of the American Medical Association* 223 : 787–89, 1973; What is medical ethics? *Annals of Internal Medicine* 80 : 657–60, 1974; Medical ethics: Some uses, abuses, and limitations. *New England Journal of Medicine* 293 : 384–87, 1975.
In these three articles, a philosopher exposes some misconceptions about medical ethics and clarifies how it can help the practitioner in practical decision making.

Fletcher, J. *Morals and Medicine.* Boston: Beacon Press, 1960.
Fletcher's was one of the first modern works on medical ethics and is the classic application of "situation ethics" to medical problems.

Gorovitz, S., et al. (Eds.). *Moral Problems in Medicine.* Englewood Cliffs, N.J.: Prentice-Hall, 1976.

This anthology contains many works by physicians, but its basic structure represents a philosophical analysis of medical ethics. The chapter introductions are especially useful. (Cited below as "Gorovitz.")

Greenberg, D. S.   Ethics and nonsense. *New England Journal of Medicine* 290 : 977–78, 1974.
A science writer reviews some then-current controversies and nicely separates the difficult questions demanding ethical analysis from the black-and-white issues that produce satisfying rhetoric but little ethical insight.

Haring, B.   *Medical Ethics.* Notre Dame, Ind.: Fides Publishers, 1973.
This text is by a well-known theologian interested in biomedical questions.

Hunt, R., and Arras, J. (eds.).   *Ethical Issues in Modern Medicine.* Palo Alto, Calif.: Mayfield, 1977.
This anthology features a nice introductory overview of ethical theory followed by representative readings on some of the major medical-ethical issues. (Cited below as "Hunt.")

Kass, L. R.   The new biology: What price relieving man's estate? *Science* 174 : 779–88, 1971.
Kass gives a comprehensive overview of the ethical challenges presented by new advances in biomedicine. (Reprinted in Beauchamp.)

Nelson, J. B.   *Human Medicine.* Minneapolis: Augsburg, 1973.
This text by a Protestant theologian looks at several ethical issues, with emphasis on reproductive decisions and genetics.

Ramsey, P.   *Ethics at the Edges of Life: Medical and Legal Intersections.* New Haven, Conn.: Yale University Press, 1978.
A conservative Protestant theologian focuses on ethical issues of life and death in medicine, with special attention to the legal issues and court cases such as *Quinlan.*

Ramsey, P.   *The Patient as Person.* New Haven, Conn.: Yale University Press, 1970.
With a strong emphasis on rights and duties, Ramsey discusses several important ethical issues; his discussions of children as research subjects and of terminal-care decisions have provoked the most controversy.

Reiser, S. J., Dyck, A. J., and Curran, W. J. (Eds.).   *Ethics in Medicine: Historical Perspectives and Contemporary Concerns.* Cambridge, Mass.: MIT Press, 1977.
This large anthology is unique for its inclusion of historical as well as modern writings, showing that there were ethical concerns in medicine before the respirator was invented. Each section ends with some sample cases for discussion. (Cited below as "Reiser.")

Rosner, F.   *Modern Medicine and Jewish Law.* New York: Yeshiva University Press, 1972.
This physician has been one of the more active writers on medical ethics as seen from the Jewish perspective.

Shannon, T. A. (Ed.).   *Bioethics.* New York: Paulist Press, 1976.
This work looks at medical ethics from a Catholic theological perspective.

Vaux, K.   *Biomedical Ethics: Morality for the New Medicine.* New York: Harper and Row, 1974.
A concise book on bioethics written by a Protestant theologian.

Veatch, R. M.   *Case Studies in Medical Ethics.* Cambridge, Mass.: Harvard University Press, 1977.
Veatch uses case studies throughout his book to develop the discussion of the various ethical issues in medicine. Veatch's book also highlights social and public policy concerns as an important area of medical ethics.

Wojcik, J.   *Muted Consent: A Casebook of Modern Medical Ethics.* West Lafayette, Ind.: Purdue University Press, 1978.

Wojcik sees medical issues such as abortion, behavior control, and genetic screening primarily as problems of absent or inadequate informed consent. He begins each chapter with sample case studies.

## Medical Ethics: Journals, Bibliographies, and Reference Works

*Bibliography of Society, Ethics, and the Life Sciences.* Hastings Center, 360 Broadway, Hastings-on-Hudson, NY 10706.

Issued more or less annually, this remains the bibliography best suited to the interested general reader. It is included in the price of membership in the Hastings Center, as is the *Report* (below).

Bioethics and the law: Bibliography, 1974–76. *American Journal of Law and Medicine* 2 : 263–81, 1977.

Duncan, A. S., Dunstan, G. R., and Welbourn, R. B.  *Dictionary of Medical Ethics.* London: Darton, Longman, and Todd, 1977.

This dictionary provides definitions of key ethical terms and short discussions of the main ethical issues.

*Ethics in Science and Medicine.* Pergamon Press, Maxwell House, Fairview Park, Elmsford, NY 10523.

This quarterly journal regularly includes articles on medical ethics.

*Hastings Center Report.* 360 Broadway, Hastings-on-Hudson, NY 10706.

The price of annual membership in the Hastings Center brings six issues of the Report. Regular features besides both brief and in-depth articles are a review of current literature and a case study with pro-and-con commentaries. This remains the best source for the medical reader who wishes to subscribe to only one medical-ethics–oriented journal.

*Journal of Medical Ethics.* Professional and Scientific Publications, 1172 Commonwealth Avenue, Boston, MA 02134.

Published by the Society for the Study of Medical Ethics in England, this quarterly journal features articles on ethical concepts, ethics teaching in medical schools, and case studies.

*Linacre Quarterly.* National Federation of Catholic Physicians' Guilds, 8430 West Capitol Drive, Milwaukee, WI 53222.

This journal has many useful articles on medical ethics, emphasizing the Catholic viewpoint.

*Man and Medicine.* 630 West 168th Street, New York, NY 10032.

Issued more or less quarterly, this journal typically features one or two main articles, each followed by commentaries by several other authors.

Reich, W. T. (Ed.).  *Encyclopedia of Bioethics.* New York: Free Press, 1978.

This massive four-volume work gives generally good, in-depth discussions of ethical concepts and issues.

Walters, L. (Ed.).  *Bibliography of Bioethics.* Detroit: Gale Research Company.

Issued annually, this is the most comprehensive bibliography of medical ethics; its price generally restricts its use to libraries.

## Chapter 1. Why Study Medical Ethics?

Carson, R. A.  What are physicians for? *Journal of the American Medical Association* 238 : 1029–31, 1977.

Carson advocates a whole-person approach to medicine, combining scientific and humanitarian goals.

Pellegrino, E. D.  Toward a reconstruction of medical morality: The primacy of the act of profession and the fact of illness. *Journal of Medicine and Philosophy* 4 : 32–56, 1979.

Medical ethics is not something extra tacked onto medical practice, but arises from the very act of "professing" the practice of medicine.

Pellegrino, E. D.   Educating the humanist physician: An ancient ideal reconsidered. *Journal of the American Medical Association* 227 : 1288–94, 1974.

Pellegrino describes the affective and cognitive domains of a "humanist" education.

Reiser, S. J.   Humanism and fact-finding in medicine. *New England Journal of Medicine* 299 : 950–53, 1978.

A historian shows how the emphasis on objective measurement in medicine has acted to downplay the importance of humanities education.

## Chapter 2. A Method of Ethical Reasoning

Aiken, H.   *Reason and Conduct.* New York: Knopf, 1962.

Aiken develops his four levels of moral discourse.

Jeffrey, R. C.   *The Logic of Decision.* New York: McGraw-Hill, 1965.

A good introduction to Bayesian decision theory.

Ladd, J.   Legalism and medical ethics. *Journal of Medicine and Philosophy* 4 : 70–80, 1979.

Ladd discusses the relationship between law and ethics.

Macklin, R.   Moral concerns and appeals to rights and duties. *Hastings Center Report* 6(October 1976) : 31–38.

Macklin gives a good discussion of the concept of rights.

Schwartz, W. B.   Decision analysis: A look at the chief complaints. *New England Journal of Medicine* 300 : 556–59, 1979.

A discussion of decision analysis and its role in clinical practice.

## Chapter 4. The Doctor–Patient Relationship

Bok, S.   *Lying: Moral Choices in Public and Private Life.* New York: Pantheon Books, 1978.

In addition to an excellent general discussion of lying and deception, Bok looks at placebos (Chapter 5) and lies to the sick and dying (Chapter 15).

Bok, S.   The ethics of giving placebos. *Scientific American* 231(November 1974): 17–23.

A philosopher reviews ethical questions in placebo use in both experimentation and clinical practice. (Reprinted in Reiser, pp. 248–52.)

Brody, H.   *Placebos and the Philosophy of Medicine.* Chicago: The University of Chicago Press, 1980.

Chapter 6 deals with the ethics of giving placebos.

Cassell, E. J.   *The Healer's Art: A New Approach to the Doctor–Patient Relationship.* Philadelphia: J. B. Lippincott, 1976.

This experienced clinician provides a sensitive exploration of the doctor–patient relationship. Some of his conclusions have paternalistic overtones.

Curran, W. J.   Confidentiality and the prediction of dangerousness in psychiatry. *New England Journal of Medicine* 293 : 285–6, 1975.

This lawyer takes a critical look at the Tarasoff case.

Gert, B., and Culver, C. M.   Paternalistic behavior. *Philosophy and Public Affairs* 6 : 45–57, 1976.

A philosopher-physician team looks at how paternalistic behavior can be justified, especially in medicine.

Guttentag, O. E.   The meaning of death in medical theory. *Stanford Medical Bulletin* 17 : 165–170, 1959.

Guttentag develops the notion of "finite freedom" to characterize the doctor–patient relationship as one primarily involving two human beings.

How well are patients' rights observed? *Hospital Practice*, March 1973, pp. 31–50. Summarizes the Patient's Bill of Rights (Appendix III) and documents the need for such a statement.

Kuschner, H., et al. Case studies in bioethics: The homosexual husband and physician confidentiality. *Hastings Center Report* 7(April 1977): 15–17.
A good case for discussion.

McIntosh, J. Patients' awareness and desire for information about diagnosed but undisclosed malignant disease. *Lancet* ii : 300–303, 1976.
Unlike most other studies, McIntosh's found a majority of patients preferring not to be told about malignancy. (The doctors on the ward studied never said "cancer" but always used euphemisms; the patients surveyed seemed to have themselves adopted that practice as their only real alternative.)

Novack, D. H., et al. Changes in physician's attitudes toward telling the cancer patient. *Journal of the American Medical Association* 241 : 897–900, 1979.
Documents the shift in behavior since Oken's study, with 97 percent of physicians responding to this questionnaire preferring a course of revealing the truth.

Oken, D. What to tell cancer patients. *Journal of the American Medical Association* 175 : 1120–28, 1961.
A classic study contrasting patients' desires to know the truth with physician unwillingness to disclose it. (Reprinted in Reiser, pp. 224–32; and Gorovitz, 109–116.)

Pemberton, L. B. A comprehensive understanding of the doctor–patient relationship. *Journal of Religion and Health* 11 : 252–261, 1972.
Pemberton arrives at a position close to the contractual model but begins from a theological view of human relations.

Reich, P., and Kelly, M. J. Suicide attempts by hospitalized medical and surgical patients. *New England Journal of Medicine* 294 : 298–301, 1976.
Summarized in the text.

Siegler, M. Pascal's wager and the hanging of crepe. *New England Journal of Medicine* 293 : 853–57, 1975.
Siegler takes note of a medical practice the opposite of withholding a terminal diagnosis – giving an overly bleak picture to cover oneself if the worst happens.

Veatch, R. M. *Death, Dying and the Biological Revolution*. New Haven, Conn.: Yale University Press, 1976.
Veatch deals with truth-telling and terminal diagnosis in Chapter 6.

Veatch, R. M. Models for ethical medicine in a revolutionary age. *Hastings Center Report* 2(June 1972): 5–7.
Veatch develops the priestly, engineering, and contractual models.

## Chapter 5. Informed Consent

Alfidi, R. J. Informed consent: A study in patient reaction. *Journal of the American Medical Association* 216 : 1325–29, 1971; and Controversy, alternatives, and decisions in complying with the legal doctrine of informed consent. *Radiology* 114 : 23134, 1975.
Alfidi bases some practical recommendations on surveys of patients' reactions to attempts at disclosing risks of invasive diagnostic studies. (Second article reprinted in Beauchamp.)

Breckler, I. A., Price, E. M., and Shore, S. Informed consent: A new majority decision. *Journal of Legal Medicine* (July–August 1973): 37–41.
The Cobbs and Canterbury court decisions are summarized.

Coleman, L. L. Terrified consent. *Physician's World* 2(May 1974): 5.
The discussion provides an example of arguing against informed consent on the

basis that such consent would necessarily frighten the patient (compare Alfidi, above).

Fellner, C. H., and Marshall, J. R.   Kidney donors — the myth of informed consent. *American Journal of Psychiatry* 126 : 1245–51, 1970.
These investigators showed that kidney donors often had emotional, rather than rational, informed reasons for agreeing to donation.

Ingelfinger, F. J.   Informed (but uneducated) consent. *New England Journal of Medicine* 287 : 465–66, 1972.
Ingelfinger is not unsympathetic to the aims of informed consent but notes practical limitations. (Reprinted in Beauchamp.)

Kaplan, S. R., Greenwald, R. A., and Rogers, A. I.   Neglected aspects of informed consent. *New England Journal of Medicine* 296 : 1127, 1977.
These authors seriously misrepresent the actual requirements of informed consent.

Katz, J., with Capron, A. M., and Glass, E. S.   *Experimentation with Human Beings.* New York: Russell Sage Foundation, 1972.
One section of this large reference book and source-book is devoted to informed consent. (A new book by Katz devoted solely to informed consent is to be published in the near future.)

Laforet, E. G.   The fiction of informed consent. *Journal of the American Medical Association* 235 : 1579–85, 1976.
This physician elucidates many of the arguments that we have applied to the so-called doctrine of omniscient decree.

Romano, J.   Reflections on informed consent. *Archives of General Psychiatry* 30 : 129–35, 1974.
Romano brings experience both as clinician and as researcher to bear on the problem.

Robinson, G., and Merav, A.   Informed consent: recall by patients tested postoperatively. *Annals of Thoracic Surgery* 22 : 209–12, 1976.
These surgeons found that patients often had little recollection of the so-called informed consent interview when tested later.

Rubsamen, D. S.   What every doctor needs to know about changes in informed consent. *Medical World News* (Feb. 9, 1973): 66–67.
This brief piece in a "throwaway" journal remains a handy synopsis of both ethical and legal requirements for informed consent.

## Chapter 6. Terminal Care and the Quality of Life

Annas, G. J.   "No-Fault Death: After Saikewicz." *Hastings Center Report* 8(June 1978): 16–18. Annas addresses cases that clarify the intent of *Saikewicz* and accuses physicians of misinterpreting the case.

Annas, G. J.   "The Incompetent's Right to Die — The Case of Joseph Saikewicz." *Hastings Center Report* 8(February 1978): 21–23. A lawyer critiques the Saikewicz decision.

Ashley, B. M., and O'Rourke, K. D.   *Health Care Ethics: A Theological Analysis.* St. Louis: The Catholic Hospital Association, 1977.
Pages 385–390 summarize an approach to the distinction between ordinary and extraordinary means.

Biomedical ethics and the shadow of nazism. *Hastings Center Report* 6(August 1976): supplement, pp. 1–20.
This symposium reviews the historical record and debates the extent to which the Nazi example applies to contemporary ethical debate.

Black, P. M.   Brain death. *New England Journal of Medicine* 299 : 338–44; 393–401, 1978.

A neurosurgeon reviews different brain–death criteria and concludes that they all reliably detect whole-brain death.

Brown, N. K., and Thompson, D. J.   Nontreatment of fever in extended-care facilities. *New England Journal of Medicine* 300 : 1246–50, 1979.
Reviews quantitatively the way quality-of-life decisions to allow death have been made in nursing homes.

Cantor, N. L.   A patient's decision to decline life-saving medical treatment: Bodily integrity versus the preservation of life. *Rutgers Law Review* 26 : 288–264, 1972.
Cantor reviews the legal basis for the right to refuse life-prolonging treatment when one is competent.

Capron, A. M., and Kass, L. R.   A statutory definition of the standards for determining human death: An appraisal and a proposal. *University of Pennsylvania Law Review* 121 : 87–118, 1972.
Discusses ambiguities in some brain-death laws and proposes a model statute, since followed in other states. (Reprinted in Beauchamp.)

Clouser, K. D.   The sanctity of life: An analysis of a concept. *Annals of Internal Medicine* 78 : 119–125, 1973.
Clouser concludes that the sanctity of life concept is either vacuous or contradictory.

Feinberg, J.   The Rights of Animals and Unborn Generations. In W. T. Blackstone (Ed.), *Philosophy and Environmental Crisis*. Athens, Ga.: University of Georgia Press, 1974.
A philosopher argues for basic characteristics that must be present before a being could meaningfully be said to possess rights.

Fletcher, J.   Elective Death. In E. F. Torrey (Ed.), *Ethical Issues in Medicine*. Boston: Little, Brown, 1968.
Joseph Fletcher was one of the first to reject the sanctity of life argument and opt for a  quality of life approach; see also Appendix VIII.

Hudson, R. P.   Death, dying and the zealous phase. *Annals of Internal Medicine* 88 : 696–702, 1978.
Hudson criticizes some excesses of the "death with dignity" movement.

Imbus, S. H., and Zawacki, B. E.   Autonomy for burned patients when survival is unprecedented. *New England Journal of Medicine* 297 : 308–11, 1977.
Patients so severely burned that death was almost inevitable were told this and given the option of dying without heroic therapy. Good cases for discussion.

Jackson, D. L., and Youngner, S.   Patient autonomy and "death with dignity": Some clinical caveats. *New England Journal of Medicine* 301 : 404–408, 1979.
Six excellent case studies reveal pitfalls in applying the principles of autonomy and dignity to patients in intensive care units.

Kass, L. R.   Death as an event: A commentary on Robert Morison. *Science* 173 : 698–702, 1971.
Replying to Morison (see below), Kass notes that Morison has confused the questions of when life is no longer worth living and of when a person is dead.

Kubler-Ross, E.   *On Death and Dying*. New York: Macmillan, 1969.
The classic work on the stages of emotional reaction to death.

McCormick, R. A.   The quality of life, the sanctity of life. *Hastings Center Report* 8(February 1978): 30–36.
A theologian argues that a proper quality-of-life approach is not inconsistent with reverence for life.

McCormick, R. A.   To save or let die: The dilemma of modern medicine. *Journal of the American Medical Association* 229 : 172–76, 1974.
Allowing to die is held appropriate when the individual is not capable of developing any meaningful interpersonal relationships. (Reprinted in Reiser, Beauchamp.)

Morison, R. S. Death: Process or event? *Science* 173 : 694–98, 1971.
Morison describes death as a biologic process, necessarily taking place over time, not at one instant; see also reply by Kass (above).

Pontoppidan, H., et al. Optimum care for hopelessly ill patients. *New England Journal of Medicine* 295 : 362–64, 1976.
Report of one hospital committee trying to develop guidelines for terminal-care decisions. Compare the work of Rabkin (below).

Rabkin, M. T., Gillerman, G., and Rice, N. R. Orders not to resuscitate. *New England Journal of Medicine* 295 : 364–66, 1976.
Proposes a hospital policy for deciding when cardiopulmonary resuscitation should not be carried out on the terminally ill.

Ramsey, P. The Saikewicz precedent: The courts and incompetent patients. *Hastings Center Report* 8(December 1978): 36–42.
Ramsey finds fault with the *Saikewicz* ruling, claiming it fails to protect vital rights of the incompetent, and offers his own decision criteria.

Ramsey, P. *The Patient as Person.* New Haven, Conn.: Yale University Press, 1970.
See Chapter 3, "On (Only) Caring for the Dying."

Supreme Court of New Jersey. *In the matter of Karen Quinlan*, 355A. 2nd 647 (N.J. 1976). (Reprinted in Reiser, Beauchamp.)

Task Force on Death and Dying, Institute of Society, Ethics and the Life Sciences. Refinements in the criteria for the determination of death: An appraisal. *Journal of the American Medical Association* 221 : 48–53, 1972.
Discusses implications of the Harvard criteria for brain death, which first appeared in the same journal, 205 : 337–40, 1968.

Tooley, M. Abortion and infanticide. *Philosophy and Public Affairs* 2 : 37–65, 1972. (Reprinted in Gorovitz, pp. 295–317.)

Veatch, R. M. Death and dying: The legislative options. *Hastings Center Report* 7(October 1977): 5–8.
Considers various attempts to legislate guidelines on living wills, such as the California Natural Death Act (Appendix VII).

Veatch, R. M. *Death, Dying and the Biological Revolution.* New Haven, Conn.: Yale University Press, 1976.
Veatch discusses many issues, notably the conceptual and legal problems of redefining death.

## Chapter 7. Determination of Ethical Participation

Blustein, J. On children and proxy consent. *Journal of Medical Ethics* 4 : 138–40, 1978.
A philosopher provides a basis for consent on behalf of children.

Duff, R. S. Guidelines for deciding care of critically ill or dying patients. *Pediatrics* 64 : 17–23, 1979.
This neonatologist's approach emphasizes family autonomy. See also the earlier paper, coauthored with A. G. M. Campbell, Moral and ethical dilemmas in the special care nursery, *New England Journal of Medicine* 289 : 890–94, 1973. (Reprinted in Reiser, Beauchamp.)

Gustafson, J. M. Mongolism, parental desires, and the right to life. *Perspectives in Biology and Medicine* 16 : 529–557, 1973.
A detailed analysis of the case in which parents refused surgery for an infant with Down's syndrome and duodenal atresia.

Hook, E. B. Behavioral implications of the human XYY genotype. *Science* 179 : 139–50, 1973.
Background information for Case 32.

Jonsen, A. R., et al.  Critical issues in newborn intensive care: A conference report and policy proposal. *Pediatrics* 55 : 756–68, 1975.
These policy guidelines emphasize the role of an ethics advisory board.

Robertson, J. A.  Involuntary euthanasia of defective newborns: A legal analysis. *Stanford Law Review* 271 : 243–269, 1975.
This attorney notes that the practice of withholding "ordinary" care from defective newborns is at odds with legal precedents, and suggests possible modifications in the law. (Reprinted in Hunt.)

Shaw, A.  Dilemmas of "informed consent" in children. *New England Journal of Medicine* 289 : 885–90, 1973.
Shaw uses several excellent case examples to sketch the spectrum of decisions on behalf of children. (Reprinted in Gorovitz, Hunt.)

Valentine, G. H., McClelland, M. A., and Sergovich, F. R.  The growth and development of four XYY infants. *Pediatrics* 48 : 583–94, 1971.
Further background data for Case 32.

## Chapter 9. Behavior Control

Breggin, P. R.  The return of lobotomy and psychosurgery. *Congressional Record* 118, Feb. 24, 1972.
Breggin traces the history of lobotomy and claims that newer techniques in psychosurgery are no better.

Breggin, P. R.  Psychotherapy as applied ethics. *Psychiatry* 34 : 59–74, 1971.

Cases of Thomas R. and Julia serve as focal points in bitter dispute about psychosurgery. *Journal of the American Medical Association* 225 : 916–20, 1973.
This report, along with Vernon Mark's reply (226 : 1121, 1973) outlines the Breggin-Mark debate on psychosurgery.

Culliton, B. J.  Psychosurgery: National Commission issues surprisingly favorable report. *Science* 194 : 299–301, 1976.
This science reporter covers not only the Commission report, but also current theories to explain the successes of psychosurgery.

Curran, W. J.  Psychiatric emergency commitments in Hawaii: Tests of dangerousness. *New England Journal of Medicine* 298 : 265–66, 1978.
Lawyer Curran uses a Hawaii court decision as an example of current trends in commitment statutes.

Delgado, J.  *Physical Control of the Mind.* New York: Harper and Row, 1969.
Delgado supports psychosurgery and electrode implantation for both therapeutic and social-control purposes.

Fish, B.  The "one child, one drug" myth of stimulants in hyperkinesis. *Archives of General Psychiatry* 25 : 193–203, 1971.
Fish reviews questionable basic assumptions about the use of drugs for behavior control.

In the service of the state: The psychiatrist as double agent. *Hastings Center Report* 8(April 1978): supplement.
Report of a conference covering the psychiatrist's role in mental institutions, prisons, and the military.

Klerman, G. L., et al.  Controlling behavior through drugs. (Special section of four articles) *Hastings Center Studies* 2, No. 1, 1974, pp. 65–112.
See especially Robert Veatch's article on the role of social values in judging drug use.

Margolis, J.  Persons and psychosurgery. In S. F. Spicker and H. T. Engelhardt (Eds.), *Philosophical Dimensions of the Neuromedical Sciences.* Holland: D. Reidel, 1976. Pp. 71–84.
This philosopher develops a concept of personhood and uses it to assess psychosurgery.

Mark, V. H.    Brain surgery in aggressive epileptics. *Hastings Center Report* 3(February 1973): 1–5.
 Mark justifies psychosurgery by arguing for an organic basis for some violent behavior.
MBD, drug research and the schools. *Hastings Center Report* 6(June 1976): supplement.
 This conference deals with an attempt to carry out research on drug use in hyperkinetic school children, and the resulting public reaction.
Platt, J.    Beyond freedom and dignity: A revolutionary manifesto. *Center Magazine* 5(March–April 1972): 34–52.
 Platt critically reviews Skinner's book and offers his own perspective on the free-will debate.
Redlich, F., and Mollica, R. F.    Overview: Ethical issues in contemporary psychiatry. *American Journal of Psychiatry* 133 : 125–36, 1976.
 A brief summary of current views on psychosurgery, social control, and other related topics.
Rhinelander, P.    *Is Man Incomprehensible to Man?* San Francisco: Freeman, 1974.
 Rhinelander's philosophical survey of views of human nature touches on Skinnerian behaviorism, which he finds flawed.
Rosenhan, D. L.    On being sane in insane places. *Science* 179 : 250–58, 1973.
 In this now notorious study, normal volunteers arriving at mental hospitals with symptoms of a nonexistent psychiatric syndrome were uniformly judged to be insane.
Rubenstein, J.    What's wrong with the "right to know"? *Medical Dimensions* February 1978, pp. 27–32.
 A psychiatrist, in this misleadingly titled article, points out unfortunate results of protecting the civil rights of mental patients.
Science, politics, and public controversy: The UCLA violence center. *Hastings Center Report* 9(April 1979): supplement.
 This proposed center to carry out research on violence ran afoul of public fears of misuse of the resulting knowledge.
Skinner, B. F.    *Beyond Freedom and Dignity.* New York: Knopf, 1972.
 Skinner presents for a general audience his philosophy of radical behaviorism.
Sweet, W. H.    Treatment of medically intractable mental disease by limited frontal leucotomy: Justifiable? *New England Journal of Medicine* 289 : 1117–25, 1973.
 A neurosurgeon defends the modern forms of psychosurgery in patients who have not responded to other treatment.
Szasz, T. S.    *The Myth of Mental Illness.* New York: Harper and Row, 1974.
 Szasz provides a classic argument that mental "illness" is really social maladjustment and that any involuntary psychiatric practices constitute social control, not therapy.
Tancredi, L. R., and Slaby, A. E.    *Ethical Policy in Mental Health Care.* New York: Prodist, 1977.
 These authors address many ethical problems in the mental health field.
Ulrich, R., Stachik, T., and Mabry, J.    *Control of Human Behavior* (3 vols.). Glenview, Ill.: Scott Foresman, 1974.
 A collection of essays on both technical and philosophical issues in behavior control, with special emphasis on applications to education.

## Chapter 10. Control of Reproduction

Ashley, B. M., and O'Rourke, K. D.    *Health Care Ethics: A Theological Analysis.* St. Louis: Catholic Hospital Association, 1978.
 Detailed discussion of the Catholic position on contraception, sterilization, and abortion is included; see especially pp. 266–75 regarding the rhythm method.

Behrman, S. J.  Artificial insemination and public policy. *New England Journal of Medicine* 300 : 619–20, 1979.

Behrman argues for the need for better guidelines for artificial insemination programs, such as for better genetic screening of donors.

Berger, L. R.  Abortion in America: The effects of restrictive funding. *New England Journal of Medicine* 298 : 1474–77, 1978.

Having lost the battle in the Supreme Court, anti-abortionists are winning the political fight to cut off public funds for abortions. A physician analyzes practical consequences of this policy.

Bok, S.  Ethical problems in abortion. *Hastings Center Studies* 2, no. 1, 1974, pp. 33–52.

This philosopher adopts a consequentialist approach to abortion. (Reprinted in Reiser.)

Callahan, D.  *Abortion: Law, Choice, and Morality.* New York: Macmillan, 1970.

A detailed discussion of social and moral issues drawing upon abortion experience in other nations; however, it was published prior to the U.S. Supreme Court abortion rulings.

Curran, W. J.  Legal abortion: The continuing battle. *New England Journal of Medicine* 290 : 1301–2, 1974.

This lawyer reviews legal issues that followed in the wake of the Supreme Court rulings.

Curran, W. J.  Sterilization of the poor: Judge Gesell's roadblock. *New England Journal of Medicine* 291 : 25–26, 1974.

Report of a court case severely restricting the use of public funds for sterilization.

Curran, W. J.  Birth of a healthy child due to negligent failure of "pill": Benefit or loss? *New England Journal of Medicine* 285 : 1063–64, 1971.

Good case for discussion.

Dyck, A. J.  Procreative rights and population policy. *Hastings Center Studies* 1, no. 1, 1973, pp. 74–82.

Dyck opposes coercive population-control policies.

Dyck, A. J.  Perplexities of the would-be liberal in abortion. *Journal of Reproductive Medicine* 8 : 351–54, 1972.

Dyck finds that so-called liberal values conflict on abortion.

Engelhardt, H. T.  Viability, abortion, and the difference between a fetus and an infant. *American Journal of Obstetrics and Gynecology* 116 : 429–34, 1973.

Engelhardt argues for the morally relevant difference between fetus and newborn, based in part on social roles.

Feinberg, J. (Ed.).  *The Problem of Abortion.* Belmont, Calif.: Wadsworth, 1973.

A collection of some of the best philosophical essays on the abortion issue.

Ingram, I. M.  Abortion games: An inquiry into the working of the act. *Lancet* ii : 969, 1971.

A "games-doctors-play" discussion of how a restrictive abortion law was manipulated by doctors in England.

Lesbian couples: Should help extend to AID? *Journal of Medical Ethics* 4 : 91–95, 1978.

Case discussion by a panel including several physicians and a lesbian spokeswoman.

McCormick, R. A.  Abortion: Rules for debate. *America* July 22, 1978, pp. 26–30.

A Catholic theologian decries the raising of political slogans and false issues instead of reasoned inquiry.

McGarrah, R. E.  Voluntary female sterilization: Abuses, risks, and guidelines. *Hastings Center Report* 4(June 1974): 5–7.

This discussion emphasizes problems in insuring informed consent.

Moore, E. C., et al.  Abortion: The new ruling. *Hastings Center Report* 3(April 1973): 4–7.

Brief immediate reactions by several experts to the Supreme Court abortion ruling.

Nelson, J. B.   *Human Medicine*. Minneapolis: Augsburg, 1973.
Chapter 3 deals with religious views on artificial insemination.

Peck, S.   Voluntary female sterilization: Attitudes and legislation. *Hastings Center Report* 4(June 1974): 8–10.
A survey of then-current practices.

Plain talk about ethics in practice. *Patient Care* March 15, 1978, pp. 186–215.
In this panel discussion about ethical problems in primary-care medicine, the first case deals with a teenager asking the family doctor for birth control pills without telling her parents.

Ramsey, P.   Abortion: A review article. *The Thomist* 37 : 174–226, 1973.
This conservative Protestant theological ethicist discusses the point at which a fetus receives a soul and so becomes human.

Robertson, J.   After Edelin: Little guidance. *Hastings Center Report* 7(June 1977): 15–17.
The Edelin case was a controversial prosecution of an obstetrician for reportedly deliberately failing to save a viable fetus during a late abortion.

*Roe v. Wade*, 410 U.S. 116, 1973.
This is the leading Supreme Court decision on abortion, in which state laws restricting early abortions were declared unconstitutional invasions of a woman's privacy. [Reprinted in Reiser, Hunt; excerpts in Feinberg (above).]

Tooley, M.   Abortion and infanticide. *Philosophy and Public Affairs* 2 : 37–65, 1972.
Tooley argues that fetuses and newborns are equally incapable of being bearers of rights. [Reprinted in Gorovitz; revised version in Feinberg (above).]

Thomson, J. J.   A defense of abortion. *Philosophy and Public Affairs* 1 : 47–66, 1971.
Thomson tries to separate the morality of abortion from the question of the rights of the fetus. [Reprinted in Reiser, Hunt, Feinberg (above), Beauchamp.]

## Chapter 11. Research on Human Subjects

Altman, L. K.   Auto-experimentation: An unappreciated tradition in medical science. *New England Journal of Medicine* 286 : 346–52, 1972.
Historical examples of scientists who experimented upon themselves, sometimes with fatal results.

Barber, B., et al.   *Research on Human Subjects*. New York: Russell Sage Foundation, 1973.
Emphasis is on social implications of research policies; includes Sullivan's study of the relation between risk-benefit ratio and the social class of subjects.

Beecher, H. K.   Ethics and clinical research. *New England Journal of Medicine* 274 : 1354–60, 1966.
Beecher's "whistle-blowing" article provides many interesting cases for discussion. (Reprinted in Reiser.)

Byar, D. P., et al.   Randomized clinical trials. *New England Journal of Medicine* 295 : 74–80, 1976.
These authors take issue with Weinstein and others, insisting that randomized trials are still the best way to get reliable data and hence to protect the research subject.

Capron, A. M.   Medical research in prisons: Should a moratorium be called? *Hastings Center Report* 3(June 1973): 4–6.
A lawyer reviews the problems of consent among prisoners.

Cardon, P. U., Dommel, F. W., and Trumble, R. J.   Injuries to research subjects. *New England Journal of Medicine* 295 : 650–54, 1976.

This survey of investigators documented the rarity of serious harm to research subjects.

Curran, W. J. Experimentation becomes a crime. *New England Journal of Medicine* 292 : 300–1, 1975.

Curran criticizes a state law prohibiting fetal research.

Curran, W. J. The Tuskegee syphilis study. *New England Journal of Medicine* 287 : 730–31, 1973.

The Tuskegee study is one of the most frequently cited examples of violations of the rights of subjects.

Department of Health, Education and Welfare, National Institutes of Health. Protection of human subjects: Policies and procedures. *Federal Register* 38 (no. 221) November 16, 1973.

The NIH proposed guidelines for research on children, prisoners, fetuses, and the mentally ill were the first major attempt to formulate national policy, prior to the creation of the National Commission.

Diamond, E. F. Redefining the issues in fetal experimentation. *Journal of the American Medical Association* 236 : 281–83, 1976.

A pediatrician proposes middle-ground approaches to fetal research.

Fletcher, J. Human experimentation: Ethics in the consent situation. *Law and Contemporary Problems* 32(Autumn 1967): 620–49.

Fletcher looks at the setting in which research occurs to discuss what makes for valid consent.

Freund, P. A. (Ed.) *Experimentation with Human Subjects.* New York: George Braziller, 1970.

This well-known collection features several classic essays, notably one by Hans Jonas (reprinted in Reiser, Hunt, and Gorovitz).

Fried, C. *Medical Experimentation: Personal Integrity and Social Policy.* New York: American Elsevier, 1974.

Fried bases his views on research on his "right to personal care," which in turn emphasizes patient dignity and autonomy.

Ingelfinger, F. J. Ethics of human experimentation defined by National Commission. *New England Journal of Medicine* 296 : 44–45, 1977.

This editorial is a useful synopsis of the Commission reports on fetuses, children, prisoners, and psychosurgery.

Jonsen, A. R. Research involving children: Recommendations of the national commission . . . *Pediatrics* 62 : 131–36, 1978.

A thorough discussion of research in children by one of the Commission members.

Katz, J., with Capron, A. M., and Glass, E. S. *Experimentation with Human Beings.* New York: Russell Sage Foundation, 1972.

A large source book, full of various codes of ethics and key court decisions as well as several important case studies.

Krugman, S., and Giles, J. P. Viral hepatitis, type B: Further observations on natural history and prevention. *New England Journal of Medicine* 288 : 755–60, 1973.

This experiment arose from the celebrated Willowbrook case in which retarded children were infected with hepatitis, with parental consent, in hopes of developing a vaccine. The editorial, 288 : 791–92, defends both the ethics of the research and the ethics of the journal in publishing it.

Levine, R. J. Clarifying the concepts of research ethics. *Hastings Center Report* 9(June 1979): 21–26.

Levine summarizes some of the conceptual conclusions that emerge from the work of the Commission in the course of ruling on the ethics of research on children, prisoners, fetuses, and psychosurgery.

Lowe, C. U., Alexander, D., and Mishkin, B. Nontherapeutic research in children: An ethical dilemma. *Journal of Pediatrics* 84 : 468–72, 1974.

These authors tried to reconcile problems of consent in minors with the benefits of research in this age group.

McCormick, R. A.   Proxy consent in the experimental situation. *Perspectives in Biology and Medicine* 18 : 2–20, 1974.
McCormick argues for a duty to aid the public welfare, and derives from this a justification for some sorts of research in children where they do not directly benefit. (Reprinted in Beauchamp.)

Murton, T.   Prison Doctors. In M. B. Visscher (Ed.), *Humanistic Perspectives in Medical Ethics*. Buffalo: Prometheus Books, 1972.
Murton describes some horror stories of exploitative research on prisoners.

Ramsey, P.   Children as research subjects: A reply to Richard McCormick. *Hastings Center Report* 6(August 1976): 21–30.
Ramsey holds that no research on children not for their therapeutic benefit is ethically justifiable. The Ramsey–McCormick debate continued in subsequent issues of this journal.

Schwartz, A. H.   Children's concepts of research hospitalization. *New England Journal of Medicine* 287 : 589–92, 1972.
Schwartz studied what children were actually told and understood about their status as research subjects.

Tiefel, H. O.   The cost of fetal research: Ethical considerations. *New England Journal of Medicine* 294 : 85–90, 1976.
This philosopher argues that fetal research (if nontherapeutic from the fetus's standpoint) is immoral, based on the rights of the fetus and other considerations.

Veterans Administration Cooperative Study Group on Antihypertensive Agents. Effects of treatment on morbidity in hypertension. *Journal of the American Medical Association* 202 : 1028, 1967.
This is the basis for Case 43.

Weinstein, M. C.   Allocation of subjects in medical experiments. *New England Journal of Medicine* 291 : 1278–85, 1974.
Weinstein proposed alternatives to randomization as valid research strategies — but see the rebuttal by Byar.

Zelen, M.   A new design for randomized clinical trials. *New England Journal of Medicine* 300 : 1242–45, 1979.
Zelen proposed research designs that would remove the need to obtain consent from some subjects, drawing sharp rebuttals (300 : 1272–73 and 301 : 786–88, 1979). Zelen erred in assuming that manipulation of the research-design component of the ethics of research could remove the need to deal with the informed-consent component.

## Chapter 12. Allocation of Scarce Resources

Childress, J. F.   Who shall live when not all can live? *Soundings* 53 : 339–362, 1970.
Childress reviews the microallocation issue and concludes in favor of random selection. (Reprinted in Reiser.)

Clouser, K. D.   Medical ethics: Some uses, abuses, and limitations. *New England Journal of Medicine* 293 : 384–87, 1975.
A philosopher outlines the scope of medical ethics, citing especially its inherent limitations.

Dukeminier, J., and Sanders, D.   Organ transplantation: A proposal for routine salvaging of cadaver organs. *New England Journal of Medicine* 279 : 413–19, 1968.
These authors deal with another scarce resource — cadaver organs for transplantation.

Engelhardt, H. T.   Rights to health care: A critical appraisal. *Journal of Medicine and Philosophy* 4 : 113–17, 1979.

Engelhardt gives an overview of the right-to-health-care issue (see also bibliography for Chapter 16).

Fried, C.   *Medical Experimentation: Personal Integrity and Social Policy.* New York: American Elsevier, 1974.
Fried develops the concept of the "right to personal care" and the two-level, decision-making process for resource allocation.

Illich, I.   *Medical Nemesis.* New York: Pantheon Books, 1976.
Illich launches the classic and controversial attack on the medical establishment for its "expropriation of health" and the social ills that result. (Excerpts in Hunt.)

Jonsen, A. R.   The totally implantable artificial heart. *Hastings Center Report* 3 (November 1973): 1–4.
The artificial-heart case provides excellent material for detailed discussion.

Kass, L. R.   The new biology: What price relieving man's estate? *Science* 174 : 779–88, 1971.
Kass outlines the microallocation and macroallocation decisions facing health care on a global basis. (Reprinted in Beauchamp.)

Lalonde, M.   *A New Perspective on the Health of Canadians.* Ottawa: Government of Canada, 1974.
This policy summary by Canada's national health minister is an excellent example of thoughtful economic analysis of health-care needs.

Leibel, R. L.   Thanatology and medical economics. *New England Journal of Medicine* 296 : 511–13, 1977.
Leibel denies that scarcity of resources is a reality, and then confuses resource-allocation decisions with decisions to stop treatment for the patient's own benefit. A primer of errors to avoid in ethical reasoning. (See also the ensuing letters to the editor, 296 : 1237–40.)

Outka, G.   Social justice and equal access to health care. *Journal of Religious Ethics* 2 : 11–32, 1974.
Outka gives alternative principles of allocation, concluding that the special features of health care favor distribution on the basis of need. (Reprinted in Reiser, Beauchamp.)

Powles, J.   On the limitations of modern medicine. *Science, Medicine and Man* 1 : 1–30, 1973.
Powles summarizes ways in which improvements in health, often attributed to medical science, in fact resulted from other social or ecological factors.

Rescher, N.   The allocation of exotic medical life-saving therapy. *Ethics* 79 : 173–86, 1969.
Rescher gives a thorough defense of the social-worth approach to microallocation on utilitarian grounds. (Reprinted in Reiser, Hunt, Gorovitz.)

Scarce medical resources. *Columbia Law Review* 69 : 620–92, 1969.
An excellent summary of legal issues and possible legislative solutions to allocation problems on the micro level.

## Chapter 13. Euthanasia

Beauchamp, T. L., and Childress, J. F.   *Principles of Biomedical Ethics.* New York: Oxford University Press, 1979.
Pages 105–17 provide an illuminating discussion of the killing–letting die distinction.

Beauchamp, T. L., and Davidson, A. I.   The definition of euthanasia. *Journal of Medicine and Philosophy* 4 : 294–312, 1979.
These philosophers develop a detailed formal definition of "euthanasia" to avoid several possible confusions.

Behnke, J. A., and Bok, S.  *The Dilemmas of Euthanasia.* New York: Anchor Press, 1975.

These editors present several essays on euthanasia, covering medical and legal issues.

Freeman, J. M.  Is there a right to die — quickly?; and R. E. Cooke, Whose suffering? *Journal of Pediatrics* 80 : 904–7, 1972.

These physicians state the positions that are paraphrased in Case 54.

Jackson, D. L., and Youngner, S.  Patient autonomy and "death with dignity": Some clinical caveats. *New England Journal of Medicine* 301 : 404–8, 1979.

This sensitive article describes six intensive care cases and analyzes pitfalls for the uncritical use of euthanasia.

Kamisar, Y.  Some nonreligious views against proposed "mercy-killing" legislation. *Human Life Review* 2 (Spring 1976): 71–114; (Summer 1976): 34–63.

A forceful summary of objections to legalizing active euthanasia. (Reprinted in Beauchamp.)

Kohl, M. (Ed.).  *Beneficent Euthanasia.* Buffalo: Prometheus Books, 1975.

Kohl gathers essays covering euthanasia from religious, philosophical, medical, and legal viewpoints.

Menzel, P. T.  Are killing and letting die morally different in medical contexts? *Journal of Medicine and Philosophy* 4 : 269–93, 1979.

This philosopher offers an excellent synthesis of the views of Rachels, Trammell and others.

Poe, W. D.  Marantology: A needed specialty. *New England Journal of Medicine* 286 : 102–3, 1972.

Poe argues that success-oriented physicians cannot humanely treat hopelessly ill patients because death, or lack of cure, is viewed as failure. A new type of physician who can accept such "failure" is needed to treat such patients with empathy and compassion.

Rachels, J.  Active and passive euthanasia. *New England Journal of Medicine* 292 : 78–80, 1975.

Rachels argues forcefully for the absence of any significant moral distinction between active and passive euthanasia. (Reprinted in Beauchamp.)

Ramsey, P.  The indignity of "death with dignity." *Hastings Center Studies* 2, no. 2, 1974, pp. 49–67.

Ramsey takes issue with the notion of "death with dignity" from a religious perspective; see also in the same issue the replies by Morison and Kass.

Relman, A. S.  Michigan's sensible "living will." *New England Journal of Medicine* 300 : 1270–1, 1979.

This medical editor endorses a bill to formalize mechanisms for medical treatment decisions, including passive euthanasia, on behalf of incompetent patients. The responses in the same journal, 301 : 788–89, 1979, include some of the same arguments that are used against active-euthanasia legislation.

Trammell, R. L.  The nonequivalency of saving life and not taking life. *Journal of Medicine and Philosophy* 4 : 251–62, 1979.

This philosopher takes a position contrary to Rachels's. However, some of his conclusions arise from a failure to make a distinction, as we have done, between "letting die" and "not saving."

## Chapter 14. Mass Screening Programs

Fletcher, J.  Moral and ethical problems of prenatal diagnosis. *Clinical Genetics* 8 : 251–57, 1975.

Fletcher relates screening to the issues of abortion and neonatal euthanasia, and also to questions of genetic "health" and social norms.

Golbus, M. S., et al. Prenatal genetic diagnosis in 3000 amniocenteses. *New England Journal of Medicine* 300 : 157–63, 1979.

This review of amniocentesis notes the variety of reasons for doing the procedure and its relative safety. (Other papers have shown a higher rate of side effects due to amniocentesis.)

Hemphill, M. Pretesting for Huntington's disease. *Hastings Center Report* 3(June 1973): 12–13.

Hemphill looks at both sides of the debate — see Case 57.

Institute of Society, Ethics and the Life Sciences, Research Group. Ethical and social issues in screening for genetic disease. *New England Journal of Medicine* 286 : 1129–32, 1972.

Offers guidelines for ethical screening programs. See also accompanying editorial, same journal, 286 : 1361–62. (Reprinted in Beauchamp.)

Lappe, M., and Roblin, R. O. Newborn genetic screening as a concept in health care delivery: A critique. *Birth Defects Original Article Series*, 10(6)1–24, 1974.

These authors cast doubt on some assumptions about the value of newborn screening, focusing particularly on PKU screening.

Leonard, C. O., et al. Genetic counseling: A consumer's view. *New England Journal of Medicine* 287 : 433–39, 1972.

An important study of the results of genetic counseling, showing how many patients fail to understand the information or fail to make use of it in their decisions.

Ramsey, P. Screening: An Ethicist's View. In B. Hilton and D. Callahan (Eds.), *Ethical Issues in Human Genetics*. New York: Plenum, 1973.

Ramsey attacks "statistical morality" as it is embodied in genetic screening followed by abortion.

Roblin, R. O. The Boston XYY case. *Hastings Center Report* 5(August 1975): 5–8.

Roblin reviews a controversial experimental screening project designed to detect the XYY chromosome abnormality. For more on XYY see Chapter 7 and Case 32.

Turner, J. H., Hayashi, T. T., and Pogoloff, D. D. Legal and social issues in medical genetics. *American Journal of Obstetrics and Gynecology* 134 : 83–99, 1979.

These authors review the state of the art of prenatal diagnosis, with special emphasis on amniocentesis and on legal issues.

Whitten, C. F. Sickle-cell programming: An imperiled promise. *New England Journal of Medicine* 288 : 318–19, 1973.

This editorial and the following editorial correspondence, 288 : 971–2, highlight especially the so-called right not to know and raise questions about the real value of knowledge of one's carrier status for a genetic disease.

## Chapter 15. Genetic Engineering

Berg, P., et al. Potential biohazards of recombinant DNA molecules. *Science* 185 : 303, 1974.

These scientists sounded the initial warnings about possible hazards of recombinant-DNA research.

Callahan, D., et al. In vitro fertilization. *Hastings Center Report* 8(October 1978): 7–17.

Paul Ramsey, Marc Lappe, and other experts comment in the wake of the Louise Brown birth.

Chargaff, E., et al. Disputations: Research on recombinant DNA. *Man and Medicine* 2(Winter 1977)77–132.

Five scientists take exception to views expressed in the text, arguing that the hazards of recombinant-DNA research are real and formidable.

Cohen, C. When may research be stopped? *New England Journal of Medicine* 296 : 1203–10, 1977.

Cohen echoes the majority view of the scientific community and argues that, with proper safeguards, there is no justification for banning recombinant-DNA research.

Crow, J. F.   Rates of genetic change under selection. *Proceedings of the National Academy of Sciences* 59 : 655–661, 1968; and   The effects of a changing environment on man's genetic future. *Bioscience* 21 : 107, 1971.
   Crow, a geneticist, offers data to demonstrate fallacies in many fears regarding the deterioration of the human gene pool.

Fletcher, J.   *The Ethics of Genetic Control.* Garden City, N.Y.: Anchor, 1974.
   Fletcher argues for increased use of genetic engineering as the best manifestation of man's rational nature.

Fletcher, J. C.   Ethics and amniocentesis for fetal sex identification. *New England Journal of Medicine* 301 : 550–53, 1979.
   Fletcher has misgivings about using amniocentesis for choosing the sex of babies, but sees no firm ground for denying this technique to parents who request it.

Friedman, T., and Roblin, R.   Gene therapy for human genetic disease? *Science* 175 : 949–55, 1972.
   These authors note the spectrum of negative-eugenics technology, and stress the need to respect our ignorance of possible deleterious consequences.

Genetics and the quality of life. World Council of Churches, Study Encounter 53, Vol. X, No. 1, 1974.
   Reports a symposium among theologians, physicians, and scientists.

Human genetic engineering: No brave new world but brand new medical potentials. *Medical World News* (May 11, 1973): 45–57.
   This account of genetic-engineering possibilities emphasizes benefits and gives short shrift to possible hazards.

Lappé, M.   Genetic knowledge and the concept of health. *Hastings Center Report* 3(September 1973): 1–3.
   Lappé tries to define a meaningful concept of genetic health.

Lappé, M.   Moral obligation and the fallacies of "genetic control." *Theological Studies* 33 : 411–27, 1972.
   Lappé reminds us of biologic facts that render some moral arguments on genetics unfounded.

Lappé, M., and Steinfels, P.   Choosing the sex of our children. *Hastings Center Report* 4(February 1974): 1–4.
   These authors focus on social and ethical consequences of sex selection.

Ramsey, P.   Shall we "reproduce"? *Journal of the American Medical Association* 220 : 1346–50, 1480–85, 1972.
   Ramsey takes a dim view of in vitro fertilization, emphasizing the "unethical means" argument.

Twiss, S. B.   Parental responsibility for genetic health. *Hastings Center Report* 4(February 1974): 9–11.
   Twiss discusses the conflict between parental procreation rights and responsibility for the unborn when parents carry known deleterious genes.

## Chapter 16. Social Responsibility

Annas, G. J.   Legalizing Laetrile for the terminally ill. *Hastings Center Report* 7(December 1977): 19–20.
   Should laetrile be made an exception to the rules prohibiting the sale of drugs scientifically held to be ineffective?

Badgley, R. F., and Wolfe, S.   The Doctor's Right to Strike. In E. F. Torrey (Ed.), *Ethical Issues in Medicine.* Boston: Little, Brown, 1968.
   These authors use the 1962 Saskatchewan strike as an introduction to the issue.

Bazell, R. J.   Health radicals: Crusade to shift medical power to the people. *Science* 173 : 506–9, 1971.
   Reviews the activities and posture of the radical health movement.
Bean, W. B.   The Medical Profession and the Drug Industry. In E. F. Torrey (Ed.), *Ethical Issues in Medicine.* Boston: Little, Brown, 1968.
   Bean looks at some Congressional hearings to characterize needs in drug regulation.
Beauchamp, T. L., and Faden, R. R.   The right to health and the right to health care. *Journal of Medicine and Philosophy* 4 : 118-31, 1979.
   These authors deny the existence of a "natural" right to health care and see such a right instead as an outgrowth of social policy.
Bruhn, J. G., and Smith, D. C.   Social Ethics for Medical Educators. In M. B. Visscher (Ed.), *Humanistic Perspectives in Medical Ethics.* Buffalo: Prometheus Books, 1972.
   A brief discussion of the social responsibilities of the medical education system.
Butler, R. N.   *Why Survive? Being Old in America.* New York: Harper and Row, 1975.
   A gerontologist attacks the inadequacies of the current health system's care of the aged.
Chapman, C. B., and Talmadge, J. M.   The Evolution of the Right-to-Health Concept in the U.S. In M. B. Visscher (Ed.), *Humanistic Perspectives in Medical Ethics.* Buffalo: Prometheus Books, 1972.
   This historical review highlights legislative initiatives and the reactions of the medical establishment. (Reprinted in Reiser.)
Childress, J. F.   A right to health care? *Journal of Medicine and Philosophy* 4 : 132–47, 1979.
   Childress notes that other moral considerations besides a moral right to health care may be used to justify the establishment of a legal right to health care.
Curran, W. J.   The "class-action" approach to protecting health care consumers — the right to psychiatric treatment. *New England Journal of Medicine* 286 : 26, 1972.
   Curran notes the role of the courts in assuring the right to treatment. A good case for group discussion.
Curran, W. J.   The right to health in national and international law. *New England Journal of Medicine* 284 : 1258, 1971.
   This lawyer reviews the legal status of the right to health care.
Daniels, N.   On the picket lines: Are doctors' strikes ethical? *Hastings Center Report* 8(February 1978): 24–29.
   A philosopher finds strikes justifiable if needed to serve patient-care needs, but not to protect doctors' autonomy or incomes.
Dubler, N. N.   Depriving prisoners of medical care: A "cruel and unusual" punishment. *Hastings Center Report* 9(October 1979)7–10.
   Prisoners are the only group with a constitutional right to health care; but in practice this right is seldom fully honored.
Engelhardt, H. T.   Rights to health care: A critical appraisal. *Journal of Medicine and Philosophy* 4 : 113–17, 1979.
   Engelhardt introduces a special issue of this journal devoted to the topic of the right to health care.
Freidson, E.   *Profession of Medicine.* New York: Harper and Row, 1970.
   A sociologist attempts to analyze the essential elements that make medicine a profession and how it functions as a social institution.
Fried, C.   Equality and rights in health care. *Hastings Center Report* 6(February 1976): 29–34.
   Fried supports a decent-minimum interpretation of the right to health care. (Reprinted in Reiser.)

Fried, C. *Medical Experimentation: Personal Integrity and Social Policy.* New York: American Elsevier, 1974.

See Chapters 3 and 4 for the development of the concept of "personal care."

Friedlies, O. P. (Letter to the editor: Holistic medicine.) *Journal of the American Medical Association* 242 : 1490, 1979.

One physician gives a limited view of the profession's social responsibilities.

Fuchs, V. R. *Who Shall Live? Health, Economics, and Social Choice.* New York: Basic Books, 1974.

A noted health economist points out that value issues, not economic efficiency judgments, underlie social policy on health expenditures.

Green, R. Health Care and Justice in Contract Theory Perspective. In R. M. Veatch and R. Branson (Eds.), *Ethics and Health Policy.* Cambridge, Mass.: Ballinger, 1976.

Green bases his view of justice in health care on John Rawls' theory of justice.

Greenberg, D. S. Kennedy urges further pharmaceutical regulation. *New England Journal of Medicine* 290 : 1211–12, 1974.

Greenberg reports on Senate hearings critical of the drug industry.

Halberstam, M. J. Liberal thought, radical theory and medical practice. *New England Journal of Medicine* 284 : 1180–85, 1971.

A physician notes that the goals of economic efficiency may conflict with the goals of personal and humane care.

Jonsen, A., and Jameton, A. L. Social and political responsibilities of physicians. *Journal of Medicine and Philosophy* 2 : 376–400, 1977.

A good overview of the different sorts of responsibilities involving health professionals.

Kaplan, H. R. The Fee-for-Service System. In M. B. Visscher (Ed.), *Humanistic Perspectives in Medical Ethics.* Buffalo: Prometheus Books, 1972.

Kaplan takes a generally critical view of the traditional American system for financing health care.

Kline, N. S., and Gordon, M. Amphetamine quotas and medical freedom. *Hastings Center Report* 3(December 1973): 8–10.

A case study of a conflict between the physician's freedom to prescribe on an individual basis, and the social desirability of restricting frequently abused drugs.

Kristein, M. M., Arnold, C. B., and Wynder, E. L. Health economics and preventive care. *Science* 195 : 457–62, 1977.

These authors argue that increased attention to preventive health care is one way to decrease health costs.

Livingston, G. Medicine and the Military. In M. B. Visscher (Ed.), *Humanistic Perspectives in Medical Ethics.* Buffalo: Prometheus Books, 1972.

An analysis of the conflict of responsibilities inherent in the role of the military physician.

Malone, P. Death row and the medical model. *Hastings Center Report* 9(October 1979): 5–6.

Should physicians cooperate with prison authorities in killing condemned convicts "humanely" by means of lethal injection?

McCullough, L. B. Rights, health care, and public policy. *Journal of Medicine and Philosophy* 4 : 204–15, 1979.

McCullough looks at both historical sources and current writings on this topic.

Mitchell, B. M., and Schwartz, W. B. Strategies for financing national health insurance: Who wins and who loses. *New England Journal of Medicine* 295 : 866–71, 1976.

Different national health-insurance plans will redistribute wealth in different ways, some favoring the poor and some the wealthy; this needs to be considered in choosing a plan.

Mechanic, D. Approaches to controlling the costs of medical care: Short-range and long-range alternatives. *New England Journal of Medicine* 298 : 249–54, 1978.

While many different approaches might keep down the cost of care in the long run, in the short run some sort of rationing plan may have to be used.

Navarro, V.  Women in health care. *New England Journal of Medicine* 292 : 398–402, 1975.
Navarro notes that women seldom occupy decision-making positions in the health-care system and calls for increased institutional democracy.

Outka, G.  Social justice and equal access to health care. *Journal of Religious Ethics* 2(1)11–32, 1974.
Outka considers different ways of distributing health care and opts for equal access as the most just. (Reprinted in Reiser, Beauchamp.)

Rosenfield, A. G.  Modern medicine and the delivery of health services: Lessons from the developing world. *Man and Medicine* 2 : 279–96, 1977.
A look at health-care problems in developing countries, where Western medical models may not be applicable.

Ruddick, W.  Doctors' rights and work. *Journal of Medicine and Philosophy* 4 : 192–203, 1979.
Ruddick argues that legitimate rights of doctors to govern their own work need not conflict with patients' rights to care.

Rutstein, D. D., et al.  Measuring the quality of medical care. *New England Journal of Medicine* 294 : 582–88, 1976.
This group outlines practical techniques for measuring the quality of medical care.

Sade, R. M.  Medical care as a right: A refutation. *New England Journal of Medicine* 285 : 1288–92, 1971.
This physician gives an extreme libertarian argument against the right to health care. See also the ensuing letters to the editor, 286 : 488–93, 1972. (Reprinted in Reiser, Gorovitz.)

Sagan, L. A., and Jonsen, A.  Medical ethics and torture. *New England Journal of Medicine* 294 : 1427–30, 1976.
These authors claim that American physicians can take some effective steps to protest participation of physicians in government-inflicted torture in other nations.

Schwartz, H.  Health care in America: A heretical diagnosis. *Saturday Review* (August 14, 1971) 14 ff.
Attacks the view that the U.S. is lagging behind European countries in guaranteeing health care to its citizens.

Sissons, P. L.  The place of medicine in the American prison: Ethical issues in the treatment of offenders. *Journal of Medical Ethics* 2 : 173–79, 1976.
Sissons notes that the "medical model" does not always apply to the role of the prison physician.

Stevens, R.  *American Medicine and the Public Interest*. New Haven, Conn.: Yale University Press, 1971.
Stevens traces the history of organized medicine in the U.S. and its often reactionary stance on social change.

Veatch, R. M.  Just social institutions and the right to health care. *Journal of Medicine and Philosophy* 4 : 170–73, 1979.
Veatch relates different views of the right to health care to theories of social justice.

Waitzkin, H., and Modell, H.  Medicine, socialism, and totalitarianism: Lessons from Chile. *New England Journal of Medicine* 291 : 171–77, 1974.
While their sympathy for the socialist Allende government of Chile brought strong rebuttals, these authors' analysis of how health policy is linked to social change is useful.

## Chapter 17. Defining Health and Disease

Akisal, H. S., and McKinney, W. T.   Depressive disorders: Toward a unified hypothesis. *Science* 182 : 20–29, 1973.
The authors review research on depression and conclude that it can be understood only by a model that takes into account its biochemical, genetic, and social aspects.

Beauchamp, T. L., and Walters, L. (Eds.).   *Contemporary Issues in Bioethics.* Encino, Calif.: Dickinson Publishing, 1978.
Chapter 3, "Health and Disease" includes four good papers on the concept of health and three important papers on the role of values in the concept of disease and the distinction between disease and illness; authors include Callahan, Engelhardt, Dubos, Kass, and Boorse.

Blum, H. L.   *Expanding Health Care Horizons.* Oakland, Calif.: Third Party Associates, 1976.
Blum develops a concept of public health policy and planning that is based on the systems-hierarchy approach used in this chapter.

Brody, H.   The systems view of man: Implications for medicine, science, and ethics. *Perspectives in Biology and Medicine* 17 : 71–92, 1973.
This paper develops the systems-hierarchy approach to health and disease.

Cassell, E. J.   Illness and disease. *Hastings Center Report* 6(April 1976): 27–37.
Cassell draws some of the important implications from the distinction between disease and illness. [For a fuller discussion see Cassell's book, *The Healer's Art* (Philadelphia, Lippincott, 1976).]

Churchman, C. W.   *The Systems Approach.* New York: Delta, 1968.
An excellent book for the non-systems-scientist on the systems approach as a tool of general inquiry.

Dubos, R.   *Man Adapting.* New Haven, Conn.: Yale University Press, 1965.
Dubos is well known for developing the evolutionary-ecological model of disease.

Engel, G. L.   The need for a new medical model: A challenge for biomedicine. *Science* 196 : 129–36, 1977.
Engel cites the weakness of traditional, reductionistic medical models and describes a "biopsychosocial model," which is in many ways similar to the systems-hierarchy model.

Engelhardt, H. T.   The roots of science and ethics. *Hastings Center Report* 6(June 1976): 35–38.
A brief review of recent work showing similarities between the scientific and the ethical modes of inquiry. See also references to the next chapter.

Engelhardt, H. T.   Explanatory models in medicine: Facts, theories, and values. *Texas Reports on Biology and Medicine* 32 : 225–39, 1974.
Engelhardt asserts that all disease ascriptions include value judgments, and that we can look at "causes" of disease in different ways depending on our therapeutic intentions.

Fabrega, H., Jr.   Concepts of disease: Logical features and social implications. *Perspectives in Biology and Medicine* 15 : 583–616, 1972.
Fabrega calls for a unified, systems view of disease and sketches some controversial implications for health-care delivery.

Fabrega, H.   The study of disease in relation to culture. *Behavioral Science* 17 : 183, 1972.
Fabrega cites examples of biologic states that are viewed very differently in different cultures.

*Hastings Center Studies,* Vol. 1, No. 3, 1973.
This journal contains five articles on the theme, "The Concept of Health." See especially Daniel Callahan's discussion of the World Health Organization

definition of health, and Peter Sedgwick on how values influence disease concepts. The essay on the "sick role" by Siegler and Osmond is a superb example of using literature (in this case, Thomas Mann's *The Magic Mountain*) to illuminate medical concepts.

Kleinman, A. M., Eisenberg, L., and Good, B.   Culture, illness, and care: Clinical lessons from anthropologic and cross-cultural research. *Annals of Internal Medicine* 88 : 251–58, 1978.

The authors extend lessons learned from studying disease in other cultures to the everyday doctor–patient encounter, emphasizing the need to elicit the meaning of the illness experience for the patient.

Meador, C. K.   The art and science of nondisease. *New England Journal of Medicine* 272 : 92–5, 1965.

Meador's classic tongue-in-cheek paper illustrates the dangers in an overly rigid acceptance of disease concepts and categories.

Snow, L.   Folk medical beliefs and their implications for the care of patients. *Annals of Internal Medicine* 81 : 82–96, 1974.

Snow, an anthropologist, reviews many of the folk medical beliefs prevalent in the modern U.S.

Temkin, O.   The Scientific Approach to Disease: Specific Entity and Individual Sickness. In A. C. Crombie (Ed.), *Scientific Change*. London: Heinemann, 1963.

This famous medical historian reviews the ontologic and the physiologic approaches to disease over time.

Veatch, R. M.   Voluntary risks to health: The ethical issues. *Journal of the American Medical Association* 243 : 50–55, 1980.

Veatch deals with questions such as: Are health-related behaviors really voluntary? What theories of justice are presupposed by schemes to make people pay extra for engaging in risky behavior? How do we balance social costs and individual rights?

Wolf, S.   Disease as a way of life: Neural integration in systemic pathology. *Perspectives in Biology and Medicine* 4 : 288–305, 1961.

Wolf reviews neurophysiologic research to demonstrate the intimate connections between thoughts and feelings and bodily functions. In a more daring extension of these concepts he attempts to tie specific diseases with specific feeling states.

## Chapter 18. The Foundations of Values

Brody, H.   *Placebos and the Philosophy of Medicine*. Chicago: The University of Chicago Press, 1980.

The Introduction and the Conclusion discuss the importance of the equilibrium model for all philosophical and ethical investigations into medicine.

Callahan, D.   Living with the new biology: Search for an ethic. *Center Magazine* 5 : 4–12, July–August 1972.

Callahan argues that the changes created by new biologic and other scientific technologies demand a radical reconstruction of culture.

Cattell, R. B.   *A New Morality From Science: Beyondism*. New York: Pergamon, 1972.

Cattell's is one of the more recent and sophisticated attempts to deduce ethical principles from scientific facts and theories. His focus is on evolutionary theory. However, he still is forced to smuggle in value consideration under the guise of "science."

Engelhardt, H. T., and Callahan, D.   *The Foundations of Ethics and Its Relationship to Science*. Hastings, N.Y., Hastings Center.

This series of volumes contains essays by philosophers and scientists on the common ground between science and ethics. (*Science, Ethics and Medicine*, Vol. I, 1976; *Knowledge, Value and Belief*, Vol. II, 1977; *Morals, Science and Sociality*, Vol. III, 1978; *Knowing and Valuing: The Search for Common Roots*, Vol. IV, 1979.)

Heilbroner, R. *An Inquiry into the Human Prospect*. New York: W. W. Norton, 1974.
An economist views the long-range consequences of present human behavior and lists changes he feels necessary for the survival of the culture.

Potter, V. R. *Bioethics: Bridge to the Future*. Englewood Cliffs, N.J.: Prentice-Hall, 1971.
Potter proposes a framework for examining the long-range consequences of holding certain values and for using science to make better value choices.

Rawls, J. *A Theory of Justice*. Cambridge, Mass.: Belknap Press, 1971.
Rawls proposes a method of "reflective equilibrium" as a way of deriving general principles — see pages 17–22 in particular.

## Appendix II. Ethics and Religion

Donagan, A. *The Theory of Morality*. Chicago: The University of Chicago Press, 1977.

## Appendix VII. "Directive to Physicians" from California Natural Death Act

Garland, M. Politics, Legislation and Natural Death. *Hastings Center Report* 6(October 1976): 5–6.

## Appendix VIII. Criteria for Determining Quality of Life

Clements, T. S. *Science and Man: The Philosophy of Scientific Humanism*. Springfield, Ill.: Charles C. Thomas, 1968.

Fletcher, J. Indicators of Humanhood: A Tentative Profile of Man. *Hastings Center Report* 2(November 1972): 1–4.

Fletcher, J. Four Indicators of Humanhood — The Enquiry Matures. *Hastings Center Report* 4(December 1974): 4–7.

Simpson, G. G. *Biology and Man*. New York: Harcourt, Brace, Jovanovich, 1969.

# Self-Evaluation

You may complete this self-test to see whether you have fulfilled the Objectives listed at the beginning of this book. Complete the test all the way through, and then compare your answers with the answers that follow.

The first group of questions refer to the case below.

---

## SELF-EVALUATION CASE

You are a pediatrician who gets a frantic call at 11:30 P.M. from the resident on duty at the local hospital, concerning your 11-month-old patient, L.K. The baby was diagnosed as having a congenital hernia, which was successfully operated on 4 days ago. L.K. seems to have been making an uneventful recovery, although he has been mostly sedated by medication.

The resident tells you that about 16 hours ago, the hospital pharmacy erred and sent up a bottle of 50 percent glucose solution for the patient's IV, instead of the 5 percent you had ordered. The nurse on the floor failed to catch the error and the bottle was hung and the fluid administered. The patient is now comatose and shows signs of severe dehydration.

You rush to the hospital, where you find that the resident has also called in an expert in fluid therapy from a nearby medical school. He tells you that the child has an extremely high blood glucose level, which is already producing severe damage to the kidneys. He will try to correct the situation, he says, but this must be done very delicately; the outlook right now for L.K. is very grim.

At this point Mr. and Mrs. K. approach you. They are very anxious and perceive from the activity that something has gone wrong; so far no one has told them anything. They urgently demand an explanation.

What do you tell Mr. and Mrs. K.?

---

1. How many alternative courses of action are open to you?
2. Which of these seems most acceptable to you? Write a formal ethical statement that expresses this choice.

Questions 3 through 9 refer to the following formal ethical statement: "When an error in therapy that has significant consequences for the patient is made, the doctor ought to inform the patient or a responsible guardian as soon as possible of the true circumstances. He should decide for each case how and when this disclosure may best be made."

3. Make as extensive a list as you can of the consequences of this formal ethical statement. For each consequence, indicate by "high," "medium," or "low" the relative probability that you attribute to this consequence actually occurring.

4. Suppose one places a high value on the terms of the doctor–patient contract as we have described it in this book. Which of the consequences are consistent with this value and which are not? Does the formal ethical statement serve this value well or poorly?

5. Suppose one places a high value also on the efficiency of the cooperation of all members of the health-care team. Which of the consequences are consistent and which are inconsistent with this value? Is this value well or poorly served by the ethical statement?

6. If, in Question 5, you found significant inconsistencies between the formal ethical statement and the value of health-care cooperation, how could you modify the formal statement to decrease them?

7. In this case, what effect does the course of action that you choose have upon L.K.?

8. Your answer to Question 6 above has some implications for how you determine the rights of ethical participation in this decision. What are your criteria for determination here?

9. Does your response to this case represent any basic modifications in the doctor–patient relationship, according to your answer to Question 6?

The remaining questions represent fragments of arguments in defense of various ethical propositions. For each one, indicate the ethical "error" that it contains, if any.

10. "It can't be ethical to deny me, as an expectant mother, the opportunity for a screening amniocentesis if I want it. Why, you're saying that I don't have a right to do everything possible to assure myself of having a normal child."

11. "You say that the man who came into the emergency room just now has a brain tumor causing increased intracranial pressure and needs an immediate craniotomy to keep him alive long enough for us to do the tests to decide if the tumor is treatable or not, and now his wife won't give consent for the operation? How am I supposed to decide what to do? Sure, I'm the doctor in charge, but I don't have all the data. We need more data."

12. "Now, Mrs. Jenkins, after all, I am your doctor. So don't worry about little things like unlikely side effects. Just have the surgery as I recommend and everything will be all right."

13. "You can't allow infertile mothers to have test-tube babies. Sure, it would be nice for them, but pretty soon everyone would want a test-tube baby instead of one born the regular way. What would become of the foundations of the sexual relationship?"

14. "How can you possibly be recommending brain surgery for that child? Have you forgotten that the doctor's first responsibility is to do no harm?"

15. "If we look at animals in the natural world, it is clear that sex is used only for purposes of procreation, and that it takes place only between members of opposite sexes. Therefore, homosexuality is unnatural and clearly wrong and deserves immediate and aggressive psychiatric treatment when detected."

16. "You say that the county medical society ought not take a stand on national health insurance because it ought to be free of political involvement. Yet in the past I have heard you encourage the society's lobbying efforts on behalf of publicly financed school vaccination programs, genetic screening, and improved sanitation. You can't accept some political involvement and reject another without giving a better reason than the one you just gave."

17. "Well, it's been 5 years now since I diagnosed that city bus driver's dangerous heart condition, and he hasn't had a heart attack. I guess that I was right in not violating confidentiality, as he requested, and in not notifying the bus company when he refused to quit his job."

18. "Abortion can't possibly be justified under any circumstances. Why, it's murder!"

19. "I make it a rule never to stop to give medical aid at the scene of an accident. I once knew a doctor who had a cousin who heard of one case where a physician stopped and gave first aid. The victim died and the poor jerk got sued for his shirt as a result."

# Self-Evaluation: Answers

Throughout this book we have avoided claiming to have any special access to "right answers," and the answers that follow should be interpreted in this light. They should be regarded as representing a minimal level of competence in fulfilling the objectives listed at the beginning of the book. If you have spent time in careful thought, you may well have come up with additional consequences, or you may possibly have thought of some more subtle distinctions beyond what is given here.

If your answer differs significantly from the one given below, you will have to decide whether your own answer is "better" than mine according to the criteria for ethical validity used in this book or whether you have misunderstood part of the material. If the latter is the case, you may wish to reread the appropriate section which is given in parentheses at the end of each answer.

1. You have been cautioned against jumping to the conclusion that there are two and only two alternatives. As was noted in connection with Case 1, when the question is "What do you say?" there are as many alternatives as there are things that could be said, up to an infinite number. On a purely practical level, there are a large number of alternatives that are significantly different from each other. Compare the following:
    "Don't worry, everything is all right with your child."
    "Your child seems to have taken a sudden turn for the worse. We don't know what caused it but we're working hard to correct it."
    "Your child is very sick now; this may be due to some of the medication he has been given."
    "We just now discovered that an error was made in the type of IV fluid the child has been getting. He's very sick now, but we shall do everything possible to correct the situation."
    "We just now discovered that an error was made in the type of IV fluid. I'm afraid that the child is going to die."
    "Well, right now the child is very sick, and it's all because the pharmacist sent up the wrong bottle of IV fluid and the nurses were too busy drinking coffee and gabbing to notice."
You can see that saying each of these would lead to a different set of consequences. With a little ingenuity you can make the list almost as long as you like, so we cannot give an exact number of alternatives. (Frames 34, 92)

2. Since there are so many alternatives, we cannot phrase a formal ethical statement for each. In order to qualify as a formal statement, yours should have included what is to be done, who is to do it and under

what circumstances; the circumstances may have been as broadly or as narrowly defined as you saw fit. (Frames 18, 36)

3. While the consequences of the ethical statement on the specific case of L.K. is a good place to start, don't forget that you are determining the consequences of the general (universalizable) ethical statement, not a specific statement about what the doctor should do in just this one case. Therefore, if your list of consequences pertains only to this one case and does not apply to possible similar cases, it is incomplete.

Your list of consequences should have included most of the following:

a. The doctor maintains his duties under the doctor–patient contract (high probability).

b. The doctor has told the truth, which we tend to view as a worthwhile exercise in general (high probability).

c. The parents will appreciate the frankness and candor of the doctor (high probability).

d. The parents will be made angry at someone, depending on exactly how the doctor phrased his account of what happened (medium probability; doctor can help parents deal with anger).

e. The parents may institute a lawsuit against the doctor (medium probability; depending on circumstances).

f. The parents may institute a lawsuit against the hospital or against other members of the health-care team (medium probability).

g. If (e) occurs, the parents may win the suit (low probability, if the circumstances are like those of the case given).

h. If (f) occurs, the parents may win the suit (high probability, under circumstances given).

i. If the error was made by another member of the team and the doctor tells the parents, the team members may feel "betrayed" by the doctor, and the team solidarity and efficiency may be weakened (high probability).

j. The doctor will avoid the consequences of not telling the parents the truth – that is, they will probably determine that something had gone wrong and will feel frustrated and left out if not told (high probability).

k. The doctor and the other team members, having suffered the embarrassment of exposure, will make fewer mistakes in the future (low probability; since such errors are already uncommon and since there are other forces acting to prevent them).

l. People in general, hearing of these errors, may lose faith in the medical professions (low probability; since it is probably known already that such mistakes can be made).

m. If (l) occurs, people may demand and get more governmental regulation of medicine (low probability; more regulation is likely, but for other reasons). (Frames 38–40)

4. Consequences (a), (b), (c), and (j) would be viewed as positive from the viewpoint of the doctor–patient contract as we have defined it: that is, giving significant information to the patient so that he can make his own ethical decisions. While instituting a lawsuit may in fact be a decision the patient may make upon receipt of the data, we would tend to regard that as indicating a breakdown of the contract, albeit a justifiable one from the patient's viewpoint. So we might say that consequences (e) and (f) are contrary to a high value in the doctor–patient contract. In all, however, the value of the contract would seem to be served well by the formal ethical statement as written. (Frames 131, 150, 160)

5. The consequence that addresses itself most directly to this value is (i), which is contradictory to the state of affairs desired. Other consequences that might contradict the stated value are (d) and (f). Consequence (k) might further the value of team performance, but it is a low-probability consequence. In sum, if one places a high value on team cooperation and efficiency, one might decide that the formal ethical statement is in need of revision.

6. The core of the problem with Consequence (i) appears to be the fact that the doctor is placing his contract with the patient above his responsibility to the other team members; the team has to shoulder the blame while the doctor has washed his hands of the matter. The team–patient contract may indeed require that the parents be told, but if so, the team, not just the doctor, ought to be in on the decision. Therefore, one might wish to alter the formal ethical statement to:

   "When an error in therapy that has significant consequences for the patient is made by a member of the health-care team, a team member, usually the doctor, ought to inform the patient or guardian as soon as possible. The health-care team should decide among themselves how and when the disclosure ought best to be made, depending on the circumstances of the individual case."

   Of course, having looked at Consequences (e) and (f) as well as (i), you might have decided that the entire ethical statement ought to be reversed and that it would be better not to tell the parents the truth. If you do this, however, you would have to be ready to accept all the consequences of withholding important information. (Frames 46–49)

7. In the case described, which course of action you choose can have little effect on L.K. Even if L.K. were conscious, and a patient in the physiologic state described, he is too young to understand what is happening. One might speculate that if L.K. were conscious, and the parents were not told what was happening and were very anxious and confused as a result, L.K. might sense this emotional atmosphere and be adversely affected by it; but that is about all the effect that the ethical decision could possibly have on him directly. The therapy that you will give him does not depend on his parents knowing the true cause of the problem.

To digress a bit, the fact that L.K. cannot be harmed in any material way by not telling the truth, while the doctor or the hospital could be hit with a lawsuit if the truth is known, might lead an ethical utilitarian to the conclusion that the true cause of the accident ought to be concealed. In that way the "greatest good for the greatest number" would best be served. On the other hand, an ethicist who places high priority on some concept of "justice" might say that the parents ought definitely to be told, and if the responsible parties are sued, they are just getting what they deserve. If you are not clear on how these ethical decision-making methods differ from the one we have been using, see Appendix I.

8. If you answered No. 6 as we did, you were extending the original concept of the doctor–patient contract to that of a team–patient contract, and you decide that therefore the entire health-care team, not just the doctor, ought to have a say in the matter. Or possibly you reasoned that while the main contract is still between patient and doctor, the pharmacist and nurses, who stood to suffer significant and deleterious consequences if the truth were told, had acquired rights of participation for that reason. (Frames 189, 391–403)

9. Again, if you were extending the contract to cover the rest of the team members as well as the doctor, this represents a basic modification in the doctor–patient relationship. (Frame 189)

10. The statement suggests that the speaker is regarding "doing everything possible to have a normal child" as something to which she is entitled by some higher authority, regardless of the consequences. Thus, she is claiming this as a "right." Since this is not a right as traditionally defined in the legal sense, the speaker is obligated to state (1) by what authority she has this right, and (2) exactly who is obligated to carry out the required actions (since this is a right requiring action instead of a right prohibiting action). She has failed to do both of these. (Frames 72–78)

11. Every ethical decision requires both data and a value judgment. The speaker here seems reluctant to make the needed value judgment, so, consciously or unconsciously, he is misstating the nature of the ethical question and confusing it with an empirical question, in order to get himself off the hook. In fact, the one-sentence case description provides nearly all the data needed to make the ethical judgment, with the exception of the psychological nature of the husband–wife relationship. (Frames 19–22)

12. The speaker here, by prefacing his remarks with "I am your doctor," seems to be assuming that because of his good motives in his role as physician, he is more competent than the patient to make the required ethical judgments. He is attributing ethical expertise to himself merely on the basis of (1) his socially "good" role and (2) his socially "good" motives — neither of which is adequate insurance that the best course of action will be chosen. These errors have led him into the priestly model of the doctor–patient relationship. (Frames 127–131, 213–218)

13. What is the actual likelihood that everyone will want to have a "manu-factured" baby when they could have a real one? On the face of it, the proposition seems highly unlikely, and the speaker has offered no evidence to the contrary. If the probability of this consequence is that low, it should be of very low weight in the ethical decision-making process, yet the speaker has based his entire argument on it. We have here the domino theory or "foot in the door" theory of ethics, which has the various flaws described in Frames 257–261.

14. Presumably the speaker is treating the injunction "do no harm" as if it settled the question definitively in favor of not doing surgery. But with the little data available, we cannot judge whether the harm done by surgery will be greater or lesser than the harm of not doing surgery. It makes a great deal of difference whether the child has a brain tumor or whether he has simply been showing signs of hyperactivity, but, by using "do no harm" as a catch phrase, the speaker has avoided these issues entirely. (Frames 346–347)

15. From an empirical statement about what animals do in the natural world, the speaker has jumped to an ethical judgment that homosexuality is "wrong" and to an ethical statement about how homosexuality should be handled. Clearly he has made a value judgment in the process, but the form of his statement has served to obscure this. The speaker is engaging in another form of confusion between ethical and empirical statements, by deriving an ethical statement purely from empirical evidence – and erroneous evidence at that. (Frames 19–22, 1173)

16. No ethical error.

17. The speaker here is indulging in retrospective ethics. It is just as likely, indeed more likely from the data available at the time of the original decision, that the bus driver would have had a heart attack, and it is possible that he would have had it on the job. The ethical decision at the time should have been based on the consequences as best they could be judged then; the ethical decision does not become right in hindsight just because the doctor "lucked out." (Frame 165)

18. The speaker here is making a moral judgment by definition of words, rather than by the consequences of actions. If it were true that (1) abortion is indeed the same as murder, and that (2) murder could be shown to have very bad consequences, which are not outweighed by good consequences, then it would indeed follow that abortion is immoral. But both these propositions require some supporting evidence, which the speaker has not provided. (Frame 582)

19. Like the speaker using the domino theory, this speaker is putting decisive weight on one possible consequence of very low probability, while ignoring relevant consequences that are much more likely to occur. In effect, this sort of person is making ethical decisions by anecdote rather than by weighing consequences according to values. This can never lead to any general agreement, since anyone can come up with an anecdote that "proves" the opposite side. (Frames 247–248)

# Index

Numbers refer to *frame* number, not *page* number. References to the Appendixes are indicated by Roman numeral.